The
Interface Between
the Psychodynamic and
Behavioral Therapies

CRITICAL ISSUES IN PSYCHIATRY
An Educational Series for Residents and Clinicians

Series Editor: **Sherwyn M. Woods, M.D., Ph.D.**
University of Southern California School of Medicine
Los Angeles, California

A RESIDENT'S GUIDE TO PSYCHIATRIC EDUCATION
Edited by Michael G. G. Thompson, M.D.

STATES OF MIND: Analysis of Change in Psychotherapy
Mardi J. Horowitz, M.D.

DRUG AND ALCOHOL ABUSE: A Clinical Guide to
Diagnosis and Treatment
Marc A. Schuckit, M.D.

**THE INTERFACE BETWEEN THE PSYCHODYNAMIC AND
BEHAVIORAL THERAPIES**
Edited by Judd Marmor, M.D. and Sherwyn M. Woods, M.D., Ph.D.

LAW IN THE PRACTICE OF PSYCHIATRY: A Handbook for Clinicians
Seymour L. Halleck, M.D.

A Continuation Order Plan is available for this series. A continuation order will bring delivery of each new volume immediately upon publication. Volumes are billed only upon actual shipment. For further information please contact the publisher.

The
Interface Between
the Psychodynamic and
Behavioral Therapies

Edited by

Judd Marmor, M.D.

Franz Alexander Professor of Psychiatry
University of Southern California School of Medicine
Supervising and Training Analyst (Emeritus)
Southern California Psychoanalytic Institute
Past President, American Psychiatric Association

and

Sherwyn M. Woods, M.D., Ph.D.

Professor in Psychiatry
University of Southern California School of Medicine
Supervising and Training Analyst
Southern California Psychoanalytic Institute
Past President, American Association of Directors of Psychiatric Residency Training

Plenum Medical Book Company · New York and London

Library of Congress Cataloging in Publication Data

Main entry under title:

The Interface between the psychodynamic and behavioral therapies.

(Critical issues in psychiatry)
Includes index.
1. Psychoanalysis. 2. Behavior therapy. I. Marmor, Judd. II. Woods, Sherwyn M.
III. Series.
RC506.I55   616.8'914   79-9197
ISBN 0-306-40251-3

© 1980 Plenum Publishing Corporation
227 West 17th Street, New York, N.Y. 10011

Plenum Medical Book Company is an imprint of Plenum Publishing Corporation

Printed in the United States of America

To Katherine and Nancy,
who for each of us prove daily that one and one
can equal much more than two.

Contributors

FRANZ ALEXANDER, M.D., formerly Clinical Professor of Psychiatry
University of Southern California School of Medicine
Los Angeles, California 90033

ANN W. BIRK, PH.D., Clinical Associate
Learning Theories, Inc.
Newton, Massachusetts 02160

LEE BIRK, M.D., Clinical Director, Learning Theories, Inc.
Associate Clinical Professor of Psychiatry
Harvard Medical School
Boston, Massachusetts 02115

EDWARD B. BLANCHARD, PH.D., Professor of Psychology
State University of New York at Albany
Albany, New York 12222

ALVIN B. BLAUSTEIN, M.D., Assistant Clinical Professor
Department of Psychiatry, Mount Sinai School of Medicine
New York City, New York 10029

JOHN PAUL BRADY, M.D., Kenneth E. Appel Professor of Psychiatry and
    Chairman of the Department
University of Pennsylvania School of Medicine
Philadelphia, Pennsylvania 19104

LOUIS BREGER, PH.D., Professor of Psychology
California Institute of Technology
Pasadena, California 91125

ALLEN T. DITTMANN, PH.D., National Institute of Mental Health
U.S. Office of Education, Bureau of Education for the Handicapped
Washington, D.C. 20202

BEN W. FEATHER, M.D., PH.D., Clinical Professor of Psychiatry
Brown University
Providence, Rhode Island 02906

MICHAEL G. GELDER, M.D., Professor
Department of Psychiatry
University of Oxford, England

MERTON M. GILL, M.D., Professor of Psychiatry
Abraham Lincoln School of Medicine, University of Illinois
Chicago, Illinois 60612

EUGENIA GULLICK, PH.D., Associate Professor of Psychiatry
Medical College of Wisconsin
Milwaukee, Wisconsin 53226

ARLENE KAGLE, PH.D., Clinical Psychologist
Private Practice
New York City, New York

HELEN S. KAPLAN, M.D., PH.D., Associate Clinical Professor of Psychiatry
Cornell University Medical College
New York, New York 10021

MARJORIE KLEIN, PH.D., Associate Professor of Psychiatry
University of Wisconsin Medical School
Madison, Wisconsin 53792

PETER LAMBLEY, PH.D.
Psychological Research Associates
901-902 Trusthouse
Foreshore, Cape Town, South Africa

ALEXANDER LEVAY, M.D., Associate Clinical Professor of Psychiatry
College of Physicians and Surgeons of Columbia University
New York, New York 10032

ISAAC M. MARKS, M.D., D.P.M., F.R.C.PSYCH., Professor of Experimental Psychopathology
Institute of Psychiatry
De Crespigny Park, Denmark Hill, London, S.E.5, England

JUDD MARMOR, M.D., Franz Alexander Professor of Psychiatry
University of Southern California School of Medicine
Los Angeles, California 90033

JAMES L. McGAUGH, PH.D., Professor of Psychobiology
University of California
Irvine, California 92717

MICHAEL E. MURRAY, PH.D., Adjunct Professor of Psychology
Southern Methodist University
Dallas, Texas 75275

MORRIS B. PARLOFF, PH.D., Chief, Psychotherapy & Behavioral Intervention Section
Clinical Research Branch, National Institute of Mental Health
Rockville, Maryland 20857

JOHN M. RHOADS, M.D., Professor of Psychiatry
Duke University Medical Center
Durham, North Carolina 27710

R. TAYLOR SEGRAVES, M.D., PH.D., Assistant Professor in Psychiatry
University of Chicago Pritzker School of Medicine
Chicago, Illinois 60637

FREDERICK A. SHECTMAN, PH.D., Faculty Member, Postdoctoral Training Program in Clinical Psychology and
The Menninger School of Psychiatry, The Menninger Foundation
Topeka, Kansas 66601

R. BRUCE SLOANE, M.D., Professor and Chairman Department of Psychiatry
University of Southern California School of Medicine
Los Angeles, California 90033

ROBERT C. SMITH, M.D., PH.D., Chief, Behavioral Neurochemistry
Texas Research Institute of Mental Sciences
Houston, Texas 77030

JOSEF H. WEISSBERG, M.D., Assistant Clinical Professor of Psychiatry
Columbia University College of Physicians and Surgeons
New York, New York 10032

BERNARD WEITZMAN, PH.D., Associate Professor of Psychology
Graduate Faculty, New School for Social Research
New York City, New York

EUGENE WOLF, M.D., M.A., F.R.C.PSYCH., Professor of Psychotherapy
Department of Psychiatry, Memorial University of Newfoundland, Health Sciences Centre
St. John's, Newfoundland A1B3V6, Canada

SHERWYN M. WOODS, M.D., PH. D., Professor in Psychiatry
University of Southern California School of Medicine
Los Angeles, California 90033

Preface

It is sobering to reflect that it has been nearly fifty years since Thomas French's article on the "Interrelations between Psychoanalysis and the Experimental Work of Pavlov," representing the first psychoanalyst to bridge the gap between the theories of conditioning, was published. In his paper French clearly delineated the manner and directions in which these two points of view might enrich each other. Regrettably, his openness to new ideas has not been characteristic of most "schools" of psychiatry thought, which have tended instead to develop an unfortunate degree of insularity. This has occurred despite the obvious reality that the bio-social-psychological nature of man is such that no one theory or discipline is likely, in the foreseeable future, to explain, much less predict, all of the complexities of human behavior. All too often disputing theoreticians, like the fabled blind men describing the elephant, assume that the whole is just a gigantic magnification of the parts with which they are in contact. When treatment strategies are extrapolated from such narrow views, more often than not they fail to achieve the parsimony of effort, the breadth of application, and the maximum of efficiency that one would hope for.

In our opinion, it is impossible adequately to conceptualize personality development, symptom formation, or responses to psychotherapy, without taking into consideration theories of conflict as well as those of learning. Similarly, the processes of adaptation and maturation, whether viewed from the perspective of coping with internal or external stimuli, cannot be adequately understood without taking into consideration the manner by which previous learning and conflict resolution have shaped the perception and responses to current circumstances.

In considering a title for this collection of essays we have chosen to use the word "psychodynamic" rather than "psychoanalytic" because the former is far broader in scope and encompasses a wider variety of therapeutic approaches. We do so because our interest is not merely with Freudian and neo-Freudian theory and therapies; it is with all clinical approaches which conceptualize human behavior as influenced by unconscious and dynamically active forces and conflicts that are derived from developmentally important antecedent experiences, and that distort the way one perceives and responds to current resonating transactions. Viewed in this fashion, behavioral obstinacy in the face of authority, for example, is seen not merely as a learned response to the stimulus of authority, but as a psychologically essential process dealing with potentially disruptive affects and anxieties that are associated with unresolved conflicts with significant authority figures in one's past. These distorted ways of dealing with authority, however, often become so strongly learned and reinforced that they may develop an "autonomy" which can result in the persistence of the behavior even after the dynamic etiological factors have been resolved. Moreover, not all maladaptive behavior is necessarily due to persistent unconscious conflict. Some faulty behavior may be extinguished either naturally or by rather simple behavioral interventions or social learning.

These facts have enormous significance both diagnostically and therapeutically. Thus, a simple diagnostic label such as "phobia" tells us very little in itself about the nature of the clinical task to be accomplished if the patient is to be freed from the debilitating symptom. An acute driving phobia following a traumatic auto accident is usually quite different from an insidious agoraphobia that over time has invaded every aspect of the patient's life.

The authors of the papers in this volume generally share this awareness that symptoms can result from relatively uncomplicated conditioned learning or from complex psychodynamic factors or both. Thus it makes sense, as many of them point out, to organize the treatment of a condition around the relative importance of the etiological factors involved. Appropriate treatment planning is not determined by the mere assignment of a correct diagnostic label, but rather through an accurate assessment of the relative importance of psychic conflict, unconscious mental processes, conditioned learning, and situational factors contributing to reinforcement or extinction of symptoms. It is clearly just as insufficient for the dynamic psychotherapist to ignore the rich literature on behavioral learning as for the behavioral therapist to ignore the manner by which unconscious processes and conflicts shape such learning. There is little doubt, for example, that a significant number of failures in behavioral therapy are the result of neglecting to recognize and deal with the unconscious dynamics and transference reactions that have been mobilized in the treatment situation.

As a number of the authors in this volume point out, often adherents of the psychodynamic and behavioral approaches merely use different terminology to describe similar concepts. For example, the analytic concept of secondary gain and the behavioral concept of reinforcement reflect different ways of describing essentially similar processes that are involved in the resistance to therapeutic change. Similarly, the concepts of transference and of conditioned learning both represent efforts to deal with the persistence of a stereotyped response to interpersonal stimuli, although in very different terms. This is not to imply that there are no important differences between psychodynamic theory and behavioral theory, or in the basic psychotherapeutic stances that are derived from these theoretical differences. Despite these differences, however, as the essays in this volume clearly indicate, in a wide variety of clinical situations the psychodynamic and behavioral approaches are neither contradictory nor antithetical but, rather, are complementary. For this reason there are often situations where an integration of these two approaches tends to enhance the clinical effectiveness of either approach used alone. For example, as a number of the papers demonstrate, symptom removal does not necessarily lead to symptom substitution; often it may bring into awareness previously repressed material and thus make underlying conflicts more accessible to dynamic intervention. Thus insight may follow rather than precede the resolution of symptoms, and this in turn may facilitate the development of transference reactions and understandings related to the unconscious material previously "bound" by the symptom. Some of the therapeutic approaches described in this volume make effective use of this phenomenon by employing behavioral techniques to facilitate dynamic psychotherapy.

The first section of this volume encompasses a group of papers that deal with various aspects of theoretical problems involved in the interface between psychodynamic and behavioral therapy. In the second section, various clinical applications of this interface are represented, reflecting a variety of approaches, employing parallel, phased, or integrated behavioral and psychodynamic techniques. Sometimes this is accomplished by the same therapist; in other instances different therapists are employed. Regardless of which approach was used, however, the widely feared consequences of "split transference" or disruptive acting-out did not become unmanageable, if they occurred at all. Although most of the papers in the clinical section are concerned with individual one-to-one therapy, several of them clearly demonstrate the usefulness of a combined psychodynamic and behavioral approach in the treatment of couples and in group psychotherapy also. The utilization of such a combined approach has probably achieved its widest acceptance in the area of the treatment of sexual dysfunctions, that is, in so-called sex therapy. That an even more creative integration of the two approaches may be possible in the future is suggested by the work of Feather and Rhoades in which behavioral techniques are addressed not to the conscious, manifest symptoms but rather to the repressed, unconscious psychodynamic conflicts underlying the symptoms. This innovative idea is an excellent example of the way in which clinical approaches to psychopathology can be enhanced by an open theoretical system which permits the integration of knowledge from other disciplines and other therapeutic approaches. It is inflexibility in the practitioner, rather than any inherent inflexibility in theory, which usually explains resistance to the evolution of new clinical techniques. Nowhere is this more apparent than in the areas of psychodynamic and behavioral theory, which are not merely "open systems," but significant and complementary approaches to the complex problems of personality development and maladaptation.

JUDD MARMOR, M.D.
SHERWYN M. WOODS, M.D., PH.D.

Acknowledgments

The Editors wish to express their appreciation and gratitude to Mary Jane Costello, Leona H. Light, and Sandra Loya for their invaluable assistance in the preparation of this manuscript. We would also like to express our appreciation to Ms. Hilary Evans, Senior Medical Editor of Plenum, for her wise counsel and assistance in the preparation of this volume.

Contents

B. PARALLEL AND ALTERNATING PSYCHODYNAMIC AND BEHAVIORAL THERAPIES

C. An Integrated Approach

D. Other Applications

The Dynamics of Psychotherapy in the Light of Learning Theory

Franz Alexander, M.D.

It is fitting that one of Franz Alexander's customarily lucid and percipient papers should introduce the material in this volume. More than any other psychoanalyst of the modern era, Alexander was a pathfinder who had the courage and the vision to integrate the newer findings of behavioral science into his theoretical and clinical perspectives without abandoning what was useful in the old.

The following paper and that of Marmor which follows it were two of the earlier psychoanalytically oriented efforts at expressly linking psychoanalytic therapy with the process of learning. Thus they created the basis for a bridge between dynamic psychotherapy and the behavioral therapies that expressly derived their techniques from learning theories.

These were not, however, the earliest attempt at such integration. As far back as 1933, Thomas French, in a lengthy and occasionally abstruse article, explored the "Interrelations between Psychoanalysis and the Experimental Work of Pavlov" (American Journal of Psychiatry 12:1165-1203). The article did not exert much influence, probably because the conditioned reflex theories of Pavlov were not as adequate to explain the complexity of learned behavior as were the later theories of Gestalt learning and Skinnerian operant conditioning, which are here emphasized by Alexander.

The Dynamics of Psychotherapy in the Light of Learning Theory

FRANZ ALEXANDER, M.D.

Most of what we know about the basic dynamic principles of psychotherapy is derived from the psychoanalytic process.

One of the striking facts in this field is that the intricate procedure of psychoanalytic treatment underwent so few changes since its guiding principles were formulated by Freud between 1912 and 1915.[7-11] Meanwhile, substantial developments took place in theoretical knowledge, particularly in ego psychology. Moreover, in all other fields of medicine, treatments underwent radical changes resulting from a steadily improving understanding of human physiology and pathology. No medical practitioner could treat patients with the same methods he learned 50 years ago without being considered antiquated. In contrast, during the same period the standard psychoanalytic treatment method as it is taught today in psychoanalytic institutes remained practically unchanged.

It is not easy to account for this conservatism. Is it due to the perfection of the standard procedure, which because of its excellence does not require reevaluation and improvement, or does it have some other cultural rather than scientific reasons?

Among several factors one is outstanding: to be a reformer of psychoanalytic treatment was never a popular role. The need for unity among the pioneer psychoanalysts, who were universally rejected by outsiders, is one of the deep cultural roots of this stress on conformity. The majority of those who had critical views became "dissenters" either voluntarily or by excommunication. Some of these became known as neo-Freudians. Some of the critics, however, remained in the psychoanalytic fold.

(Some analysts jocularly expressed the view that the stress on con-

From *American Journal of Psychiatry*, 120:440-448, November 1963. Copyright 1963 by the American Psychiatric Association. Reprinted by permission.

formity was a defense against the analyst's unconscious identification with Freud, each wanting to become himself a latter-day Freud and founder of a new school. Conformity was a defense against too many prima donnas.) Another important factor is the bewildering complexity of the psychodynamic processes occurring during treatment. It appears that the insecurity which this intricate field necessarily provokes creates a defensive dogmatism which gives its followers a pseudosecurity. Almost all statements concerning technique could be legitimately only highly tentative. "Tolerance of uncertainty" is generally low in human beings. A dogmatic reassertion of some traditionally accepted views—seeking for a kind of consensus—is a common defense against uncertainty.

In spite of all this, there seems to be little doubt that the essential psychodynamic principles on which psychoanalytic treatment rests have solid observational foundations. These constitute the areas of agreement among psychoanalysts of different theoretical persuasion. Briefly, they consist in the following observations and evaluations:

1. During treatment unconscious (repressed) material becomes conscious. This increases the action radius of the conscious ego: the ego becomes cognizant of unconscious impulses and thus is able to coordinate (integrate) the latter with the rest of conscious content.

2. The mobilization of unconscious material is achieved mainly by two basic therapeutic factors: interpretation of material emerging during free association and the patient's emotional interpersonal experiences in the therapeutic situation (transference). The therapist's relatively objective, nonevaluative, impersonal attitude is the principal factor in mobilizing unconscious material.

3. The patient shows resistance against recognizing unconscious content. Overcoming this resistance is one of the primary technical problems of the treatment.

4. It is only natural that the neurotic patient will sooner or later direct his typical neurotic attitude toward his therapist. He develops a transference which is the repetition of interpersonal attitudes, mostly the feelings of the child to his parents. This process is favored by the therapist encouraging the patient to be himself as much as he can during the interviews. The therapist's objective, nonevaluative attitude is the main factor, not only in mobilizing unconscious material during the process of free association, but also in facilitating the manifestation of transference. The original neurosis of the patient, which is based on his childhood experiences, is thus transformed in an artificial "transference neurosis" which is a less intensive repetition of the patient's "infantile neurosis." The resolution of these revived feelings and behavior patterns—the resolution of the transference neurosis—becomes the aim of the treatment.

There is little disagreement concerning these fundamentals of the treatments. Controversies, which occur sporadically, pertain primarily to the technical means by which the transference neurosis can be resolved. The optimal intensity of the transference neurosis is one of the points of contention.

This is not the place to account in detail the various therapeutic suggestions which arose in recent years. Most of these modifications consisted in particular emphases given to certain aspects of the treatment. There are those who stressed interpretation of resistance (Wilhelm Reich, Helmuth Kaiser), while others focused on the interpretation of repressed content. Fenichel stated that resistance cannot be analyzed without making the patient understand what he is resisting.[6]

It is most difficult to evaluate all these modifications because it is generally suspected that authors' accounts about their theoretical views do not precisely reflect what they are actually doing while treating patients. The reasons for this discrepancy lies in the fact that the therapist is a "participant observer" who is called upon constantly to make decisions on the spot. The actual interactional process between therapist and patient is much more complex than the theoretical accounts about it. In general there were two main trends: (1) emphasis on cognitive insight as a means of breaking up the neurotic patterns and (2) emphasis upon the emotional experiences the patient undergoes during treatment. These are not mutually exclusive, yet most controversies centered around emphasis on the one or the other factor: cognitive versus experiential.

While mostly the similarity between the transference attitude and the original pathogenic childhood situation has been stressed, I emphasized the therapeutic significance of the difference between the old family conflicts and the actual doctor-patient relationship. This difference is what allows "corrective emotional experience" to occur, which I consider as the central therapeutic factor both in psychoanalysis proper and in analytically oriented psychotherapy. The new settlement of an old unresolved conflict in the transference situation becomes possible not only because the intensity of the transference conflict is less than that of the original conflict, but also because the therapist's actual response to the patient's emotional expressions is quite different from the original treatment of the child by the parents. The fact that the therapist's reaction differs from that of the parent, to whose behavior the child adjusted himself as well as he could with his own neurotic reactions, makes it necessary for the patient to abandon and correct these old emotional patterns. After all, this is precisely one of the ego's basic functions—adjustment to the existing external conditions. As soon as the old neurotic patterns are revived and brought into the realm of consciousness, the ego has the opportunity to readjust them to the changed external and internal conditions. This is the essence of the corrective influence of those series of experiences which occur during treatment.[2,3] As will be seen, however, the emotional detachment of the therapist turned out under observational scrutiny to be less complete than this idealized model postulates.

Since the difference between the patient-therapist and the original child-parent relationship appeared to me a cardinal therapeutic agent, I made technical suggestions derived from these considerations. The therapist in order to increase the effectiveness of the corrective emotional experiences should attempt to create an interpersonal climate which is suited to highlight the discrepancy between the patient's transference attitude and the actual situation as it exists between patient and therapist. For example, if the original childhood situation which the patient repeats in the transference was between a strict punitive father and a frightened son, the therapist should behave in a calculatedly permissive manner. If the father had a doting, all-forgiving attitude toward his son, the therapist should take a more impersonal and reserved attitude. This suggestion was criticized by some authors, that these consciously and purposefully adopted attitudes are artificial and will be recognized as such by the patient. I maintained, however, that the therapist's objective, emotionally not participating attitude is itself artificial inasmuch as it does not exist between human beings in actual life. Neither is it as complete as has been assumed. This controversy will have to wait to be decided by further experiences of practitioners.

I made still other controversial technical suggestions aimed at intensifying the emotional experiences of the patient. One of them was changing the number of interviews in appropriate phases of the treatment in order to make the patient more vividly conscious of his dependency needs by frustrating them.

Another of my suggestions pertains to the ever-puzzling question of termination of treatment. The traditional belief is that the longer an analysis lasts, the greater is the probability of recovery. Experienced analysts more and more came to doubt the validity of this generalization. If anything, this is the exception; very long treatments lasting over many years do not seem to be the most successful ones. On the other hand, many so-called transference cures after very brief contact have been observed to be lasting. A clear correlation between duration of treatment and its results has not been established. There are no reliable criteria for the proper time of termination. Improvements observed during treatment often prove to be conditioned by the fact that the patient is still being treated. The patient's own inclination to terminate or to continue the treatment is not always a reliable indication. The complexity of the whole procedure and our inability to estimate precisely the proper time of termination induced me to employ the method of experimental temporary interruptions, a method which in my experience is the most satisfactory procedure. At the same time it often reduces the total number of interviews. The technique of tentative temporary interruptions is based on trusting the natural recuperative powers of the human personality, which are largely underestimated by many psychoanalysts. There is an almost general trend toward "overtreatment." A universal regressive trend in human beings has been generally recognized by psychoanalysts. Under sufficient stress everyone tends to regress to the helpless state of infancy and seek help from others. The psychoanalytic treatment situation caters to this regressive attitude. As Freud stated, treatments often reach a point where the patient's will to be cured is outweighed by his wish to be treated.

In order to counteract this trend a continuous pressure on the patient is needed to make him ready to take over his own management as soon as possible. During temporary interruptions patients often discover that they can live without their analyst. When they return, the still not worked out emotional problems come clearly to the forefront.*

Furthermore, I called attention to Freud's distinction between two forms of regression. He first described regression to a period of ego-development in which the patient was still happy, in which he functioned well. Later he described regressions to traumatic experiences, which he explained as attempts to master subsequently an overwhelming situation of the past. During psychoanalytic treatment both kinds of regression occur. Regressions to pretraumatic or preconflictual periods—although they offer excellent research opportunity for the study of personality development—are therapeutically not valuable. Often we find that the patient regresses in his free associations to preconflictual early infantile material as a maneuver to evade the essential pathogenic conflicts. This material appears as "deep material" and both patient and therapist in mutual self-deception spend a great deal of time and effort to analyze this essentially evasive material. The recent trend to look always for very early emotional conflicts between mother and infant as the most common source of neurotic disturbances is the result of overlooking this frequent regressive evasion of later essential pathogenic conflicts. Serious disturbances of the early symbiotic mother-child relation occur only with exceptionally disturbed mothers. The most common conflicts begin when the child has already a distinct feeling of being a person (ego-awareness) and relates to his human environment, to his parents and siblings as to individual persons. The oedipus complex and sibling rivalry are accordingly the common early sources of neurotic patterns.

*This type of "fractioned analysis," which was practiced in the early days of the Outpatient Clinic of the Berlin Institute, is an empirical experimental way to find the correct time for termination.

There are many exceptions, of course, where the personality growth is disturbed in very early infancy.

Another issue which gained attention in the post-Freudian era is the therapist's neglect of the actual present life situation in favor of preoccupation with the patient's past history. This is based on the tenet that the present life circumstances are merely precipitating factors, mobilizing the patient's infantile neurosis. In general, of course, the present is always determined by the past. Freud in a rather early writing proposed the theory of complementary etiology. A person with severe ego defects acquired in the past will react to slight stress situations in his present life with severe reactions; a person with a relatively healthy past history will require more severe blows of life to regress into a neurotic state.[12] Some modern authors like French, Rado, myself, and others feel that there is an unwarranted neglect of the actual life circumstances.[1,15] The patient comes to the therapist when he is at the end of his rope, is entangled in emotional problems which have reached a point when he feels he needs help. These authors feel that the therapist never should allow the patient to forget that he came to him to resolve his present problem. The understanding of the past should always be subordinated to the problems of the present. Therapy is not the same as genetic research. Freud's early emphasis upon the reconstruction of past history was the result of his primary interest in research. At first he felt he must know the nature of the disease he proposes to cure. The interest in past history at the expense of the present is the residue of the historical period when research in personality dynamics of necessity was a prerequisite to develop a rational treatment method.

These controversial issues will have to wait for the verdict of history. Their significance cannot yet be evaluated with finality. One may state, however, that there is a growing inclination to question the universal validity of some habitual practices handed down by tradition over several generations of psychoanalysts. There is a trend toward greater flexibility in technique, attempting to adjust the technical details to the individual nature of the patient and his problems. This principle of flexibility was explicitly stressed by Edith Weigert, Thomas French, myself, and still others.

While there is considerable controversy concerning frequency of interviews, interruptions, termination, and the mutual relation between intellectual and emotional factors in treatment, there seems to be a universal consensus about the significance of the therapist's individual personality for the results of the treatment. This interest first manifested itself in several contributions dealing with the therapist's own emotional involvement in the patient—"the countertransference phenomenon." Freud first used the expression, countertransference, in 1910. It took,

however, about 30 years before the therapist's unconscious, spontaneous reactions toward the patient were explored as to their significance
for the course of the treatment. The reasons for this neglect were both
theoretical and practical. Originally Freud conceived the analyst's role in
the treatment as a blank screen who carefully keeps his incognito and
upon whom the patient can project any role, that of the image of his
father (father transference), of mother (mother transference), or of any
significant person in his past. In this way the patient can reexperience
the important interpersonal events of his past undisturbed by the specific personality of the therapist. The phenomenon called "countertransference," however, contradicts sharply the "blank screen" theory.

It is now generally recognized that in reality the analyst does not
remain a blank screen, an uninvolved intellect, but is perceived by the
patient as a concrete person. There is, however, a great deal of difference
among present-day authors in the evaluation of the significance of the
therapist's personality in general and his countertransference reactions
in particular.

Some authors consider countertransference as an undesirable impurity just as the patient's emotional involvement with his therapist
(transference) originally was considered as an undesirable complication.
The ideal model of the treatment was that the patient should freely associate and thus reveal himself without controlling the train of his ideas,
and should consider the therapist only as an expert who is trying to help
him. Later, as is well known, the patient's emotional involvement
turned out to be the dynamic axis of the treatment. So far as the therapist's involvement is concerned, it is considered by most authors as
an unwanted impurity. The therapist should have only one reaction to
the patient, the wish to understand him and give him an opportunity for
readjustment through the insight offered to him by the therapist's interpretations. The latter should function as a pure intellect without being
disturbed by any personal and subjective reactions to the patient.

The prevailing view is that the analyst's own emotional reactions
should be considered as disturbing factors of the treatment.

Some authors, among them Edith Weigert, Frieda Fromm-Reichmann, Heimann, Benedek, and Salzman, however, mention certain assets of the countertransference; they point out that the analyst's understanding of his countertransference attitudes may give him a particularly valuable tool for understanding the patient's transference reactions.[5,13,14,16] As to the therapeutic significance of the countertransference, there is a great deal of disagreement. While Balint and Balint consider this impurity as negligible for the therapeutic process,[4] Benedek
states in her paper on countertransference that the therapist's personality is the most important agent of the therapeutic process.[5] There is,

however, general agreement that a too intensive emotional involvement on the therapist's part is a seriously disturbing factor. Glover speaks of the "analyst's toilet" which he learns in his own personal analysis, which should free him from unwanted emotional participation in the treatment. This is, indeed, the most important objective of the training analysis; it helps him to know how to control and possibly even to change his spontaneous countertransference reactions.

I believe that the countertransference may be helpful or harmful. It is helpful when it differs from that parental attitude toward the child which contributed to the patient's emotional difficulties. The patient's neurotic attitudes developed not in a vacuum but as reactions to parental attitudes. If the therapist's reactions are different from these parental attitudes, the patient's emotional involvement with the therapist is not realistic. This challenges the patient to alter his reaction patterns. If, however, the specific countertransference of the therapist happens to be similar to the parental attitudes toward the child, the patient's neurotic reaction patterns will persist and an interminable analysis may result. There is no incentive for the patient to change his feelings. I recommended therefore that the therapist should be keenly aware of his own spontaneous—no matter how slight—feelings to the patient and should try to replace them by an interpersonal climate which is suited to correct the original neurotic patterns.

One of the most systematic revisions of the standard psychoanalytic procedure was undertaken by Sandor Rado, published in several writings, beginning in 1948.[15] His critical evaluation of psychoanalytic treatment and his suggested modifications deserve particular attention because for many years Rado has been known as one of the most thorough students of Freud's writings.

As years went on, Rado became more and more dissatisfied with the prevailing practice of psychoanalysis, and proposed his adaptational technique based on his "adaptational psychodynamics." As it is the case with many innovators, some of Rado's formulations consist in new terminology. Some of his new emphases, however, are highly significant. He is most concerned, as I am, with those features of the standard technique of psychoanalysis which foster regression without supplying a counterforce toward the patient's progression, that is to say, to his successful adaptation to the actual life situation. He raises the crucial question: Is the patient's understanding of his past development sufficient to induce a change in him? "To overcome repressions and thus be able to recall the past is one thing; to learn from it and be able to act on the new knowledge, another."[15]

Rado recommends, as a means to promote the goal of therapy, raising the patient from his earlier childlike adaptations to an appropriate adult level—"to hold the patient as much as possible at the adult level of cooperation with the physician." The patient following his regressive trend "parentifies" the therapist but the therapist should counteract this trend and not allow himself to be pushed by the patient into the parent role. Rado criticizes orthodox psychoanalytic treatment as furthering the regressive urge of the patient by emphasizing the "punitive parentify-ing" transference (the patient's dependence upon the parentalized image of the therapist).[15] Rado points out that losing self-confidence is the main reason for the patient to build up the therapist into a powerful parent figure. Rado's main principle, therefore, is to "bolster up the pa-tient's self-confidence on realistic grounds." He stresses the importance of dealing with the patient's actual present life conditions in all possible detail. Interpretations must always embrace the conscious as well as un-conscious motivations. In concordance with mine and French's similar emphasis[1] Rado succinctly states: "Even when the biographical mate-rial on hand reaches far into the past, interpretation must always begin and end with the patient's present life performance, his present adap-tive task. The significance of this rule cannot be overstated."

Rado considers his adaptational technique but a further develop-ment of the current psychoanalytic technique, not something basically contradictory to it. It should be pointed out that while criticizing the standard psychoanalytic procedure, Rado in reality criticizes current practice, but not theory. According to accepted theory, the patient's de-pendent—in Rado's term—"parentifying" transference should be re-solved. The patient during treatment learns to understand his own motivations; this enables him to take over his own management. He assimilates the therapist's interpretations and gradually he can dispense with the therapist, from whom he has received all he needs. The therapeutic process thus recapitulates the process of emotional matura-tion; the child learns from the parents, incorporates their attitude and eventually will no longer need them for guidance. Rado's point becomes relevant when one points out that the current procedure does not al-ways achieve this goal, and I may add, it unnecessarily prolongs the procedure. The reason for this is that the exploration of the past became an aim in itself, indeed the goal of the treatment. The past should be subordinated to a total grasp of the present life situation and serve as the basis for future adaptive accomplishments.

At this point my emphasis is pertinent, that it is imperative for the therapist to correctly estimate the time when his guidance becomes not only unnecessary but detrimental, inasmuch as it unnecessarily fosters the very dependency of the patient on the therapist which the latter tries to combat. I stated that deeds are stronger than words; the treatment should be interrupted at the right time in order to give the patient the experience that he can now function on his own and thus gain that self-confidence which Rado tries to instill into the patient by "positive interpretations." No matter, however, what technical devices they emphasize, the goal of these reformers is the same: to minimize the danger implicit in the psychotherapeutic situation, namely, encouraging undue regression and evasion of the current adaptive tasks. It is quite true that regression is necessary in order to give the patient opportunity to reexperience his early maladaptive patterns and grapple with them anew to find other more appropriate levels of feeling and behavior. The key to successful psychoanalytic therapy is, however, not to allow regression in the transference to become an aim in itself. It is necessary to control it.

In view of these controversies the need for a careful study of the therapeutic process became more and more recognized. Different research centers initiated programs from grants given by the Ford Foundation to study the therapeutic process. At the Mount Sinai Hospital in Los Angeles, under my direction, we undertook a study of the therapeutic process, in which a number of psychoanalysts observed the therapeutic interaction between therapist and patient in several treatment cases. All interviews were sound-recorded and both the participant observer—that is the therapist—and the nonparticipant observers recorded their evaluation of the process immediately after each interview. Our assumption was that the therapist, being an active participant in the interactional process, is not capable of recognizing and describing his own involvements with the same objectivity as those who observe him. His attention is necessarily focused on patient's material and, being himself involved in this complex interaction, cannot fully appreciate his own part in it. This expectation was fully borne out by our study.

As was expected the processing of the voluminous data thus collected proved to be a prolonged affair, which will require several years of collaborative work. Yet even at the present stage of processing, several important conclusions emerge. The most important of these is the fact that the traditional descriptions of the therapeutic process do not adequately reflect the immensely complex interaction between therapist and patient. The patient's reactions cannot be described fully as transference reactions. The patient reacts to the therapist as to a concrete person and not only as a representative of parental figures. The therapist's reactions also far exceed what is usually called countertransference. They include, in addition to this, interventions based on conscious deliberations and also his spontaneous idiosyncratic attitudes. Moreover, his own values are conveyed to the patient even if he consistently tries to protect his incognito. The patient reacts to the therapist's overt but also to his nonverbal hidden intentions and the therapist reacts to the patient's reaction to him. It is a truly transactional process.

In studying this transactional material I came to the conviction that the therapeutic process can be best understood in the terms of learning theory. Particularly the principle of reward and punishment and also the influence of repetitive experiences can be clearly recognized. Learning is defined as a change resulting from previous experiences. In every learning process, one can distinguish two components. First the motivational factor, namely, the subjective needs which activate the learning process and second, certain performances by which a new behavioral pattern suitable to fill the motivational need is actually acquired. In most general terms unfulfilled needs no matter what their nature may be — hunger for food, hunger for love, curiosity, the urge for mastery — initiate groping trial and error efforts which cease when an adequate behavioral response is found. Adequate responses lead to need satisfaction which is the reward for the effort. Rewarding responses are repeated until they become automatic and their repetition no longer requires effort and further experimentation. This is identical with the feedback mechanisms described in cybernetics. Every change of the total situation requires learning new adequate responses. Old learned patterns which were adequate in a previous situation must be unlearned. They are impediments to acquiring new adequate patterns.

I am not particularly concerned at this point with the controversy between the more mechanistic concepts of the older behaviorist theory and the newer Gestalt theory of learning. The controversy pertains to the nature of the process by which satisfactory behavior patterns are acquired. This controversy can be reduced to two suppositions. The older Thorndike and Pavlov models operate with the principle of contiguity or connectionism. Whenever a behavioral pattern becomes associated with both a specific motivating need and need satisfaction, the organism will automatically repeat the satisfactory performance whenever the same need arises. This view considers the organism as a passive receptor of external and internal stimuli, which become associated by contiguity. The organism's own active organizing function is neglected. The finding of the satisfactory pattern, according to the classical theory, takes place through blind trial and error.

In contrast, the Gestalt theoretical model operates with the supposition that the trials by which the organism finds satisfactory behavioral responses are not blind but are aided by cognitive processes. They are intelligent trials which are guided by certain generalizations arrived at with the aid of the memory of previous experiences. They imply an active organization of previous experiences. This organizational act amounts to a cognitive grasp of the total situation. I am not concerned at this juncture with the seemingly essential difference between the connectionistic and Gestalt theories of learning. Probably both types of

learning exist. The infant learns without much help from previous experiences. In this learning blind trials and errors must of necessity prevail. Common basis in all learning, whether it takes place through blind trials and errors or by intelligent trials, is the forging of a connection between three variables: a specific motivating impulse, a specific behavioral response, and a gratifying experience which is the reward.

Accepting Freud's definition of thinking as a substitute for acting, that is to say, as acting in phantasy, the reward principle can be well applied to intellectual solutions or problems. Groping trials and errors in thought—whether blind or guided by cognitive processes—lead eventually to a solution which clicks. Finding a solution which satisfies all the observations without contradictions is accompanied by a feeling of satisfaction. After a solution is found—occasionally it may be found accidentally—the problem-solving urge, as everyone knows who has tried to solve a mathematical equation or a chess puzzle, ceases and a feeling of satisfaction ensues. The tension state which prevails as long as the problem is not solved yields to a feeling of rest and fulfillment. This is the reward for the effort, whether it consists of blind or intelligent trials. The principle of reward can be applied not only to a rat learning to run a maze, but to the most complex thought processes as well. The therapeutic process can be well described in these terms of learning theory. The specific problem in therapy consists in finding an adequate interpersonal relation between therapist and patient. Initially this is distorted because the patient applies to this specific human interaction feeling-patterns and behavior-patterns which were formed in the patient's past and do not apply either to the actual therapeutic situation or to his actual life situation. During treatment the patient unlearns the old patterns and learns new ones. This complex process of relearning follows the same principles as the more simple relearning process hitherto studied by experimental psychologists. It contains cognitive elements as well as learning from actual interpersonal experiences which occur during the therapeutic interaction. These two components are intricately interwoven. They were described in psychoanalytic literature with the undefined, rather vague term *emotional insight*. The word *emotional* refers to the interpersonal experiences; the word *insight* refers to the cognitive element. The expression does not mean more than the recognition of the presence of both components. The psychological process to which the term refers is not yet spelled out in detail. Our present observational study is focused on a better understanding of this complex psychological phenomenom—emotional insight—which appears to us as the central factor in every learning process including psychoanalytic treatment. Every intellectual grasp, even when it concerns entirely nonutilitarian preoccupations, such as playful puzzle-solving efforts, is motivated by some

kind of urge for mastery and is accompanied with tension resolution as its reward. In psychotherapy the reward consists in less conflictful, more harmonious interpersonal relations, which the patient achieves first by adequately relating to his therapist, then to his environment, and eventually to his own ego ideal. At first he tries to gain the therapist's approval by living up to the supreme therapeutic principle—to the basic rule of frank self-expression. At the same time he tries to gain acceptance by living up to the therapist's expectations of him, which he senses in spite of the therapist's overt nonevaluating attitude. And finally, he tries to live up to his own genuine values, to his cherished image of himself. Far-reaching discrepancy between the therapist's and the patient's values is a common source of therapeutic impasse.

This gradually evolving dynamic process can be followed and described step by step in studies made by nonparticipant observers. Current studies give encouragement and hope that we shall eventually be able to understand more adequately this intricate interpersonal process and to account for therapeutic successes and failures. As in every field of science, general assumptions gradually yield to more specific ones which are obtained by meticulous controlled observations. The history of sciences teaches us that new and more adequate technical devices of observation and reasoning are responsible for advancements. In the field of psychotherapy the long overdue observation of the therapeutic process by nonparticipant observers is turning out to be the required methodological tool. This in itself, however, is not sufficient. The evaluation of the rich and new observational material calls for new theoretical perspectives. Learning theory appears to be at present the most satisfactory framework for the evaluation of observational data and for making valid generalizations. As it continuously happens at certain phases of thought development in all fields of science, different independent approaches merge and become integrated with each other. At present, we are witnessing the beginnings of a most promising integration of psychoanalytic theory with learning theory, which may lead to unpredictable advances in the theory and practice of the psychotherapies.

REFERENCES

1. Alexander, F., and French, T. M.: *Psychoanalytic Therapy. Principles and Application*. New York: Ronald Press, 1946.
2. Alexander, F.: *Psychoanalysis and Psychotherapy*. New York: W. W. Norton, 1956.
3. Alexander, F.: *Behav. Sci., 3*; Oct. 1958.
4. Balint, A., and Balint, M.: *Int. J. Psychoanal., 20*; 1939.
5. Benedek, T.: *Bull. Menninger Clin., 17*:6, 1953.
6. Fenichel, O.: *The Psychoanalytic Theory of Neurosis*. New York: W. W. Norton, 1945.

7. Freud, S.: The Dynamics of the Transference (1912). Collected Papers, Vol. II. London: Hogarth Press, 1924.
8. Freud, S.: Recommendations for Physicians on the Psychoanalytic Method of Treatment (1912). *Collected Papers, Vol. II.* London: Hogarth Press, 1924.
9. Freud, S.: Further Recommendations in the Technique of Psychoanalysis on Beginning the Treatment. The question of the first communications. The Dynamics of the Cure (1913). *Collected Papers, Vol. II.* London: Hogarth Press, 1924.
10. Freud, S.: Further Recommendations in the Technique of Psychoanalysis. Recollection, Repetition and Working Through (1914). *Collected Papers, Vol. II.* London: Hogarth Press, 1924.
11. Freud, S.: Further Recommendations in the Technique of Psychoanalysis. Observations on Transference-Love (1915). *Collected Papers, Vol. II.* London: Hogarth Press, 1924.
12. Freud, S.: *New Introductory Lectures on Psychoanalysis.* New York: W. W. Norton, 1933.
13. Fromm-Reichmann, F.: *Principles of Intensive Psychotherapy.* London: Allen & Unwin, 1957.
14. Heimann, P.: *Int. J. Psychoanal.,* 31: 1950.
15. Rado, S.: *Psychoanalysis of Behavior: Collected Papers.* Vol. I (1922-1956); Vol. II (1956-1961). New York: Grune and Stratton, Vol. I, 1956, Vol. II, 1962.
16. Weigert, E.: *J. Am. Psychoanal. Ass.,* 2: 4, 1954.

Dynamic Psychotherapy and Behavior Therapy

Are They Irreconcilable?

JUDD MARMOR, M.D.

The following article by Marmor is noteworthy because it constituted one of the earliest recognitions by an experienced psychoanalyst of the legitimacy and efficacy of behavioral therapy for certain clinical conditions. Marmor, like others before him, is critical of simplistic theoretical explanations of the behavioral therapeutic process. By focusing on the therapist-patient transactions in three different behavioral techniques—Wolpe's reciprocal inhibition therapy, aversive conditioning in homosexuality, and the Masters-Johnson approach to sexual dysfunction—Marmor demonstrates that what actually goes on in these techniques is much more complex than behavioral therapy implies. He suggests that common denominators are involved in the therapeutic processes of both behavior therapy and dynamic psychotherapy but with differences of emphasis. Thus he considers them to be complementary, rather than antithetical, approaches to therapy.

Dynamic Psychotherapy and Behavior Therapy

Are They Irreconcilable?

JUDD MARMOR, M.D.

In the course of psychiatric training and practice our professional iden-
tities become so intimately linked to what we have learned and how we
practice that we are prone to extol uncritically the virtues of our own
techniques and to depreciate defensively those techniques that are different. The dialogue that has gone on between most behavior therapists
and dynamic psychotherapists has been marred by this kind of bias, and
claims as well as attacks have been made on both sides that are exaggerated and untenable. Science is not served by such emotional polemics
but rather by objective efforts to evaluate and extend our knowledge.

Part of the confusion that exists in discussing these two basic approaches to therapy is that they are often dealt with as though each
group represents a distinct entity when, in fact, they are anything but
monolithic. The various schools of thought among dynamic psychotherapists are too well known to require elaboration. They cover a wide
range from classical Freudians to adherents of other major theorists to
eclectics who borrow from all of them to still others who try to adapt
their concepts to correspond with modern learning theories, information
theory, game theory, or general systems theory.

What is less well known is that among behavior therapists also there
is a broad range of differences, from adherents of Pavlov and Hull to
Skinnerians to eclectics and to those who lean toward information
theory and general systems theory. At one end of each spectrum the
theories of behavioral and dynamic psychotherapists tend to converge,
while at the other end their divergence is very great. It is because adherents of these two approaches tend to define each other stereotypically
in terms of their extremes that so much misunderstanding and heat are
often generated between them.

Reprinted by permission from *Archives of General Psychiatry*, 24:22-28, January 1971.
Copyright 1971 by the American Medical Association.

It would further serve to clarify the discussion of this problem if we distinguish between investigative methods, therapeutic techniques, and theoretical formulations. A good investigative technique is not necessarily a good therapeutic technique, nor is the reverse true. By the same token, as we have long known, the success of a psychotherapeutic method for any particular condition does not in itself constitute a validation of its theoretical framework; indeed, exactly why and how any particular psychotherapeutic method works and what it actually accomplishes within the complex organization of drives, perception, integration, affect, and behavior that we call personality is itself a major research challenge.

In the remarks that follow, therefore, I shall not concern myself with the knotty issues of the comparison of results between behavior and psychodynamic therapies or of their validation. The problem of how to measure or evaluate psychotherapeutic change is still far from clear, and a matter for much-needed research. Moreover, comparisons of results between these two approaches are unsatisfactory because different criteria of efficacy are applied, and different techniques of investigation are employed, even if complete objectivity on the part of the various protagonists could be assumed—which is doubtful!

In addition, I shall not get into the oft-argued issue of whether or not simple symptom removal inevitably leads to symptom substitution. Long before behavior therapists began to question this hoary assumption, hypnotherapists had presented evidence that symptom substitution did not always take place when a symptom was removed by hypnosis.[1] Indeed, I would agree, on purely theoretical grounds, that symptom substitution is *not* inevitable. Earlier psychoanalytic assumptions concerning symptom substitution were based on what we now know was an erroneous closed-system theory of personality dynamics. If the conflictual elements involved in neurosis formation are assumed to be part of a closed system, it follows logically that removal of the symptomatic consequences of such an inner conflict without altering the underlying dynamics should result in some other symptom manifestation. If, however, personality dynamics are more correctly perceived within the framework of an open system, then such a consequence is not inevitable. Removal of an ego-dystonic symptom may, on the contrary, produce such satisfying feedback from the environment that it may result in major constructive shifts within the personality system, thus leading to modification of the original conflictual pattern. Removal of a symptom also may lead to positive changes in the perception of the self, with resultant satisfying *internal* feedbacks, heightening of self-esteem, and a consequent restructuring of the internal psychodynamic system.

Psychodynamic theorists have been aware of this possibility for many years, dating back at least to 1946 when Alexander and French[2] published their book entitled *Psychoanalytic Therapy*. In this volume a number of cases of brief psychotherapy are described, some of them involving only one to three interviews, following which the patients were not only dramatically relieved of their presenting symptoms but were then able to go on to achieve more effective adaptive patterns of functioning than they had previously displayed. In the years that followed this important publication, dynamic psychotherapists have become increasingly involved with techniques of brief psychotherapy and of crisis intervention, with a growing body of evidence that in many instances such interventions can have long-lasting positive consequences for personality integration.

Where I part company with most behavior therapists is not in questioning their therapeutic claims—although I would offer the caution that many of them are repeating the error of the early psychoanalysts of promising more than they can deliver—but in what I consider to be their oversimplified explanations of what goes on in the therapeutic transaction between patient and therapist. The explanations to which I refer are those which assume that the essential and central core of their therapeutic process rests on pavlovian or skinnerian conditioning and, incidentally, is therefore more "scientific" than the traditional psychotherapies. With these formulations often goes a conception of neurosis that seems to me to be quite simplistic. Thus, according to Eysenck, "Learning theory [note that he uses the singular—actually there are many theories of learning] regards neurotic symptoms as simply learned habits; there is no *neurosis* underlying the symptom but merely the symptom itself. *Get rid of the symptom and you have eliminated the neurosis.*"[3] Such an explanation is like evaluating the contents of a package in terms of its wrapping, and represents a regrettable retrogression from the more sophisticated thinking that has begun to characterize dynamic psychiatry in recent years; an approach that recognizes that "psychopathology" does not reside solely in the individual but also has significant roots in his system of relationships with his milieu and with other persons within his milieu. Hence the growing emphasis on family therapy, on conjoint marital therapy, on group therapy, and on dealing with the disordered socioeconomic conditions which constitute the matrix of so many personality disorders. To see the locus of psychopathology only in the individual leads to an emphasis on techniques of adjusting the individual to his environment regardless of how distorted, intolerable, or irrational that environment might be. Such an emphasis brings us uncomfortably close to the dangerous area of thought and behavior control.

However, I do not wish to overemphasize this ethical issue. The fact that a technical method may lend itself to being misused does not constitute an argument against its scientific validity. My major point is that the *theoretical* foundation of Eysenck's formulation is scientifically unsound. Even if we deliberately choose to restrict our focus only to what goes on within the individual himself, the eysenckian point of view has profound limitations. It overlooks all of the complexities of thought, symbolism, and action which must be accounted for in any comprehensive theory of psychology and psychopathology. To assume that what goes on subjectively within the patient is irrelevant and that all that matters is how he behaves is to arbitrarily disregard all of the significant psychodynamic insights of the past 75 years. In saying this, I am not defending all of psychoanalytic theory. I have been as critical as anyone of certain aspects of classical freudian theory and I am in full accord with those who argue that psychodynamic theory needs to be reformulated in terms that conform more closely to modern theories of learning and of neurophysiology. Current researches strongly suggest that the brain functions as an extremely intricate receiver, retriever, processor, and dispatcher of information. A stimulus-response theory of human behavior does not begin to do justice to this complex process. It is precisely what goes on in the "black box" *between* stimulus and response that is the central challenge of psychiatry, and no theory that ignores the complexities of the central processes within that "black box" can be considered an adequate one. It is to Freud's eternal credit, regardless of the limitations of some of his hypotheses, that he was the first to develop a rational investigative technique for, and a meaningful key to, the understanding of this uncharted realm that exerts so profound an influence on both our perceptions and our responses.

Evidence from learning theories themselves reveals that neurotic disorders are not necessarily the simple product of exposure to traumatic conditioning stimuli or to the operant conditioning of responses. The work of Pavlov, Liddell, Masserman, and others has clearly demonstrated that neurotic symptoms can ensue when an animal is faced with incompatible choices between simultaneous approach and avoidance reactions, or with confusing conditioned stimuli which it is unable to differentiate clearly. This corresponds to the psychodynamic concept of conflict as being at the root of the vast majority of human neurotic disorders. Once such a neurotic conflict is set up in a human being, secondary elaborations, defensive adaptations, and symbolic distortions may become extensively and indirectly intertwined with almost every aspect of the individual's perceptual, cognitive, and behavioral process.

A behavioral approach alone cannot encompass these complexities. Granting that skinnerians include verbal speech as an aspect of behavior that may require modification, what shall we say about subjective *fantasies*, concealed *thoughts*, and hidden *feelings*? Are they totally irrele-

vant? What about problems involving conflicts in value systems, disturbances in self-image, diffusion of identity, feelings of anomie, or even
concealed delusions and hallucinations? Are they less important than
specific symptom entities of a behavioral nature? No comprehensive
theory of psychopathology or of the nature of the psychotherapeutic
process can properly ignore these aspects of man's subjective life.

To illustrate my point that much more goes on between therapist
and patient than most behavior therapists generally recognize, I should
like now to briefly focus on three contrasting behavioral therapeutic approaches: (1) Wolpe's technique of reciprocal inhibition, (2) aversive
conditioning treatment of homosexuality, and (3) the Masters and
Johnson technique of treating sexual impotence and frigidity. In discussing these three approaches, I wish to emphasize that it is not my intention to denigrate their usefulness as therapeutic modalities or to question their results, but solely to present some of the diverse variables that
I believe are involved in their therapeutic effectiveness.

Wolpe has elaborated his technique in many publications as well as
in at least one film that I have seen. Although he considers the crux of
his technique to be the development of a hierarchical list of graded anxieties which are then progressively dealt with by his technique of "reciprocal inhibition," the fact is that a great deal more than this takes
place in the patient-therapist transaction in the Wolpe technique. Most
significantly, in the orientation period of the first session or two the
patient is informed not only of the treatment method per se, but also of
the fact that it has yielded successful results with comparable patients,
and it is indicated implicitly, if not explicitly, that the patient can expect
similar success for himself if he is cooperative. Wolpe, moreover, is
warm, friendly, and supportive. At the same time he is positive and
authoritative in such a way as to reinforce the patient's expectations of
therapeutic success. During this introductory period a detailed history is
taken and even though the major emphasis is on the symptom with all
of its manifestations and conditions for appearance, a detailed genetic
history of personality development is usually taken also.

Following this a hierarchical list of the patient's anxieties is established. The patient is then taught a relaxation technique which is remarkably similar to what is traditionally employed in inducing hypnosis. After complete relaxation is achieved, the patient is instructed to
create in fantasy these situations of graded anxiety beginning at the lowest level of anxiety, and is not permitted to go to the next level until he
signals that he is completely relaxed. This procedure is repeated over
and over again in anywhere from 12 to 60 or more sessions until the
patient is able to fantasy the maximally phobic situation and still achieve
muscular relaxation. Throughout this procedure the patient receives the

strong implication, either explicitly or implicitly, that this procedure will cause his symptoms to disappear.

Wolpe attributes the success of his technique to "systematic desensitization" and explains it on the basis of pavlovian counterconditioning. He asserts that any "activities that might give any grounds for imputations of transference, insight, suggestion, or de-depression," are either "omitted or manipulated in such a way as to render the operation of these mechanisms exceedingly implausible."[4] This kind of claim that Wolpe repeatedly makes in his writings clearly reflects his failure to appreciate the complexity of the variables involved in the patient-therapist transaction. I cannot believe that anyone who watches Wolpe's own film demonstration of his technique would agree that there are no elements of transference, insight, or suggestion in it. Indeed, one could make as plausible a case for the overriding influence of suggestion in his technique as for the influence of desensitization. In saying this I am not being pejorative about Wolpe's technique. Suggestion, in my opinion, is an integral part of every psychotherapeutic technique, behavioral or psychodynamic. It need not be overt; indeed, it probably works most potently when it is covert. Suggestion is a complex process in which elements of transference, expectancy, faith, and hope all enter. To the degree that a patient is receptive and perceives the therapist as a powerful help-giving figure, he is more likely to accept the suggestions he is being given and to try to conform to them. This process is most obvious in hypnosis but it is equally present in all psychotherapeutic techniques, where the suggestion is usually more covert. Wolpe's technique abounds in covert as well as overt suggestion. It is questionable, moreover, whether the fantasies that Wolpe has his patients create are actual substitutes for the phobic reality situations, as he would have us believe. It may well be that what is really taking place is not so much desensitization to specific stimuli as repeated reassurance and strong systematic suggestion, within a setting of heightened expectancy and faith.

However, even the combination of *desensitization* (assuming that it is taking place) and *suggestion* do not begin to cover all the elements that are present in the Wolpe method. There is also the *direct transmission of values* as when Wolpe says to a young patient, "You must learn to stand up for yourself." According to Ullmann and Krasner,[5] Wolpe hypothesizes that if a person can assert himself, anxiety will automatically be inhibited. (Parenthetically, one might question whether this is inevitably so. One frequently sees patients who assert themselves regularly, but always with enormous concomitant anxiety.) In any event, Ullmann and Krasner say: "The therapist provides the motivation by pointing out the irrationality of the fears and encouraging the individual to insist on his legitimate human rights."[5] Obviously this is not very different from what goes on in dynamic psychotherapy and it is not rendered different by virtue of the fact, according to Ullmann and Krasner, that it is "given a physiological basis by Wolpe, who refers to it as excitatory."[5] Still another variable which cannot be ignored is Wolpe's manner, which, whether he realizes it or not, undoubtedly facilitates a "positive transference" in his patients. In his film he is not only kindly and empathic to his female patient, but occasionally reassuringly touches her. Does Wolpe really believe that a programmed computer repeating his instructions to a patient who had had no prior contact with the doctor himself would achieve the identical therapeutic results?

The second behavioral technique that I would like to briefly consider is that of the aversion treatment of homosexuals. I had occasion to explore this technique some time ago with Dr. Lee Birk, of the Massachusetts Mental Health Center, who was kind enough to demonstrate his technique and go over his results with me.

Dr. Birk's method is based on the anticipatory avoidance conditioning technique introduced by Feldman and MacCulloch.[6] The patient is seated in a chair in front of a screen with an electrode cuff attached to his leg. The method involves the use of patient-selected nude and seminude male and female pictures which are flashed onto the screen. The male pictures (and presumably the fantasies associated with them) become aversive stimuli by linkage with electric shocks which are administered to the leg whenever these pictures appear on the screen. On the other hand, the female pictures become discriminative stimuli signaling safety, relief, and protection from the shocks.

In Dr. Birk's hands, as in others, the use of this method has apparently produced a striking reversal of sexual feelings and behavior in more than one-half of the male homosexuals so treated. On the face of it, this would seem to be the result of a relatively simple negative conditioning process to aversive "male" stimuli, with concomitant positive conditioning to "female" stimuli.

Closer inspection will reveal, however, that the process is considerably more complex. I wonder whether most psychiatrists realize what is actually involved in such aversive conditioning. I know that I, for one, did not, until I asked Dr. Birk to permit me to experience the kind of shock that he administered to his patients—the least intense, incidentally, of the graded series that he employed. I can only say that if that was a "mild" shock, I never want to be subjected to a "severe" one! I do not have a particularly low threshold for pain, but it was a severe and painful jolt—much more than I had anticipated—and it made me acutely aware of *how strongly motivated toward change a male homosexual would have to be to subject himself to a series of such shocks visit after visit.*

The significance of this variable cannot be ignored. Once it is recognized, the results of aversive therapy, although still notable, become less remarkable. The fact is that if other forms of psychotherapy were limited only to such a select group of exceptionally motivated homosexuals, the results also would be better than average. Although one might assume that in dynamic psychotherapies the cost of therapy in itself should insure equally good motivation, this is not always the fact. Costs of therapy may not be sacrificial, or they may be borne or shared by others, but no one else can share the pain involved in the aversive conditioning process.

Again, then, it becomes clear that we are dealing with something that is much more complicated than a simple conditioning process. The patient's intense wish to change, and his faith and expectation that this very special technique will work for him—as the doctor himself implicitly or explicitly suggests—are important factors in the total therapeutic gestalt of this aversive technique, as they are in successful dynamic psychotherapies also.

But more than this, the transference-countertransference transaction between therapist and subject is also of paramount importance. Dr. Birk communicated two interesting experiences he had which underline this point. Two of his subjects who had had very favorable responses to the "conditioning" procedure suffered serious relapses immediately after becoming angry at him. The first patient became upset because of what he considered a breach in the privacy of his treatment. Before this, he had not only been free from homosexual contacts for the first time in many years, but also free of conscious homosexual urges. When he became angry, he immediately went and sought out a homosexual partner because he wanted to see "how really good" the treatment was. Dr. Birk was aware that his patient obviously wanted to show him up and prove that the treatment was no good. Although the patient remained improved as compared to his previous homosexual behavior, *he was never again,* despite many more conditioning treatments, completely free from conscious homosexual urges and continued to act them out although less frequently than in the past. The second patient became angry with Dr. Birk because he concluded that the therapist seemed to be more interested in the results he was obtaining than he was in the patient as a person. Immediately after expressing this irritation the patient regressed to a series of homosexual encounters.

These striking examples illustrate that a simple conditioning explanation does not fit the complex process that goes on in such techniques of therapy. Aversive conditioning that has been solidly established would not be expected to disappear on the basis of such experiences unless there is something that goes on centrally in the patient that is a very important factor in the therapeutic modifications achieved. A basic aspect of this central process is in the patient-physician interpersonal relationship and it cannot and must not be ignored even in behavior therapies. I have recently encountered a number of instances where patients who were referred to behavior therapists failed to return to them after the initial sessions because the behavior therapists involved ignored this essential factor and related to the patients as though they were dealing with experimental animals.

Let us now turn to a consideration of the Masters and Johnson[7] technique of treating disorders of sexual potency. In many ways this technique falls midway between a behavioral and a psychodynamic approach and illustrates one of the ways in which a fusion of both can be successfully employed. The Masters and Johnson technique is behavioral in the sense that it is essentially symptom-focused, and that one of its most important technical tools is desensitization of the performance anxieties of the patients.

Conceptually, however, the Masters and Johnson approach to their patients goes considerably beyond simple conditioning or desensitization processes. For one thing, Masters and Johnson recognize that the problem of impotency or frigidity does not exist merely in the symptomatic individual but in his relationship with his partner. Therefore, they insist on treating the couple as a unit, and the symptom as a problem of the unit. This constitutes a systems approach in contrast to a strictly intrapsychic or behavioral one.

Secondly, Masters and Johnson are acutely aware of the influence of psychodynamic factors on the sexual behavior of their couples. In their preliminary interviews they carefully assess and evaluate the importance of these factors, and if they consider the neurotic components or interpersonal difficulties to be too great, they may refuse to proceed with their method and will refer the couple back to their physicians for appropriate psychotherapy.

This kind of selective procedure has an effect, of course, on their percentage of successful results, as does the high degree of motivation that their patients must have to come to St. Louis (who, after all, goes to St. Louis for a two-week vacation?) and to commit themselves to the considerable expense and inconvenience that is involved.

The fact, also, that Masters and Johnson insist that the therapeutic team consist of a man and a woman reveals their sensitivity to the transference implications of their relationship to their couples. They function as a sexually permissive and empathic mother-surrogate and father-surrogate who offer not only valuable technical advice and suggestions concerning sexual behavior, but also a compassion and understanding that constitute a corrective emotional experience for their patients.

Finally, the tremendous charisma and authority of this highly publicized therapeutic team must inevitably have an enormous impact on the expectancy, faith, and hope with which their patients come to them. This cannot help but greatly accentuate the suggestive impact of the given instructions in facilitating their patients' therapeutic improvement. This improvement is then reinforced by subsequent follow-up telephone calls which, among other things, confirm to the patient the empathic interest, concern, and dedication of these parent-surrogates.

I am all too aware that these brief and summary remarks cannot begin to do justice to the three above-mentioned behavioral techniques. I hope, however, that I have succeeded in making the point that in each of these instances, complex variables are involved that go beyond any simple stimulus-response conditioning model.

The research on the nature of the psychotherapeutic process in which I participated with Franz Alexander beginning in 1958 has convinced me that all psychotherapy, regardless of the techniques used, is a learning process.[8-10] Dynamic psychotherapies and behavior therapies simply represent different teaching techniques, and their differences are based in part on differences in their goals and in part on their assumptions about the nature of psychopathology. Certain fundamental elements, however, are present in both approaches.

In any psychotherapeutic relationship, we start with an individual who presents a problem. This problem may be in the form of behavior that is regarded as deviant, or it may be in the form of subjective discomfort, or in certain distortions of perception, cognition, or affect, or in any combination of these. Usually, but not always, these problems motivate the individual or someone in his milieu to consider psychiatric treatment. This decision in itself establishes an *expectancy* in the individual which is quite different than if, say, "punishment" rather than "treatment" were prescribed for his problems. This expectancy is an essential part of *every* psychotherapeutic transaction at its outset, regardless of whether the patient presents himself for behavioral or dynamic psychotherapy. The patient, in other words, is *not* a neutral object in whom certain neurotic symptoms or habits have been mechanically established and from whom they can now be mechanically removed.

Expectancy is a complex process. It encompasses factors that Frank[11] has demonstrated as being of major significance in psychotherapy—the degree of faith, trust, and hope that the patient consciously or unconsciously brings into the transaction. It is based in large part on previously established perceptions of authority or help-giving figures, perceptions that play a significant role in the degree of receptivity or nonreceptivity that the patient may show to the message he receives from the psychotherapist. Psychoanalysts have traditionally referred to these presenting expectations as aspects of "transference," but regardless of what they are called, they are always present. Transference is not, as some behavior therapists seem to think, something that is "created" by the therapist—although it is true that transference distortions may be either increased or diminished by the technique the therapist employs. The way in which the therapist relates to the patient may reinforce certain maladaptive perceptions or expectations, or it may teach the patient that his previously learned expectations in relation to help-giving or authority figures are incorrect. The latter teaching is part of what Alexander and French[2] called the "corrective emotional experience."

Even in "simple" conditioning studies, experimenters like Liddell, Masserman, and Pavlov have called attention to the significance of the relationship between the experimental animal and the experimenter. In humans the problem is more complex, however. Thus, a therapist who behaves in a kindly but authoritarian manner may confirm the patient's expectancies that authority figures are omnipotent and omniscient. This increases the patient's faith and may actually facilitate his willingness to give up his symptoms to please the powerful and good parent-therapist, but it does *not* alter his childlike self-image in relation to authority figures. Depending on the therapist's objectives, this may or may not be of importance.

What I am indicating, in other words, is that a positive transference facilitates symptom removal, but if the patient's *emotional maturation, rather than just symptom removal, is the goal of therapy,* what is necessary eventually is a "dissolution" of this positive transference—which means teaching the patient to feel and function in a less childlike manner, not only in relation to the therapist but also to other authority figures.

Closely related and interacting with the patient's motivations and expectancies is the therapist's social and professional role, by virtue of which the help-seeking patient endows him with presumptive knowledge, prestige, authority, and help-giving potential. These factors play an enormous role in strengthening the capacity of the therapist to influence the patient, and constitute another element in the complex fabric that makes up the phenomenon of positive transference.

Also, the *real persons* of both patient and therapist, their actual physical, intellectual, and emotional assets and liabilities, and their respective *value systems* enter into the therapeutic transaction. Neither the patient nor the therapist can be regarded as a stereotype upon whom any particular technique will automatically work. Their idiosyncratic variables are always an important part of their transaction.

Given the above factors, a number of things begin to happen more or less simultaneously, in varying degrees, in behavior therapies as well as in dynamic psychotherapies. I have discussed these factors in detail elsewhere and will merely summarize them here. They are: (1) *Release of tension* through catharsis and by virtue of the patient's hope, faith, and expectancy; (2) *cognitive learning*, both of the trial-and-error variety and of the gestalt variety; (3) reconditioning by virtue of *operant conditioning*, by virtue of subtle reward-punishment cues from the therapist, and by corrective emotional experiences; (4) identification with the therapist; (5) repeated *reality testing*, which is the equivalent of *practice* in the learning process. These five elements encompass the most significant factors on the basis of which change takes place in a psychotherapeutic relationship.[10]

As I have mentioned above, suggestion takes place in all of these, covertly or overtly. Furthermore, as can be seen, a conditioning process takes place in dynamic psychotherapies as well as in behavior therapies, except that in the latter this process is intentional and more structured, while in the former it has not been generally recognized. In focusing on this conditioning process, behavior therapists have made a valuable contribution to the understanding of the therapeutic process. It is the thrust of this paper, however, that in so doing they have tended to minimize or ignore other important and essential elements in the therapeutic process, particularly the subtle but critical aspects of the patient-therapist interpersonal relationship.

In the final analysis, the technique of therapy that we choose to employ must depend on what aspect of man's complex psychic functioning we address ourselves to. If we choose to focus on the patient's overt symptoms or behavior patterns, some kind of behavior therapy may well be the treatment of choice. On the other hand, if the core of his problems rests in symbolic distortions of perception, cognition, affect, or subtle disturbances in interpersonal relationships, the source and nature of which he may be totally unaware, then the more elaborate reeducational process of dynamic psychotherapy may be necessary.

Moreover, indications for one approach do not necessarily rule out the other. Marks and Gelder[12,13] and Brady,[14] among others, have demonstrated that the use of both behavior therapy and dynamic therapy in the same patient either concurrently or in sequence often brings about better therapeutic results than the use of either approach alone. Indeed, many dynamic psychotherapists have for years been unwittingly using such a combination of approaches when they prescribe drugs for the direct control of certain symptoms while concurrently pursuing a psychotherapeutic approach.

To conclude, then, in my opinion behavior therapies and dynamic psychotherapies, far from being irreconcilable, are complementary psychotherapeutic approaches. The line of demarcation between them is by no means a sharp one. As Breger and McGaugh[15] and others have shown, behavior therapists do many things in the course of their conditioning procedures that duplicate the activities of dynamic psychotherapists including "discussions, explanation of techniques and of the unadaptiveness of anxiety and symptoms, hypnosis, relaxation, 'nondirective cathartic discussions,' and 'obtaining an understanding of the patient's personality and background.' "[15] The process in both approaches is best explicable in terms of current theories of learning which go beyond simple conditioning explanations and encompass central cognitive processes also. The fact that in some disorders one or the other approach may be more effective should not surprise us and presents no contradiction. Just as there is no single best way of teaching all pupils all subjects, there is no single psychotherapeutic technique that is optimum for all patients and all psychiatric disorders.

Within this total context, it seems to me that behavior therapists deserve much credit for having opened wide the armamentarium of therapeutic strategies. By so doing, they have forced dynamic psychotherapists into a reassessment of their therapeutic techniques and their effectiveness—a reassessment that in the long run can only be in the best interests of all psychiatrists and their patients. The psychotherapeutic challenge of the future is to so improve our theoretical and diagnostic approaches to psychopathology as to be able to most knowledgeably and flexibly apply to each patient the particular treatment technique and the particular kind of therapist that together will most effectively achieve the desired therapeutic goal.

Since completing this paper, I have come across the excellent article by Klein et al.[16] in which many of the conclusions I have set forth are confirmed by them as a result of five days of direct observation of the work of Wolpe and his group at the Eastern Pennsylvania Psychiatric Institute. The authors also point out that as a consequence of their increasing popularity, behavior therapists are now beginning to treat a broader spectrum of more "difficult" patients (complex psychoneurotic problems, character neuroses, or borderline psychotic problems) with the result that their treatment procedures are "becoming longer and more complicated, with concomitant lowering of success rates."

References

1. Wolberg LR: Hypnotherapy, in McCary JL (ed): *Six Approaches to Psychotherapy*. New York, Dryden Press, 1955, pp 63-126.
2. Alexander F, French TM, et al: *Psychoanalytic Therapy*. New York, Ronald Press Co, 1946.
3. Eysenck HJ (ed): *Behavior Therapy and the Neuroses*. New York, Pergamon Press, 1960.
4. Wolpe J: *Psychotherapy by Reciprocal Inhibition*. Stanford, Calif, Stanford University Press, 1958.

5. Ullmann LP, Krasner L (eds): *Case Studies in Behavior Modification*. New York, Holt Rinehart & Winston Inc, 1965.
6. Feldman MP, MacCulloch MI: The application of anticipatory avoidance learning to the treatment of homosexuality. *Behav Res Ther* 2:165-183, 1965.
7. Masters WH, Johnson VE: *Human Sexual Response*. Boston, Little, Brown & Co, 1965.
8. Marmor J: Psychoanalytic therapy as an educational process, in Masserman J, Salzman L (eds): *Modern Concepts of Psychoanalysis*. New York, Philosophical Library Inc, 1962, pp 189-205.
9. Marmor J: Psychoanalytic therapy and theories of learning, in Masserman J (ed): *Science and Psychoanalysis*. New York, Grune and Stratton Inc, 1964, vol 7, pp 265-279 [See also Chapter 3, this volume.]
10. Marmor J: The nature of the psychotherapeutic process, in Usdin G (ed): *Psychoneurosis and Schizophrenia*. New York, JB Lippincott Co, 1966, pp 66-75.
11. Frank JD: *Persuasion and Healing*. Baltimore, Johns Hopkins Press, 1961.
12. Marks IM, Gelder MG: A controlled retrospective study of behavior therapy in phobic patients. *Brit J Psychiat* 111: 561-573, 1965.
13. Marks IM, Gelder MG: Common ground between behavior therapy and psychodynamic methods. *Brit J Med Psychol* 39:11-23, 1966. [See also Chapter 10, this volume.]
14. Brady JP: Psychotherapy by a combined behavioral and dynamic approach. *Compr Psychiat* 9:536-543, 1968. [See also Chapter 15, this volume.]
15. Breger L, McGaugh JL: Critique and reformulation of learning theory approaches to psychotherapy and neurosis. *Psychol Bull* 63:338-358, 1965. [See also Chapter 4, this volume.]
16. Klein MH, Dittman AT, Parloff MB, et al: Behavior therapy: Observations and reflections. *J Consult Clin Psychol* 33:259-266, 1969. [See also Chapter 14, this volume.]

Psychoanalytic Therapy and Theories of Learning

JUDD MARMOR, M.D.

In this paper, published a year later than Alexander's but written before Alexander's paper was published (which is why no reference is made to Alexander's paper), Marmor pursues the same line of thought that Alexander does in his paper, but discusses some of the pertinent theories of learning in somewhat greater detail and elaborates on the kinds of learning that take place in psychoanalysis and dynamic psychotherapy.

It is noteworthy that Alexander's and Marmor's articles were both outgrowths of their experiences in the Ford Foundation research project described by Alexander in the preceding paper. The use of nonparticipant observers made it possible for the first time to begin to appreciate what Alexander called "the immensely complex interaction between therapist and patient" and the learning process that was involved in it.

Psychoanalytic Therapy and Theories of Learning

JUDD MARMOR, M.D.

In a previous communication[14] I advanced the suggestion that psychoanalytic therapy is a learning procedure and that its underlying *modus operandi* is essentially the same in the various "schools" of psychoanalysis despite their ideological differences. Today I wish to look more closely at some contributions of learning theory which have relevance to psychoanalytic therapy, and to consider more thoroughly some of the inherent problems.

Learning has been defined by Hilgard[8] as "the process by which an activity originates or is changed through reacting to an encountered situation, provided that the characteristics of the change in activity cannot be explained on the basis of native response tendencies, maturation, or temporary (physiological) states of the organism." It should be noted that in human beings such a definition encompasses all behavior which cannot be attributed to the exclusive effects of biological drives (i.e., instincts), growth and maturation, or transitory states caused by drugs, fatigue, infections, etc. Clearly, all neurotic and deviant behavior which is not entirely physiologically determined falls within the scope of this definition; it is "learned" through experiential vicissitudes with parents, siblings, peers, and all of the other people, objects, and relationships which are encountered by an individual in the course of his development. Together these constitute the infinite variety of unconditioned and conditioned stimuli which subtly shape his adaptive responses from the moment of birth on.

Over the past half century an enormous body of experimental work has accumulated, representing the efforts of behavioral scientists to elucidate the nature of this learning process, and although there are at least as many schools of learning theory as there are of psychoanalysis, certain basic points of agreement have gradually emerged which ought

Reprinted by permission from *Science and Psychoanalysis*, 7:265-279, Grune & Stratton, Inc., New York, 1964.

not to be disregarded in our efforts to refine the core of our own psycho-analytic theories and practices.

As Hilgard[9] points out, learning theories fall into two major families: *stimulus-response* theories—represented by those of Thorndike, Guthrie, Skinner and Hull—and *cognitive* theories—exemplified by those of Tolman, Kurt Lewin, and the gestalt psychologists. The former tend to regard most learned behavior as a process of gradual accretion acquired through conditioning and trial-and-error sequences in which responses are reinforced by reward or success, or inhibited by punishment or fail-ure. The cognitive group, on the other hand, tends to emphasize the greater importance in learning of more rapid perceptual "insights" or understanding.

The eclectic learning theorist recognizes that both types of learning take place in life. Trial-and-error learning is more apt to take place when the essence of the adaptive problem is beyond the immediate cognitive grasp of the learner and where imitation is not possible; even here, how-ever, one has to make a distinction between random fumbling and an intelligent search for solutions. On the other hand, where cognitive so-lutions are possible, human beings tend to learn by insight and, in social situations, to a considerable extent by imitation.[17] Freud's concept of the reality principle clearly refers to patterns of thought and behavior which are learned partly through cognitive insights and partly through trial and error—all influenced by experienced rewards and punishments.

With regard to personality development in general, early psychoan-alytic theory tended to emphasize "libidinal" pleasure-strivings and *de-fenses* against anxiety as the primary shaping forces. It has been only in the past 25 years that more adequate recognition has been given in psy-choanalytic theory to the "nonlibidinal," "nondefensive," *adaptive*, and maturational strivings of the organism, as well as to indirect effects of the social and cultural environment. Over the same quarter century, psychologists too, particularly Skinner and Hull, have laid increasing stress upon "reinforcing" stimuli in the environment, and particularly upon positive or rewarding reinforcers, as primary motivating factors in the acquisition of new behavior patterns.

In general it can be said that psychoanalytic theory has tended to focus more strongly on the *internal* motivational aspects of personality development, while learning theories have tended to focus their atten-tion more strongly on the nature of the *external* conditions which facili-tated or retarded the acquisition of new behavioral patterns. In this re-spect the effect of each has been to enhance and deepen the understand-ing of the total learning situation in humans.

The fundamental problem with which we are faced in psychoana-lytic therapy is that of how we can enable or cause the patient to give up certain acquired patterns of thought, feeling, or behavior in favor of others which are considered more "mature," "adaptive," "productive," or "self-realizing." The learning theorist, if he is a member of the stimulus-response school, structures this as an effort to teach the patient new habit patterns; or, if he belongs to the cognitive school, as an effort to teach the patient new patterns of perception and new cognitive "insights."

Psychoanalytic theories have generally favored the latter conception as the essential model for what happens in therapy. In his earlier papers, Freud assumed that the insights involved were related to repressed memories of childhood traumata[6] and that the mere recovery of these memories would *ipso facto* result in altered patterns of behavior very rapidly. Subsequently,[7] Freud modified these expectations and placed emphasis instead upon the more arduous and prolonged task of the "working through" of the patient's "resistances."

It is clear that an important difference between the analytic situation and any *de novo* learning situation is that in the treatment of personality disorders the task is complicated by the fact that the previously learned behavior—the neurotic pattern—is particularly resistant to change. Learning theorists have suggested various reasons for this "resistance" that differ from the usual psychoanalytic explanation of repression. One of the major explanations offered is that the neurotic behavioral pattern had adaptive value originally or still does. On the basis of the original adaptive value, it is thought that the neurotic habit patterns tended to become "overlearned," as a result of which they have become more resistant to extinction. In terms of their current adaptive value the learning theorist suggests that there are conflicting environmental stimuli in which the pain or discomfort of some aspects of the neurotic behavior is constantly being offset by the positive reinforcement of its benefits to the patient. This corresponds to what analysts call the "secondary gain" of the neurosis.

In any event, there is little doubt that the problem of overcoming the resistance to change in the neurotic patient—in whatever conceptual framework this resistance is seen—remains the basic challenge of the psychoanalytic and psychotherapeutic process. Let us consider the contributions of learning theories to two major aspects of this problem: (1) the role of cognitive insights and (2) the role of the patient-therapist interaction.

In the aforementioned communication, I suggested[14] that since the insight given by therapists from differing psychoanalytic schools differed in content and yet their patients were all capable of showing favorable therapeutic responses, the specific insight given could not logically be the only or exclusive basis for the therapeutic response. I would like, however, to elaborate upon this problem.

A rather important distinction needs to be made first, it seems to me, between the "insight" *given* by the analyst and the "insight" which is *perceived* by the patient. I have suggested that insight, as given by a therapist, "is essentially the conceptual framework by means of which a therapist establishes, or attempts to establish, a logical relationship between events, feelings, or experiences that seem unrelated in the mind of the patient," and that "in terms of the analyst's objectives, insights constitute the *rationale* by which the patient is persuaded to accept the model of more 'mature' or 'healthy' behavior which analysts of all schools, implicitly or explicitly, hold out to him."[14] In looking back upon this formulation, however, it occurs to me that it is subject to the misinterpretation that insights given by analysts of different schools may be capriciously different, and that they do not necessarily have any relationship to the actual realities of the patient's life and behavior. Such an interpretation would be misleading. *The insights given by psychoanalysts of different schools all bear a definite relationship to clinical reality* and all fit the observable facts reasonably well, although the proponents of each theory, of course, believe theirs to be the most valid and fruitful way of organizing these facts.

Consider a specific clinical example. A young man, descriptively, is passively dependent in his interpersonal relationships. A Freudian might organize the observable data of the patient's life around the fact that he was either excessively indulged or excessively frustrated in the early years of childhood, that he is consequently fixated at an "oral-receptive" level of libidinal development, with an unresolved Oedipus complex, etc. An Adlerian might organize the same data around the patient's having developed expectations of being taken care of, with a consequent "life-style" of passivity and helplessness as a way of achieving this objective. A member of the Horney school might interpret the same material in terms of a neurotic need for affection and a basic pattern of "moving toward" people. A Rankian might derive his interpretations from the basic problem of separation anxiety and defenses against it. A Jungian might bring in the concept of the archetypal Mother and the patient's deep strivings for reunion with her. A follower of Erich Fromm might think in terms of "receptive orientation," "symbiotic relationships," and "nonproductivity" in dealing with the same data. A Sullivanian might theorize in terms of "oral dynamisms" and emphasize the patient's "interpersonal relationships" in his interpretations; while a student of Rado might speak of "emergency controls" and "adaptational mechanisms." *The critical point, however, is that fundamentally they are all dealing with the same data, and that there is a central core of common reality underlying all of these "insights"* — they all refer to observed or inferred patterns of passivity, dependency, and immaturity in the patient, and the implicit or explicit message which is inherent in the various interpretations is essentially the same—namely that the patient's behavior ought to become more mature, self-assertive, and autonomous.*

What I have sketchily set forth with passive dependency can be done equally with any other specific clinical pattern of behavior, whether it be aggressiveness, competitiveness, fearfulness, withdrawal, compulsiveness, etc. In each instance proponents of different schools may explain these phenomena with theoretical constructs which represent different ways of organizing the same data but which are fundamentally saying the same thing to the patient. The relative merit of each theory, then, is not a matter of which is more "true" but rather a matter of which is more parsimonious, and which has the greater heuristic and predictive value. One should not even rule out the possibility that for certain kinds of data one theoretical approach seems more meaningful while for other kinds, another might be. This would correspond to Bohr's theory of "complementarity" in the field of physics.

But what about "insight" on the part of the patient? Is it the same thing? Unfortunately the term *insight*, as applied to what goes on in the patient, is used very ambiguously in psychoanalysis. Occasionally it refers merely to a cognitive awareness of the analyst's interpretation. It is then usually described as "intellectual insight." If, on the other hand, the cognitive awareness is accompanied by a simultaneous display or "release" of emotion, the insight is believed to be "deeper" and is then referred to as "emotional insight." The latter is considered to be more efficacious than the former in changing neurotic behavior, yet every analyst knows that frequently even emotional insight does not result in alterations of the neurotic pattern. Under such circumstances, the analyst who is convinced that insight is the key to therapeutic change will sometimes argue that the insight is still not sufficiently deep or thorough, and that resistance to a full awareness still has to be overcome. This is implicitly utilizing a behavioral criterion for insight without making it explicit. Presumably, when the patient *really* understands, he will behave differently; which is merely another way of saying that

---

*Subsequently, patients of each school, as a result of the suggestive impact of their analyst's interpretations, inevitably tend to bring out data in their dreams and "free associations" which appear to confirm the theoretical frame of reference of their analysts. This is why each theory seems to be self-validating and this is what makes the "dialogue" between members of differing schools so difficult. For this reason, too, the relative validity of the various psychoanalytic theories can never be established from their respective analytic data, but must be sought for in phenomena and experimental findings which can be reproduced and objectively verified by members of all schools, as well as by nonanalysts.

when he begins to behave adaptively, it will then be assumed that his insight is genuine!*

It is of interest in this context to consider what the Gestalt theorists, who more than any other school of learning theory concerned themselves with the problem of insight, had to say about it. Hilgard,[10] in summarizing the experimental work of the Gestaltists, describes three distinctive criteria of insight in an experimental subject: (1) a period of survey, inspection and attention which is then followed by the critical solution, (2) the ready repetition of the solution after a single critical solution, (3) the ability to generalize the insight to new situations that require mediation by common principles or awareness of common relationships. Exemplifying these criteria, once Kohler's or Yerkes's apes grasped the gestalt of the experimental problem, they were able, immediately and thereafter, not only to solve the problem, but also to generalize the insight to new problems based on similar principles.[20]

It is worth noting that by these criteria, the definition of insight is linked to the ability of the subject to solve a previously unsolved problem. Such a sequence of events can and occasionally *does* take place following a psychoanalytic interpretation or confrontation. The patient may have what Karl Buhler has called an "a-ha" experience[4] and from that point on no longer reacts with the neurotic pattern, the maladaptive nature of which has now become clear to him.

More often, however, the mere acquisition of intellectual or even emotional insight does not result in any immediate alteration of the neurotic patterns. There still remains the arduous and time-consuming task of (1) overcoming the patient's tendency to cling tenaciously to his previously learned patterns of perception and behavior, and (2) enabling him to generalize the acquired "insights" to all situations in which similar principles are operative. These two tasks are essentially what is involved in the concept of "working through."

It is with regard to the nature of this "working through" process that proponents of the Skinner and Hull schools of learning theory in recent years have come up with some particularly interesting findings. A host of experimental studies[2,11,12,18] seem to indicate that the nonverbal as well as the verbal reactions of the therapist act as positive and negative reinforcing stimuli to the patient, encouraging certain kinds of responses and discouraging others. According to these investigators, what seems to be going on in the working through process is a kind of conditioned learning, in which the therapist's overt or covert approval and

---

*E.g., Zilboorg: "Insight is a state of personality or ego functioning as much as a neurosis is a special state of ego functioning. It should be considered the ultimate and crowning point of integration of ego functioning."[21]

disapproval—expressed in his nonverbal reactions as well as in his verbal confrontations, and in what he interprets as neurotic or healthy —act as reward-punishment cues or conditioning stimuli.* The analyst's implicit or explicit approval acts as a positive reinforcer to the more "mature" patterns of reacting, while his implicit or explicit disapproval tends to inhibit the less "mature" patterns. As with experimental studies in animals, this process requires frequent repetition before the previous overlearned conditioned responses become extinguished, and the new conditioned-responses ("habit patterns") become firmly established.†

Interestingly enough, experimental studies have demonstrated that intermittent and irregular reinforcements are more effective than frequent or regular ones in changing patterns of behavior or maintaining desired ones.[19] This would appear to bear out Franz Alexander's claim[1] that variations in the frequency of analytic visits as well as intermittent vacations from analysis appear to have a beneficial effect on the course of therapy. This is a fruitful area for further research, not only with regard to the question of frequency and regularity of visits but also with regard to the question of the length of therapeutic sessions. There is no reason to assume *a priori* that the traditional 50-minute hour which is a historical carry-over from what Freud found personally convenient necessarily represents an optimum time arrangement for all patients.

Some interesting findings on the relative value of positive (rewarding) reinforcers and negative (punitive) ones in effecting behavioral changes also have a bearing on certain problems of analytic and psychotherapeutic technique. Kurt Lewin[13] was the first to point out the differences in the field situation that exist between reward techniques and punishment techniques. If a subject is kept at an intrinsically disliked task by the threat of punishment, he is being forced to choose between two disagreeable alternatives, and his impulse then will be to "leave the field" altogether, to avoid both alternatives. To prevent him from leaving, usually some kind of policing, authoritarian measures become

---

*As I have pointed out elsewhere,[15] the so-called neutrality of the analyst is a fiction, and constitutes an attitude which invariably affects the patient either positively or negatively, depending on his needs.

†It is of interest to note that in the course of this therapeutic transaction, the therapist, as well as the patient, undergoes a learning experience. By the end of an analysis it can usually be observed that the analyst's perceptions of and relationship to his patient are quite different from what it was originally. The patterns of *mutual* trust and understanding that develop between therapist and patient are important ingredients in the therapeutic process. One must also recognize that self-correcting mechanisms within the patient himself, as well as fortuitous events in his life outside of the analyst's office, also enter into the complex of forces which produce change in the patient.

necessary. In this connection one is reminded of the classical psychoanalytic assumption that an atmosphere of frustration favors the analytic
process—thus the patient may be forbidden to smoke, his questions may
go unanswered, the analyst maintains an aloof attitude, etc. Now it is
true that moderate anxiety often increases a learner's motivation, but it
is also true that too much anxiety disrupts the learning process. The
usual consequence of too frustrating a technique in psychoanalysis is
either that the patient leaves the field altogether—i.e. breaks off the
treatment—or else that he regresses into more primitive patterns of behavior. Although this so-called reactivation of the "infantile neurosis" is
considered to be an essential aspect of classical analysis and an important desideratum, it is by no means proved that this is either the only or
the best route to the eventual establishment of more mature patterns of
behavior.

Another example of the rule of frustration is the common assumption that the patient must make a sacrifice—generally a financial one—if
he is really to benefit from therapy. The implicit rationale here is that the
pain of having to give up substantial portions of his security will help to
overcome his inner resistances to change. As Lewin's work indicates,
however, if both of these alternatives are sufficiently disagreeable, the
more likely outcome is that the patient will quit the therapeutic field
altogether. As I have stated elsewhere[16] the patient's motivation in
therapy depends "on how much the suffering from his illness outweighs
any secondary gains which he obtains from it. While the amount of
money he is willing to pay to get rid of his illness may *reflect* the degree
of his motivation, it is not the *source* of it. . . There is by now a vast body
of experience which indicates that patients in free and low-cost psychoanalytic clinics can respond to therapy just as well as patients in private
offices."

In contrast to a punitive situation, the attractiveness of a reward
situation tends to keep the learned in the field rather than drive him out
of it. Lewin's work indicates, however, that the reward must be obtain-
able only by the performance of the desired task; otherwise the learner
will simply short-circuit the feared or disliked activity and fail to change.
Assuming the immediate rewards which the patient seeks in the transference situation is the therapist's "love" and approval, then Lewin's
findings suggest that the common psychological assumption that "love
should be unconditional," if it is interpreted to mean an unconditional
positive reaction to anything the patient says or does, may be neither
good psychology nor good therapy. The approach which is most likely
to effect changes in behavior, according to him, would be to give approval when the desired behavior takes place, but to withhold it when it

does not take place. Furthermore, as indicated previously, intermittent approval is more effective than constant approval, even when the desired behavior is forthcoming.*

Lewin also makes a significant distinction between reward and success, particularly when the desired goals are intrinsic, as they are in the analytic situation. The reward of approval enables a patient to make progress toward his goals, but only the achieving of a goal constitutes a success experience. Success leads to the development of a sense of mastery which is one of the chief objectives of the therapeutic process. This underlines the importance for both the therapist and the patient of setting realistic and attainable goals.

Estes, a follower of Skinner, did a number of experiments on the effects of punishment on learning which also have a bearing on psychotherapeutic techniques.[5] Estes's experiments demonstrated that a response cannot be eliminated from an organism's repertoire by the action of punishment alone—i.e., punishment alone suppressed the response, but the tendency toward the response continued to exist.† Moreover, he found, punishment not only did not hasten the elimination of a response, but actually retarded its elimination. Permanent weakening of a response came about only when it failed to elicit any reinforcement at all, positive or negative, and this weakening process was prevented if the punishment did not permit the response to occur at all! To put this in a familiar clinical context, a child's tantrums are more likely to stop occurring if they elicit no response at all than if they incur punishment. Within the therapeutic situation this implies that apart from the positive reinforcing value of approval, the simple withholding of approval may be a more potent therapeutic instrument for changing the patient than the direct expression of disapproval. This, it seems to me, confirms the value of the traditional psychoanalytic technique of avoiding attitudes of moral condemnation toward socially dystonic behavior in the patient. To carry over this "neutrality," however, to avoiding a show of approval toward desirable behavior patterns may not be equally therapeutic.

Still another experimental finding was that punishment tends to suppress other responses in addition to the one punished. In analytic parlance we would say that it leads to ego restriction, while reward tends to lead toward expansion of ego function.

---

*This should not be misunderstood as negating the paramount importance in the therapeutic transaction of the therapist's genuine interest in the patient's welfare and belief in his fundamental worth as a human being. It may be useful, however, to make a distinction between such basic *acceptance* of the patient and *approval* of his behavior.

†This is a validation of the psychoanalytic concept that if an impulse is repressed it will nevertheless continue to exist in the unconscious.

One of the consequences of the increased awareness of psychotherapy as a learning process is the emergence of a school of therapists which lays stress on techniques of modifying the *behavior* of the patient without reference to his subjective cognitive or emotional processes and without recourse to interview psychotherapy. This school utilizes theoretical constructs of learning theory and stresses principles of counterconditioning, extinction, discrimination, operant conditioning, reciprocal inhibition, and social limitation. Significantly, most of the clinical examples dealt with in their case reports are phobias and circumscribed symptom complexes, rather than personality disorders.

Bandura, in a recent book entitled *Behavioristic Psychotherapy*,[3] attacks the prevailing theories of psychopathology as essentially an amalgam of "medical and demonology models, which have in common the belief that the underlying pathology and not the symptomatic manifestations must be treated." "Consequently," he says, "therapeutic attention is generally focused not on the deviant behavior itself, but on the presumably influential internal processes." He argues further that what is called a symptom is merely a learned reaction which is regarded as deviant, and that "when the actual social learning history of maladaptive behavior is known, 'psychodynamic' explanations become superfluous." Moreover, he contends, once the maladaptive *behavior* is altered by the application of appropriate social learning procedures it is unnecessary to modify or remove "an underlying pathology," and symptom substitution will not occur. He emphasizes that concepts such as ego strength or emotional maturity or mental health are hypothetical constructs which in the final analysis can be inferred only from observable behavior. He regards behavior as the only modifiable reality available to the psychotherapist.

I have quoted Bandura's views in some detail not only because they are representative of this new movement in psychotherapy, but also because they reflect a basic blind spot which is characteristic of this school of therapists. Although my central thesis in this paper has been to stress the value of an understanding of learning theory for psychoanalytic therapy, and although I am in agreement with some of the criticisms leveled by the members of this school against certain aspects of psychoanalytic theory and practice, I believe that people like Bandura, Wolpe, and Eysenck are making the serious error of throwing the baby out with the bath water, and of returning to a kind of oversimplified behaviorism which cognitive learning theorists, no less than Freud, have demonstrated long ago to be inadequate. To assume that what goes on subjectively within the patient is irrelevant and that all that matters is how he behaves is to discard a half century of psychodynamic insights. We know that two people may behave in externally identical ways for en-

tirely different internal reasons. A socially adjusted schizophrenic whose outward behavior is apparently normal is nevertheless a considerably different individual from one with identical outward behavior but without the inner delusional system. Moreover, symptoms are obviously not always behavioral, and the "free-floating" panic reactions of a person with an anxiety state may have no objective stimulus precipitating them against which the patient can be counterconditioned. In addition, certain behavioral symptoms, like those in conversion hysteria, are clearly only symbolic expressions of an underlying psychological conflict, and the mere removal of the symptom, which is often a simple matter, does not touch the underlying conflict at all. This is a clinical fact which decades of clinical experience have repeatedly verified. It is precisely the vast and complex area *between* stimulus and response that constitutes the major concern of modern dynamic psychiatry. It is what *cannot* be objectively seen or measured that is our chief challenge and preoccupation. It was Freud's genius, regardless of whatever limitations some of his theoretical assumptions have turned out to have, that he was the first to present us with a technique and a key to a rational understanding of this vast subjective, symbolic, and largely unconscious realm which exerts so profound an influence upon both our perceptions and our actions.

Bandura quotes with obvious approval the case of a fetishist with an impulse to smear mucus on ladies' handbags, who was treated by the counterconditioning technique of the paired presentation of a collection of handbags with the onset of nausea produced by injections of apomorphine; and claims that an 18-month follow-up study revealed not only that the fetish had been successfully eliminated but that the patient showed a "vast improvement" in his social, legal, vocational, and sexual relationships. I have no way of evaluating the validity of this particular case report, but certainly there have been many years of experience with similar counterconditioning therapies in cases of alcoholism; and the ineffectiveness of such an approach, when used exclusively, in modifying the inner psychodynamic problems of the alcoholic is a matter of common knowledge. When Bandura asserts that no symptom substitution occurs in such cases he seems to be assuming that symptoms must be behaviorally manifested since the persistence of tension and anxiety states in alcoholics treated by counterconditioning therapy is a matter of common observation and is the basis for the general recommendation that any such therapy, if utilized, must be combined with psychotherapy aimed at the patient's underlying inner conflicts.

Moreover, the evidence of learning theory itself reveals that neurotic disorders are not the simple product of an exposure to a painful conditioned stimulus. The work of Pavlov, Liddell, Masserman, and others

has clearly demonstrated that neurotic symptoms ensue when an animal is faced with incompatible choices eliciting simultaneous approach and avoidance reactions, or with confusing conditioned stimuli which it is unable clearly to differentiate. This corresponds to the psychoanalytic concept of conflict which is at the root of the vast majority of neurotic disorders in humans. Once such a neurotic conflict is set up, the secondary elaborations, defensive adaptations, and symbolic distortions become extensively involved in every aspect of the individual's thought and behavioral processes.

I am not attempting to deny the potential usefulness of counterconditioning techniques as a part of our total psychotherapeutic armamentarium. I believe that the proponents of these views have a contribution to make and that there may well be types of behavioral disorders, particularly those which have been induced by a single traumatic experience or series of such experiences, in which such forms of therapy have a great deal to offer. It should not surprise us that certain techniques work better than others with different patients and different problems. Just as there is no single best way of teaching all people and all subjects, there is no single best way of treating all patients. To assume, however, that behavioral disorders and personality distortions which have been subtly inculcated by 5, 10, or 20 years of daily disturbances in interpersonal experience, by an entire climate of faulty relationships, confused communications, inconsistent disciplinary cues, etc., can be totally eradicated by the application of a dozen or two counterconditioning sessions aimed at some specific behavioral symptom is to simply misjudge the complexity of the problems that are being dealt with.

For such problems I believe there is still no satisfactory substitute for the time-consuming process of patiently reeducating the patient concerning the nature of his perceptual, emotional, symbolic, and behavioral distortions and of enabling him, by the working-through process, to generalize and apply his increased understanding to many different life situations. The therapeutic techniques of all the current psychoanalytic "schools," regardless of their conceptual differences, operate upon this basis, either explicitly or implicitly. In this process cognitive learning, imitation (identification with the analyst), and a subtle conditioning procedure all usually take place, in varying degrees.* Precisely because this is a learning process we as analysts have much to gain

*That therapeutic change *can* take place with hardly any cognitive insight is a matter of common experience. Not infrequently, successfully analyzed patients report that their feelings and functioning have improved enormously, but that they have no idea of what it was that made them better! In such instances unconscious identification processes, subtle conditioning, and corrective emotional experiences have probably been the chief sources of the therapeutic modifications.

by a better acquaintance with the contributions of the various theories of learning to see what application we can make of their findings in our own work. I shall not pretend that I have made more than a bare beginning in this direction with this paper; I have not even touched, for example, on the possible applications of communications theory, cybernetics, game theory, and general systems theory to psychoanalytic theory and practice. I would hope, however, that this effort may encourage others to explore these fruitful areas.

References

1. Alexander, F.: The principle of flexibility. *In* F. Alexander and T. M. French (Eds.), *Psychoanalytic Therapy*. New York, Ronald Press, 1946, Ch. 3.
2. Bandura, A.: Psychotherapy as a learning process. *Psychol. Bull.* 58:143, 1961.
3. Bandura, A.: *Behavioristic Psychotherapy*. New York, Holt, Rinehart & Winston, 1963.
4. Buhler, K.: *Die Krise der Psychologie*, 2nd Ed., Jena, Gustav Fischer, 1929, p. 136.
5. Estes, W. K.: An experimental study of punishment. *Psychol. Monogr.* 57, No. 263, 1944.
6. Freud, S.: *Collected Papers*, London, Hogarth Press, 1933, Vol.2, p. 362.
7. Freud, S.: Ibid., p. 376.
8. Hilgard, E. R.: *Theories of Learning*, 2nd Ed., New York, Appleton-Century-Crofts, 1956.
9. Hilgard, E. R.: Ibid., p. 8.
10. Hilgard, E. R.: Ibid., p. 238.
11. Krasner, L.: Studies of the conditioning of verbal behavior. *Psychol. Bull.* 55:148, 1958.
12. Krasner, L.: The therapist as a social reinforcement machine. *In* H. H. Strupp and L. Luborsky (Eds.), *Research in Psychotherapy*, Washington, D.C., Am. Psychol. Assoc., 1963.
13. Lewin, K.: Field theory and learning. *In The Psychology of Learning*. Nat. Soc. Stud. Educ., 41st Yearbook, 1942, Ch. 4.
14. Marmor, J.: Psychoanalytic therapy as an educational process. *In* J. H. Masserman (Ed.), *Psychoanalytic Education*, New York, Grune and Stratton, 1962, p. 286.
15. Marmor, J.: A reevaluation of certain aspects of psychoanalytic theory and practice. *In* L. Salzman and J.H. Masserman (Eds.), *Modern Concepts of Psychoanalysis*, New York, Philosophical Library, 1962, p. 191.
16. Marmor, J.: Ibid., p. 203.
17. Miller, N. E. and Dollard, J. C.: *Social Learning and Imitation*. New Haven, Yale University Press, 1941.
18. Shoben, E. J., Jr.: Psychotherapy as a problem in learning theory. *Psychol. Bull.* 46:366, 1949.
19. Skinner, B. F.: *The Behavior of Organisms: An Experimental Analysis*. New York, Appleton-Century-Crofts, 1938.
20. Yerkes, R. M.: The mind of a gorilla. *Genetic Psychol. Monogr.* 1927, p. 156.
21. Zilboorg, A.: The emotional problem and the therapeutic role of insight. *Psychoanal. Quart.* 21:1, 1952.

Critique and Reformulation of "Learning-Theory" Approaches to Psychotherapy and Neurosis

LOUIS BREGER, PH.D., AND
JAMES L. MCGAUGH, PH.D.

This classic paper by Breger and McGaugh was the first within the field of clinical psychology to critically review and elegantly dissect the overly simplistic theoretical explanations of the process of behavioral therapy. Without denying the clinical usefulness of certain behavioral therapies, the authors cogently demonstrate that the explanations given by their proponents of how they work are quite inadequate. Particularly open to criticism are (a) the emphasis on the peripheral response, (b) the assumption that concepts taken from Pavlovian and operant conditioning can be utilized as explanatory principles, and (c) the use of the concept of reinforcement. Breger and McGaugh, in addition, demonstrate the inadequacy of a conception of neurosis that is couched only in terms of discrete symptoms. Finally, they offer a reformulation of the learning process in which it is seen as the acquisition and storage of information, with emphasis on the role of central processes. Thus they construct a theoretical structure that can more adequately explain what goes on in both behavioral therapies and dynamic psychotherapies.

Critique and Reformulation of "Learning-Theory" Approaches to Psychotherapy and Neurosis

4

LOUIS BREGER, PH.D., AND
JAMES L. McGAUGH, PH.D.

A careful look at the heterogeneous problems that are brought to psychotherapy points up the urgent need for new and varied theories and techniques. While some new methods have been developed in recent years, the field is still characterized by "schools"—groups who adhere to a particular set of ideas and techniques to the exclusion of others. Thus, there are dogmatic psychoanalysts, Adlerians, Rogerians, and, most recently, dogmatic behaviorists.

It is unfortunate that the techniques used by the behavior-therapy group (Bandura, 1961; Eysenck, 1960; Grossberg, 1964; Wolpe, 1958) have so quickly become encapsulated in a dogmatic "school," but this seems to be the case. Before examining the theory and practice of behavior therapy, let us first distinguish three different positions, all of which are associated with the behaviorism or "learning-theory" label. These are: (a) Dollard and Miller (1950) as represented in their book, (b) the Wolpe-Eysenck position as represented in Wolpe's work (1958; Wolpe, Salter, and Reyna, 1964) and in the volume edited by Eysenck (1960), and (c) the Skinnerian position as seen in Krasner (1961) and the work that appears in the *Journal of the Experimental Analysis of Behavior.*

Dollard and Miller present an attempt to translate psychoanalytic concepts into the terminology of Hullian learning theory. While many recent behavior therapists reject Dollard and Miller because of their identification with psychoanalysis and their failure to provide techniques distinct from psychoanalytic therapy, the Dollard-Miller explanation of neurotic symptoms in terms of conditioning and secondary anxiety drive is utilized extensively by Wolpe and his followers. Wolpe's position seems to be a combination of early Hullian learning theory and various active therapy techniques. He relies heavily on the idea of recip-

Reprinted by permission from *Psychological Bulletin,* 63:338-358, May 1965. Copyright 1965 by the American Psychiatric Association.

rocal inhibition, which is best exemplified by the technique of counter-conditioning. In line with this Hullian background, Wolpe, Eysenck, and others in this group use explanations based on Pavlovian conditioning. They define neurosis as "persistent unadaptive habits that have been conditioned (that is, learned)" (Wolpe et al., 1964, p. 9), and their explanation of neurosis stresses the persistence of "maladaptive habits" which are anxiety reducing.

The Skinnerian group (see Bachrach in Wolpe et al., 1964) have no special theory of neurosis; in fact, following Skinner, they tend to disavow the necessity of theory. Their approach rests heavily on *techniques* of operant conditioning, on the use of "reinforcement" to control and shape behavior, and on the related notion that "symptoms," like all other "behaviors," are maintained by their effects.

Our discussion will be directed to the Wolpe-Eysenck group and the Skinnerians, keeping in mind that some of the points we will raise are not equally applicable to both. Insofar as the Skinnerians disavow a theory of neurosis, for example, they are not open to criticism in this area.

It is our opinion that the current arguments supporting a learning-theory approach to psychotherapy and neurosis are deficient on a number of grounds. First, we question whether the broad claims they make rest on a foundation of accurate and complete description of the basic data of neurosis and psychotherapy. The process of selecting among the data for those examples fitting the theory and techniques while ignoring a large amount of relevant data seriously undermines the strength and generality of the position. Second, claims for the efficacy of methods should be based on adequately controlled and accurately described evidence. And, finally, when overall claims for the superiority of behavioral therapies are based on alleged similarity to laboratory experiments and alleged derivation from "well-established laws of learning," the relevance of the laboratory experimental findings for psychotherapy data should be justified and the laws of learning should be shown to be both relevant and valid.

In what follows we will consider these issues in detail, beginning with the frequently voiced claim that behavior therapy rests on a solid "scientific" base. Next, we will examine the nature and adequacy of the learning-theory principles which they advocate. We will point out how their learning theory is unable to account for the evidence from laboratory studies of learning. That is to say, the laws or principles of conditioning and reinforcement which form the basis of their learning theory are insufficient explanations for the findings from laboratory experiments, let alone the complex learning phenomena that are encountered in psychotherapy. Then we will discuss how the inadequate conception of learning phenomena in terms of conditioned responses is paralleled by an equally inadequate conception of neurosis in terms of discrete symptoms. Within learning theory, conceptions of habit and response have been shown to be inadequate and are giving way to conceptions emphasizing "strategies," "plans," "programs," "schemata," or other complex central mediators. A central point of this paper is that conceptions of habit and response are also inadequate to account for neuroses and the learning that goes on in psychotherapy and must here too be replaced with conceptions analogous to strategies. Next we will turn our attention to an evaluation of the claims of success put forth by the proponents of behavior therapy. Regardless of the adequacy of their theory, the claims that the methods work are deserving of careful scrutiny. Here we shall raise a number of questions centering around the issue of adequate controls. Finally, we shall attempt a reformulation in terms of more recent developments within learning, emphasizing the role of central processes.

Science Issue

Claims of scientific respectability are made with great frequency by the behavior therapists. Terms such as *laboratory-based, experimental, behavioral, systematic,* and *control* are continually used to support their position. The validity of a theory or method must rest on empirical evidence, however. Thus, their use of scientific-sounding terminology does not make their approach scientific but rather seems to obscure an examination of the evidence on which their claims are based.

Let us examine some of this evidence. Bandura (1961) provides the following account of a typical behavior-therapy method (Wolpe's counterconditioning):

> On the basis of historical information, interview data, and psychological test responses, the therapist constructs an anxiety hierarchy, a ranked list of stimuli to which the patient reacts with anxiety. In the case of desensitization based on relaxation, the patient is hypnotized, and is given relaxation suggestions. He is then asked to imagine a scene representing the weakest item on the anxiety hierarchy and, if the relaxation is unimpaired, this is followed by having the patient imagine the next item on the list, and so on. Thus, the anxiety cues are gradually increased from session to session until the last phobic stimulus can be presented without impairing the relaxed state. Through this procedure, relaxation responses eventually come to be attached to the anxiety evoking stimuli. (p. 144)

Without going into great detail, it should be clear from this example that the use of the terms stimulus and response are only remotely allegorical to the traditional use of these terms in psychology. The "imagination of a scene" is hardly an objectively defined stimulus, nor is something as general as "relaxation" a specifiable or clearly observable response. What the example shows is that counterconditioning is no more objective, no more controlled, and no more scientific than classical psychoanalysis, hypnotherapy, or treatment with tranquilizers. The claim to scientific respectability rests on the misleading use of terms such as *stimulus, response,* and *conditioning,* which have become associated with some of the methods of science because of their place in experimental psychology. But this implied association rests on the use of the same *words* and not on the use of the same *methods*.

We should stress that our quarrel is not with the techniques themselves but with the attempt to tie these techniques to principles and concepts from the field of learning. The techniques go back at least as far as Bagby (1928), indicating their independence from "modern learning theory." Although techniques such as these have received little attention in recent years (except from the behavior therapists) they are certainly worth further consideration as potentially useful techniques.*

The use of the term *conditioning* brings us to a second point, that the claims to scientific respectability rest heavily on the attempts of these writers to associate their work with the prestigious field of learning. They speak of something called modern learning theory, implying that psychologists in the area of learning have generally agreed upon a large number of basic principles and laws which can be taken as the foundation for a "scientific" approach to psychotherapy. For example, Eysenck (1960) states:

> Behavior therapy . . . began with the thorough experimental study of the laws of learning and conditioning in normal people and in animals; these well-established principles were then applied to neurotic disorders. . . . It may be objected that learning theorists are not always in agreement with each other and that it is difficult to apply principles about which there is still so much argument. This is only very partially true; those points about which argument rages are usually of academic interest rather than of practical importance. . . . The 10% which is in dispute should not blind us to the 90% which is not—disagreements and disputes naturally attract more attention, but agreements on facts and principles are actually much more common. Greater familiarity with the large and rapidly growing literature will quickly substantiate this statement. (pp. 14-15)

As we shall show in the next section, this assertion is untenable. "Greater familiarity with the large and rapidly growing literature" shows that the very core of "modern learning theory," as Eysenck describes it, has been seriously questioned or abandoned in favor of alter-

---

*Another early application of behavioral techniques has recently been brought to our attention: Stevenson Smith's use of the Guthrie approach to learning in his work at the children's clinic at the University of Washington. Guthrie's interpretation of reinforcement avoids the pitfalls we discuss shortly, and contemporary behaviorists might learn something from a review of his work (see Guthrie, 1935).

native conceptualizations. For example, the notion that the discrete response provides an adequate unit of analysis, or that reinforcement can be widely used as an explanation of both learning and performance, or that mediational processes can be ignored is being or has been rejected. Eysenck's picture of the field as one with 90% agreement about basic principles is quite simply untrue. The references that Eysenck himself gives for this statement (Hilgard, 1956; Osgood, 1953) do not support the claim. Hilgard presented many theories, not one "modern learning theory," some of which (Gestalt, Tolman, Lewin) might just as easily be said to be in 90% disagreement with behavioristic conditioning approaches. In the same vein, Osgood's text was one of the first to give heavy emphasis to the role of mediation, in an attempt to compensate for the inadequacies of a simple conditioning or one-stage S-R approach. Eysenck seems largely unaware of the very problems within the field of learning which necessitated the introduction of mediational concepts, even by S-R theorists such as Osgood.

These inadequacies center, in part, around the problem of generalization. The problem of generalizing from the level of conditioning to the level of complex human behavior has been recognized for a long time (Lewin, 1951; Tolman, 1933). It is a problem that is crucial in simple laboratory phenomena such as maze learning where it has resulted in the introduction of a variety of mediational concepts, and it is certainly a problem when complex human behavior is being dealt with. For example, Dollard and Miller (1950) began their book with an attempt to explain neurosis with simple conditioning principles. A careful reading of the book reveals, however, that as the behavior to be explained became more and more complex, their explanations relied more and more on mediational concepts, including language. The necessity for these mediators arises from the inadequacy of a simple *peripheral* S-R model to account for the generality of learning, the equivalence of responses, and the adaptive application of behavior in novel situations. We shall return to these points shortly; here we just wish to emphasize that the field of learning is not "one big happy family" whose problems have been solved by the widespread acceptance of a simple conditioning model. The claim to scientific respectability by reference back to established laws of learning is, thus, illusory.

Learning and Learning Theories

We have already noted the differences between the Wolpe-Eysenck and the Skinnerian approaches; let us now examine the similarities. Three things stand out: the focus on the overt response, the reliance on a conditioning model, and the notion of reinforcement. First, there is the belief that the response, consisting of some discrete aspect of overt behavior, is the most meaningful unit of human behavior. While this should ideally refer to a specific contraction of muscles or secretion of glands, with the possible exception of Guthrie (1935), traditional S-R theorists have tended to define response in terms of an effect on the environment rather than as a specific movement of the organism. The problems raised by the use of the response as a basic unit, both in traditional learning phenomena and in the areas of neuroses and psychotherapy, will be discussed in the section entitled "What Is Learned?" A second common assumption is that the concepts taken from conditioning, either as described by Pavlov or the operant conditioning of Skinner, can be used as explanatory principles. The assumption in question here is that conditioning phenomena are the simplest kinds of learning and that all other behavior can be explained in terms of these "simple" principles. We shall deal with the problems that arise from this source in a second section. The third assumption is that rewards play an essential role in all learning phenomena. We shall consider the problems that stem from this assumption in a third section.

WHAT IS LEARNED?

Since its inception in the early twentieth century, behaviorism has taken overt stimuli and responses as its core units of analysis. Learning, as the behaviorist views it, is defined as the tendency to make a *particular response* in the presence of a *particular stimulus*; what is learned is a discrete response. Almost from its inception, however, this view has been plagued by a number of problems.

First, findings from studies of perception, particularly the fact of perceptual constancy, provide embarrassment for a peripheral S-R theory. Perceptual constancy findings show, for example, that the stimulus is much more than peripheral receptor stimulation. For example, once we have learned a song in a particular key (i.e., particular stimulus elements), we can readily recognize it or sing it in other keys. We are amazingly accurate in recognizing objects and events as being "the same" or equivalent, even though the particular stimulation they provide varies considerably on different occasions (Gibson, 1950). Although the bases of perceptual constancies (size, shapes, brightness, etc.) are not yet well understood, the facts of perceptual constancy—invariance in percept with variation in perceptual stimulation—are not in question. The related phenomenon of transposition has received considerable attention in animal experimentation. Animals, infrahuman as well as human, respond to relations among stimuli (Köhler, 1929). For a number of years, transposition was not considered to pose a serious problem for a peripheral S-R theory since it was thought that it could be adequately handled by principles of conditioning and stimulus generalization (Spence, 1937). This view has not been supported by later experiments, however (Lawrence and DeRivera, 1954; Riley, 1958). It now appears more likely that stimulus generalization is but a special case of the more general complex phenomenon of stimulus equivalence. The absolute theory of transposition was important and instructive because it revealed in clear relief the nature and limitations of a peripheral S-R approach to behavior. The effective stimulus is clearly more "central" than receptor excitation. The chapters on learning in the recent Koch series make it clear that workers in this area have seen the need for coming to terms with the facts of perception (Guttman, 1963; Lawrence, 1963; Leeper, 1963; Postman, 1963).

Second, the facts of response equivalence or response transfer posed the same kind of problem for a peripheral S-R view. A learned response does not consist merely of a stereotyped pattern of muscular contraction or glandular secretion. Even within the S-R tradition (e.g., Hull, Skinner), there has been a tendency to define responses in terms of environmental achievements. Anyone who has trained animals has recognized that animals can achieve the same general response, that is, make the same environmental change, in a variety of different ways once the response is learned. "What is learned," then is not a mechanical sequence of responses but rather, *what needs to be done in order to achieve some final event*. This notion is not new; Tolman stressed it as early as 1932 when he wrote of "purposive behavior," and it has been strongly supported by a variety of experimental findings (e.g., Beach, Hebb, Morgan, and Nissen, 1960; Ritchie, Aeschliman, and Peirce, 1950). As this work shows, animals somehow seem to be able to bypass the execution of specific responses in reaching an environmental achievement. They can learn to go to particular places in the environment in spite of the fact that to do so requires them to make different responses from trial to trial. The learning of relatively specific responses to specific stimuli appears to be a special case which might be called stereotyped learning (canalization) rather than a basic prototype on the basis of which all other learning may be explained.

It should be noted further that even the stereotyped learning that forms the basic model of S-R conditioning does not hold up under closer scrutiny. First, once a subject has learned a stereotyped movement or response, he is still capable of achieving a goal in other ways when the situation requires it. Thus, while we all learned to write our names with a particular hand in a relatively stereotyped fashion, we can switch to the other hand, or even write our name with a pencil gripped in our teeth if we have to, in spite of the fact that we may not have made this specific response in this way before. Second, even a response that is grossly defined as constant, stable, or stereotyped does not appear as such a stereotyped pattern of muscular contractions when it is closely observed.* These findings in the area of response transfer indicate that a response seems to be highly variable and equipotential. This notion is, of course, quite old in the history of psychology, and it has been stressed repeatedly by numerous investigators including Lashley (see Beach et al., 1960), Osgood (1953), Tolman (1932), and Woodworth (1958).

The facts of both response transfer and stimulus equivalence seem much more adequately handled if we assume that what is learned is a *strategy* (alternatively called cognitive maps, programs, plans, schemata, hypotheses, e.g., Krechevsky, 1932) for obtaining environmental achievements. When we take this view, habits, in the traditional behaviorist sense, become a later stage of response learning rather than a basic explanation (building block) for later, more complex learning.

Perhaps this whole problem can be clarified if we look at a specific example such as language learning. As Chomsky (1959) has demonstrated in his excellent critique of Skinner's *Verbal Behavior* (1957), the basic facts of language learning and usage simply cannot be handled within an S-R approach. It seems clear that an adequate view of language must account for the fact that humans, at a rather early age, internalize a complex set of rules (grammar) which enable them to both recognize and generate meaningful sentences involving patterns of words that they may never have used before. Thus, in language learning, what is learned are not only sets of responses (words and sentences) but, in addition, some form of internal strategies or plans (grammar). We learn a grammar which enables us to generate a variety of English sentences. We do not merely learn specific English sentence habits. How this grammar or set of strategies is acquired, retained, and used in language comprehension and generation is a matter for serious research effort; but it is clear that attempts to understand language learning on the basis of analogies from bar-pressing experiments are doomed before they start. To anticipate, we will argue shortly that if we are to make an attempt to understand the phenomena of neurosis using analogies from the area of learning, it will be much more appropriate to take these analogies from the area of psycholinguistics and language learning rather than, as has typically been done, from studies of classical and operant conditioning. That is, the focus will have to be on response transfer, equipotentiality, and the learning of plans and strategies rather than on stereotyped response learning or habituation.

*G. Hoyle, personal communication, 1963.

USE OF A CONDITIONING MODEL

As we indicated earlier, when writers in the behaviorist tradition say "learning theory," they probably mean a conditioning theory; most of the interpretations of clinical phenomena are reinterpretations in terms of the principles of conditioning. Thus, a phobic symptom is viewed as a conditioned response, maintained by the reinforcement of a secondary fear drive or by a Skinnerian as a single operant maintained by reinforcement. Two types of conditioning are involved in these explanations by reduction. The first is Pavlovian or classical conditioning, frequently used in conjunction with later Hullian concepts such as secondary drive; the second is operant conditioning of the kind proposed by Skinner. The use of both of these models to explain more complex phenomena such as transposition, response transfer, problem solving, language learning, or neurosis and psychotherapy poses a number of difficulties.

The basic assumption that underlies the use of either kind of conditioning as an explanation for more complex phenomena is that basic laws of behavior have been established in the highly controlled laboratory situation and may thus be applied to behavior of a more complex variety. When we look at the way conditioning principles are applied in the explanation of more complex phenomena, we see that only a rather flimsy analogy bridges the gap between such laboratory-defined terms as *stimulus, response,* and *reinforcement* and their referents in the case of complex behavior. Thus, while a stimulus may be defined as an electric shock or a light of a certain intensity in a classical conditioning experiment, Bandura (1961) speaks of the "imagination of a scene"; or, while a response may consist of salivation or a bar-press in a conditioning experiment, behavior therapists speak of anxiety as a response. As Chomsky (1959) puts it, with regard to this same problem in the area of language:

> He [Skinner in *Verbal Behavior*] utilizes the experimental results as evidence for the scientific character of his system of behavior, and analogic guesses (formulated in terms of a metaphoric extension of the technical vocabulary of the laboratory) as evidence for its scope. This creates the illusion of a rigorous scientific theory with a very broad scope, although in fact the terms used in the description of real-life and of laboratory behavior may be mere homonyms, with at most a vague similarity of meaning. (p. 30)

A second and related problem stems from the fact that the behavior-therapy workers accept the findings of conditioning experiments as basic principles or laws of learning. Unfortunately, there is now good reason to believe that classical conditioning is no more simple or basic than other forms of learning. Rather, it seems to be a form of learning that is in itself in need of explanation in terms of more general principles. For example, a popular but naive view of conditioning is that of stimulus substitution—the view that conditioning consists merely of the substitution of a conditioned stimulus for an unconditioned stimulus. Close examination of conditioning experiments reveals that this is not the case, however, for the conditioned response is typically *unlike* the unconditioned response (Zener, 1937). Apparently, in conditioning, a new response is learned. Most of the major learning theorists have taken this fact into account in abandoning the notion of conditioning as mere stimulus substitution.

More than this, the most important theoretical developments using essentially Pavlovian conditioning principles have not even stressed overt behavior (Osgood, 1953). Hull and the neo-Hullians, for example, have relied quite heavily on Tolman's (1932) distinction between learning and performance, performance being what is observed while learning (conditioning) is but one essential ingredient contributing to any instance of observed performance. The most important, and perhaps the most sophisticated, developments in Hullian and neo-Hullian theory concern the attempts to explain complicated goal-directed behavior in terms of the conditioning of fractional responses. Unobserved, fractional responses (already we see the drift away from the overt behavior criteria of response) are assumed to serve a mediating role in behavior. Once a fractional response is conditioned in a particular situation, it is assumed to occur to the stimuli in that situation when those stimuli recur. The stimulus consequences of the fractional response referred to as the r_g are assumed to serve as guides to behavior either by serving as a cue or by activating responses or by serving to reinforce other responses by secondary reinforcement. The latter-day proponents of a conditioning point of view (Bugelski, 1956; Osgood, 1953) have come to rely more and more heavily on concepts like the fractional response to bridge the gap between stimulus and overt behavior and to account for the facts of response transfer, environmental achievements, and equipotentiality. What this indicates is that a simple conditioning paradigm which rests solely on observable stimuli and responses has proved inadequate even to the task of encompassing simple conditioning and maze-learning phenomena, and the workers within this tradition have come to rely more and more heavily on mediational (central, cognitive, etc.) concepts, although they still attempt to clothe these concepts in traditional conditioning garb. To add to the problem, a number of recent papers (Deutsch, 1956; Gonzales and Diamond, 1960) have indicated that the r_g interpretations of complex behavior are neither simple nor adequate.

When we look again at the way conditioning principles have been applied to clinical phenomena we see an amazing unawareness of these problems that have been so salient to experimental and animal psychologists working with conditioning.

While the above discussion has been oriented primarily to classical conditioning, the general argument would apply equally well to those attempts to make the principles of learning derived from operant conditioning the basis of an explanation of neurosis and psychotherapy (as in Krasner, 1961). The Skinnerians have been particularly oblivious to the wide variety of problems that are entailed when one attempts to apply concepts and findings from laboratory learning experiments to other, and particularly more complex, phenomena. While we will deal more directly with their point of view shortly, a few comments might be in order now concerning their use of the operant-conditioning paradigm as a basis for the handling of more complex data. When Skinnerians speak of laws of learning, they have reference to the curves representing rate of responding of rats pressing bars (Skinner, 1938) and pigeons pecking (Ferster and Skinner, 1957), which are, in fact, a function of certain highly controlled contingencies such as the schedule of reinforcement, the amount of deprivation, the experimental situation itself (there is very little else to do in a Skinner box), and the species of animals involved. These experiments are of some interest, both as exercises in animal training under highly restricted conditions, and for what light they may shed on the more general question of partial reinforcement. It is dubious that these findings constitute laws of learning that can be applied across species (see Breland and Breland, 1961) or even to situations that differ in any significant way from the Skinner box.

Use of Reinforcement

Advocates of the application of learning theory to clinical phenomena have relied heavily on the "law of effect" as perhaps their foremost established principle of learning. We shall attempt to point out that a good deal of evidence from experimental animal studies argues strongly that, at the most, the law of effect is a weak law of performance.

Essentially, the controversy can be reduced to the question of whether or not reward is necessary for learning. The initial source of evidence indicating that it was not came from the findings of latent learning studies (Blodgett, 1929; Tolman and Honzik, 1930), in which it was found, for example, that rats who were allowed to explore a maze without reward made fewer errors when learning the maze than controls who had no opportunity for exploration. Thus, these early latent learning studies, as well as a variety of more recent ones (Thistlethwaite, 1951) indicate that learning can take place without reward but may not be revealed until a reward situation makes it appropriate to do so (or to put it another way, the reward elicits the performance but plays little role during learning). Other sources which point to learning without reward come from studies of perceptual learning (Hebb, 1949), imitation (Herbert and Harsh, 1944), language learning (Chomsky, 1959), and imprinting (Moltz, 1960).

Defenders of the point of view that reinforcement is necessary for learning have attempted to handle results such as these in a variety of ways. One has been by appealing to the concept of secondary reinforcement (e.g., a maze has secondary reinforcing properties which account for the learning during exploration). When this sort of thing is done, even with respect to experiments where attempts were made to minimize secondary reinforcements (Thistlethwaite, 1951), it seems clear that this particular notion of reinforcement has become incapable of disproof. Another way of handling these potentially embarrassing results has been by the invention of a new set of drives (curiosity drive, exploratory drive, etc.) but this too has a post hoc flavor to it, and one wonders what kind of explanation is achieved by postulating an "exploratory drive" to account for the fact that animals and humans engage in exploration. In fact, the assumption that exploration reduces an exploratory drive makes it difficult to explain why a rat's tendency to enter an alley of a maze *decreases* after he has explored the alley (Watson, 1961). Finally, there are those (particularly the Skinnerians) who tend to define reinforcement so broadly that neither the findings from latent learning nor any other source can prove embarrassing, since whenever learning has taken place this "proves" that there has been reinforcement. To better understand this problem, however, we had best look for a moment at the general problem of defining reinforcement in a meaningful way.

Obviously, if the view that reinforcement is necessary for learning is to have any meaning, what constitutes a reinforcement must be defined independently from the learning situation itself. There has been a great deal of difficulty in getting around a circular definition of the law of effect, and it might be worthwhile to examine some of the attempts that have been made in the past.

One of the best known was the attempt to relate the reinforcing properties of stimuli to their drive-reducing characteristics (Hull, 1951). The drive-reduction model has had to be abandoned, however, because of evidence from a variety of areas including latent learning, sensory preconditioning (Brogden, 1939), and novelty and curiosity (Berlyne, 1960). Other evidence such as that of Olds and Milner (1954) on the effect of direct brain stimulation has strengthened the conviction that the drive-reduction interpretation of reinforcement is inadequate; and, in fact, original adherents of this view have begun to abandon it (e.g., Miller, 1959).

The other most frequent solution to the circularity problem has been by way of the "empirical law of effect," an approach typified by Skinner's definition of reinforcement as any stimulus that can be demonstrated to produce a change in response strength. Skinner argues that this is not circular since some stimuli are found to produce changes and others are not, and they can subsequently be classified on that basis. This seems to be a reasonable position if it is adhered to; that is, if care is taken to define reinforcement in terms of class membership *independently* of the observations that show that learning has taken place. When we examine the actual use of the term *reinforcement* by Skinner (see especially *Verbal Behavior*, 1957) and by other Skinnerians (Lundin, 1961), we find that care is only taken in this regard within the context of animal experiments, but that when the jumps are made to other phenomena, such as language and psychotherapy, care is usually *not* taken to define reinforcement independently from learning as indicated by response strength. This leads to a state of affairs where any observed change in behavior is said to occur *because of* reinforcement, when, in fact, the change in behavior is itself the only indicator of what the reinforcement has been. Chomsky (1959) reviews the use of the concept of reinforcement by Skinner with regard to language and reaches the following conclusion:

> From this sample, it can be seen that the notion of reinforcement has totally lost whatever objective meaning it may ever have had. Running through these examples, we see that a person can be reinforced though he emits no response at all, and the reinforcing "stimulus" need not impinge on the reinforced person or need not even exist (it is sufficient that it be imagined or hoped for). When we read that a person plays what music he likes (165), says what he likes (165), thinks what he likes (438-9), reads what books he likes (163), etc., *because* he finds it reinforcing to do so, or that we write books or inform others of facts *because* we are reinforced by what we hope will be the ultimate behavior of reader or listener, we can only conclude that the term "reinforcement" has a purely ritual function. The phrase "X is reinforced by Y (stimulus, state of affairs, event, etc.)" is being used as a cover term for "X wants Y," "X likes Y," "X wishes that Y were the case," etc. Invoking the term "reinforcement" has no explanatory force, and any idea that this paraphrase introduces any new clarity or objectivity into the description of wishing, liking, etc., is a serious delusion. (pp. 37-38)

This problem is exemplified in the area of psychotherapy by the attempts to use the studies of verbal conditioning (Krasner, 1958) as analogues to psychotherapy. First we should note that if these studies are taken at face value (i.e., if subjects are conditioned to increase the emission of certain responses because of reinforcement, without their awareness of this fact) it appears that a simple conditioning model is inadequate since subjects are presumably responding in terms of a class of responses (e.g., plural nouns, etc.) rather than in terms of a specific response (e.g., bar press), such classes implying response transfer and mediation. Second, and more to the point, a number of recent investigators (Eriksen, 1962) have begun to question whether verbal conditioning does occur without the subject's awareness. If it does not, the whole phenomenon begins to look like nothing more than a rather inefficient way to get subjects to figure out what the experimenter wants them to do (telling them directly to emit plural nouns would probably be much more efficient), after which they can decide whether they want to do it or not. In any case, there seems to be enough question about what goes on in verbal conditioning itself to indicate that it cannot be utilized as a more basic explanation for complex phenomena such as psychotherapy. Psychotherapists of many persuasions would agree that rewards of some kind are important in work with patients. Thus, the view that the psychotherapist is a "reinforcement machine" is trivial. The difficult problems are in specifying just what therapist activities are rewarding, in what ways, to what sorts of patients, and with what effects.

The above discussion should make clear that the use of the concept of reinforcement is only of explanatory usefulness when it is specified in some delimited fashion. As an empirical law of performance almost everyone in and out of psychology would accept it, including Lewin, Freud, Tolman, and others outside the traditional S-R movement. But this amounts to saying nothing more than that some events, when presented, tend to increase the probability of responses that they have followed. The hard job, but the only one that will lead to any meaningful use of the concept of reinforcement, is specifying what the various events called reinforcers have in common. Some have argued that since this is such a difficult task, we should restrict ourselves to listing and cataloging so-called reinforcers. But this is nearly impossible, in a general way, because reinforcers differ from individual to individual, from species to species, from situation to situation, and from time to time (the saying "one man's meat is another man's poison" is trite but true). Meaningful analysis must stem from a comprehensive study of the particular learning phenomena in question, whether it is language learning, the development of perceptual and perceptual-motor skills (Fitts, 1964; Hebb, 1949), the acquisition of particular species behavior patterns during critical periods of development (Scott, 1962), the learning of a neurosis, or the learning that takes place during psychotherapy. Experience with all of these phenomena has revealed that different kinds of events seem to be involved and that these can only be understood in the context of the phenomena in question. Lumping all these events together under the single term *reinforcement* serves to muddle rather than to clarify understanding.

The staunch reinforcement adherent might respond that all these complicated arguments may be true but we can ignore them, since all we are really interested in is predicting what the organism will do, and we can do this when we know the organism's reinforcement history. The answer to this is that the experimental literature does not support such a claim; rather, it shows that, in many instances, performance *cannot* be predicted on the basis of a knowledge of the history of reinforcement.

Latent learning studies indicate this quite cearly. Perhaps of more interest are the findings of discrimination-reversal learning studies (Goodwin and Lawrence, 1955; Mackintosh, 1963). Here we find that subjects that have been trained on a series of discrimination reversals learn to select the correct stimulus with very few errors even though they may have been rewarded *much more frequently and more recently for responding to another stimulus*. Similarly, in the double drive discrimination studies (Thistlethwaite, 1951) animals chose alleys leading to food when they were hungry and water when they were thirsty, even though they have been rewarded equally frequently on the alleys on previous trials. In other words, "what is learned" was not equivalent with "reinforcement history." The law of effect is not disproved by these studies; it is merely shown to be irrelevant.

To summarize: The "law of effect," or reinforcement, conceived as a *"law of learning,"* occupies a very dubious status. Like the principles of conditioning, it appears to be an unlikely candidate as an explanatory principle of learning. As a strong law of learning it has already been rejected by many of the theorists who previously relied on it. As an empirical "law of *performance*" it is noncontroversial, but usually so generally stated as to be of little explanatory value.

CONCEPTION OF NEUROSIS

In this section we will explicate the conception of neurosis that forms the basis of the behavior-therapy approach (particularly of the Wolpe-Eysenck group) and attempt to demonstrate its inadequacies both in terms of learning theory and as a way of accounting for the observed facts of neurosis. Our argument in the first instance will be that the conception of neurosis in terms of symptoms and anxiety parallels the general conception of learning in terms of overt responses, conditioning, and secondary drives, and suffers from the same inadequacies that we have outlined in the preceding section. With regard to the facts of neurosis, we will argue that the behavior-therapy position is inadequate at a descriptive level as well as being conceptually incorrect. It should be pointed out again that we are discussing the explanation or theory of neurosis here and not the techniques used by the behavior therapists. The strict Skinnerian may excuse himself at this point if he adheres to a "no-theory" position and is only concerned with the effects of environmental manipulation. Furthermore, certain techniques themselves may be useful and have some of the effects attributed to them regardless of the theory.

In its essence, the conception of neurosis put forth by the behavior therapists is that neuroses are conditioned responses or habits (including conditioned anxiety) and *nothing else*, though it should be noted that they do not adhere to this argument when they describe the success of their methods. Wolpe, for example, while ostensibly treating overt symptoms, describes his patients as becoming more productive, having improved adjustment and pleasure in sex, improved interpersonal relationships, and so forth. The argument that removal of a troublesome symptom somehow "generalizes" to all of these other areas begs the question. Their conception is typically put forth as an alternative to a psychodynamic viewpoint, which they characterize as resting on a distinction between symptoms and underlying causes (unconscious conflicts, impulses, defenses, etc.). They stress the point that inferences about underlying factors of this sort are unnecessary and misleading and that a more parsimonious explanation treats symptoms (which are typically equated with behavior or that which can be objectively observed) as the neurosis per se. They argue that by equating neurosis with symptoms, and symptoms, in turn, with habits (conditioned responses), they are able to bring "modern learning theory" with its "well-established laws" to bear on the understanding and treatment of neurosis.

As we have labored to show in the preceding section, the well-established laws of learning to which they refer have considerable difficulty within the area of simple animal behavior. More specifically, it seems clear that a wide variety of behaviors (from maze learning to more complex forms) cannot be adequately dealt with when the overt response and conditioned habit are the units of analysis. Furthermore, their learning position leads the behavior therapists into postulating an isomorphic relationship between antecedent learning and present behavior in which observed differences are accounted for in terms of principles of generalization. This is a key issue, and we shall explore it a little further at this time.

Much of the behaviorist conception of neurosis rests on a rejection of the distinction between symptoms and underlying causes (Eysenck, 1960) as typified by Yates's (1958) argument against "symptom substitution." By focusing attention on overt symptoms and banishing all underlying causes, however, the behavior therapists are faced with the same problem that has long confronted behaviorism; namely, the difficulty of explaining how *generality* of behavior results from specific learning experiences. The problem of *generality* (i.e., as exemplified by the facts of transposition and response transfer) has, in fact, brought about the downfall of peripheral S-R learning, of the conditioned habit as a basic unit, and tangentially, is leading to the dethroning of the law of effect. With regard to neurosis, this view has led the behavior therapists into the position where they must posit a specific learning experience for each symptom of a neurosis. They have partly avoided this problem by focusing their attention on those neuroses that can be described in terms of specific symptoms (bed-wetting, if this is a neurosis, tics, specific phobias, etc.) and have tended to ignore those conditions which do not fit their model, such as neurotic depressions, general unhappiness, obsessional disorders, and the kinds of persistent interpersonal entanglements that characterize so many neurotics. This leaves them free to explain the specific symptom in terms of a specific learning experience, as, for example, when a fear of going outdoors is explained in terms of some previous experience in which the stimulus (outdoors) has been associated with (conditioned to) something unpleasant or painful and has now, through generalization, spread to any response of going outdoors. As our previous analysis should make clear, however, even a simple conceptualization such as this, in terms of stimuli, responses, and conditioning is extremely cumbersome and begs the important questions. Within an S-R framework, in which generalization occurs along the dimension of physical stimulus similarity, it is difficult, if not impossible, to show how a previous experience such as being frightened in the country as a child could generalize to the "stimulus" outdoors without a great deal of *mediation* in which the concept of "outdoors" carried most of the burden of generalization. As we have pointed out, most workers in the field of learning recognize this and rely heavily on mediational concepts in their explanations of complex behavior. Dollard and Miller (1950), for example, return again and again to mediational explanations once they move beyond the "combat neuroses" which lend themselves more readily to a simple isomorphic explanation.

A second important facet of the behaviorist conception of neurosis is the use of the concept of anxiety as a secondary drive. Here, Wolpe and Eysenck and some others seem to follow the explanatory model laid down by Dollard and Miller. Anxiety is viewed as the main motivating force for symptoms and, in general, occupies a central place in their thinking. Briefly, it is worth pointing out that the concept of drive reduction, the distinction between primary drives and secondary drives, as well as the early thinking about the uniquely persistent qualities of fear-motivated behavior have had serious difficulty within learning theory (Watson, 1961; Solomon, 1964). The use of these concepts to explain clinical phenomena thus rests on an exceedingly shaky foundation.

Let us turn our attention now to the phenomena of neuroses. We shall try to point out that underlying the dispute over symptoms versus underlying causes is a real difference in definition that arises at the descriptive level, which, in a sense, antedates disagreements at the level of theory and explanation.

To keep the presentation simple, we will adopt the term *psychodynamic* to refer to all those theorists and therapists, following Freud, whose view of neurosis and its treatment deals with motives (conscious and unconscious), conflict, etc. This covers a wide variety of workers, in addition to the more or less traditional followers of Freud, including Sullivan and his adherents (Fromm-Reichman, 1950), other neo-Freudians, and that broad group of psychiatrists and clinical psychologists who have been strongly influenced by the Freudian and neo-Freudian viewpoints even though they may not claim allegiance to any of the formal schools.

The point we wish to make here is that disagreement between the behaviorist and psychodynamic viewpoints seems to rest on a very real difference at the purely descriptive or observational level. The behaviorist looks at a neurotic and sees specific symptoms and anxiety. The psychodynamicist looks at the same individual and sees a complex intra- and interpersonal mode of functioning which may or may not contain certain observable fears* or certain behavioral symptoms such as compulsive motor acts. When the psychodynamicist describes a neurosis, his referent is a cohering component of the individual's functioning, including his characteristic ways of interacting with other people (e.g., sweet and self-effacing on the surface but hostile in covert ways), his characteristic modes of thinking and perceiving (e.g., the hysteric who never "remembers" anything unpleasant, the obsessive whose memories are overelaborated and circumstantial, etc.), characteristic modes of fantasy and dreaming, a variety of secondary gain features, and the like. Specific or isolatable symptoms may sometimes be a part of such an integrated neurotic pattern, but, even viewed descriptively, they in no sense constitute the neurosis per se.

So far, we have considered the behavior therapists' position at face value. In actuality, a good case can be made that they *behave* in a way which is quite inconsistent with their own position. A specific example, taken from one of Wolpe's own case descriptions, will illustrate this point and, at the same time, show what the psychodynamicist sees when he looks at a neurotic. Wolpe (1960) presents the following case:

Case 5. An attractive woman of 28 came for treatment because she was in acute distress as a result of her lovers' casual treatment of her. Everyone of very numerous love affairs had followed a similar pattern—first she would attract the man, then she would

---

*The term *anxiety* is frequently used as a theoretical inference, i.e., a patient deals with personal material in an overly intellectual fashion, and this is described as a defense mechanism—intellectualization—whose purpose is to ward off anxiety.

offer herself on a platter. He would soon treat her with contempt and after a time leave her. In general she lacked assurance, was very dependent, and was practically never free from feelings of tension and anxiety.

What is described here is a complex pattern of interpersonal relationships, psychological strategies, and misunderstandings (such as the way she became involved with men, the way she communicated her availability to them, her dependency, etc.), expectations that she had (presumably that men would not react with contempt to her generosity, that being dependent might lead to being taken care of, etc.), and thoughts and feelings about herself (lack of assurance, acute distress, etc.). Many of the statements about her (e.g., the description of the course of her love affairs) are abbreviations for very complex and involved processes involving two people interacting over a period of time. It is this, the psychodynamicist would argue, that *is* the neurosis. The tension and anxiety may be a part of it in this particular case (though there might be other cases in which there is no complaint of anxiety but, rather, its reverse—seeming inability to "feel" anything)—but it is secondary and can be understood only in relation to the other aspects of the patient's functioning. Wolpe's case histories are classic testaments to the fact that he cannot, and does not, apply the symptom approach when working with actual data. As a further example, consider the argument against a symptom-substitution point of view (Yates, 1958) in which it is implied that anything other than symptoms is some sort of metaphysical inference. While it may be true that theories such as psychoanalysis deal with a number of inferential and higher-order constructs in their attempts to integrate the complex mass of data that constitutes a neurosis, it is also true that much more than symptoms exist at the level of observation. Secondary-gain features of a neurosis, in which it is apparent that a variety of goals may be served by a set of interchangeable symptoms, are the rule in most neurotic individuals. We are not defending the view (attributed to psychoanalysis by Yates) that if one symptom is removed another pops up to take its place; rather, we are arguing that the empirical phenomena of neurosis do not fit the symptom or response theory, but are much more compatible with a theory built around central mediators. Whether unconscious conflicts and defense mechanisms are adequate ways of conceptualizing the problem is an entirely separate question. What is clear is that a view stressing central mediators in which specific responses are seen as equipotential means of reaching certain goals is necessary to encompass the data of neurosis just as it has proven necessary to encompass the phenomena of animal learning.

To sum up, it would seem that the behaviorists have reached a position where an inadequate conceptual framework forces them to adopt an inadequate and superficial view of the very data that they are concerned with. They are then forced to slip many of the key facts in the back door, so to speak, for example, when all sorts of fantasy, imaginary, and thought processes are blithely called responses. This process is, of course, parallel to what has gone on within S-R learning theory where all sorts of central and mediational processes have been cumbersomely handled with S-R terminology (e.g., Deutsch, 1956). Thus, we have a situation where the behavior therapists argue strongly against a dynamic interpretation of neurosis at some points and at other points behave as if they had adopted such a point of view. This inconsistency should be kept in mind in reading the next section in which we evaluate the claims of success put forth by the behaviorist group. Insofar as there is disagreement as to what constitutes the descriptive facts of neurosis, it makes little sense to compare the effectiveness of different methods. However, since the behaviorist group adopts very broad (or psychodynamic, if you will) criteria for improvement, and since their *techniques* may have some effectiveness, in spite of theoretical and conceptual inadequacies, it is crucial that we look carefully at the empirical results that they lay claim to.

CLAIMS OF SUCCESS

While much of the writing of the behavior therapists consists of arguments and appeals to principles of science and learning, the claims that are made for the success of the methods seem open to empirical analysis. No doubt a great deal of the appeal of behavior therapy lies right here. Here seems to be methods whose application can be clearly described (unlike such messy psychodynamic methods as "handling countertransference" or "interpreting resistance"), whose course is relatively short, and which seem to achieve a large number of practical results in the form of removal of symptoms. Wolpe (1960), for example, presents the following data: of 122 cases treated with behavioral techniques, 44% were "apparently cured," 46% were "much improved," 7% were "slightly or moderately improved," and 3% were "unimproved." Combining categories, he claims 90% "apparently cured or much improved," and 10% "improvement moderate, slight or nil." (Criteria of improvement consist of "symptomatic improvement, increased productiveness, improved adjustment and pleasure in sex, improved interpersonal relationships and ability to handle ordinary psychological conflicts and reasonable reality stresses.")

He compares this with data from the Berlin Psychoanalytic Institute (Knight, 1941) which shows 62-40.5% in the first category and 38-59.5% in the second. Wolpe concludes, as have others (Bandura, 1961; Eysenck, 1960; Lazarus, 1963), that this demonstrates the superiority of the behavior therapy methods. The fact that the psychoanalytic method showed as much as 62% improvement is explained as being due to whatever accidental "reciprocal inhibition" occurred during the therapy. (There is, however, no analysis or description of how this might have happened.) The behavioral methods achieve superior results presumably because of the more explicit application of these techniques.

It is fair to say that if these results can be substantiated they present a very strong argument in favor of behavioral *techniques* — even granting the theoretical and empirical inconsistencies we have discussed. However, we must ask if these claims are any better substantiated than those made by the practitioners of other methods of psychotherapy. Insofar as claims such as Wolpe's are based on uncontrolled case histories, they may reflect the enthusiasm of the practitioner as much as the effect of the method. History shows that new methods of therapy (ECS, tranquilizing drugs, as well as various schools of psychotherapy) have been oversold by their original proponents. Thus, a careful look at what lies behind the claims of the behavior-therapy group is in order.

The following does not purport to be a comprehensive review of the behavior-therapy literature. Rather, it is based on a survey of all the studies reported in the two reviews that have appeared (Bandura, 1961; Grossberg, 1964). The most striking thing about this large body of studies is that they are almost all case studies. A careful reading of the original sources reveals that only one study (Lang and Lazovik, 1963) is a controlled experiment, and here the subjects were not neurotics but normal college students. Thus, most of the claims (including those of Wolpe, which have been widely quoted) must be regarded as no better substantiated than those of any other enthusiastic school of psychotherapy whose practitioners claim that their patients get better. Behavior therapy has appeared to differ on this score because of its identification with experimental psychology and with "well-established laws of learning." We have already dealt with this issue, so let us now turn to some problems in evaluating psychotherapy as a technique.

The problems here are essentially those of control, and they may be broken down into three areas: (a) sampling biases, (b) observer bias, and (c) problems of experimental control. While research in psychotherapy presents particular difficulties in controlling "experimental input," more sophisticated workers (Frank, 1959) have attempted to deal with at least the sampling and observer problems. It thus comes as somewhat of a surprise that the behavior-therapy workers, despite their identification with experimental psychology, base their claims on evidence which is almost totally lacking in any form of control. Let us examine these issues in greater detail.

Sampling Biases. Obviously a claim such as Wolpe's of 90% success has meaning only when we know the population from which the sample of patients was drawn and the way in which they were selected. Ideally, a comparison of treatment techniques would involve the random assignment of patient from a common population pool to alternative treatments. Since, in practice, this is rarely feasible, it is essential for anyone making comparisons of different treatment methods to, at the very least, examine the comparability of the populations *and* of the methods used in selecting from these populations. Neither Wolpe's data nor those of Lazarus (1963) contain this evidence. Wolpe reports, for example:

> Both series (70 patients reported on in 1952 and 52 patients reported on in 1954 on which the 90% figure is based) include only patients whose treatment has ceased after they have been afforded a reasonable opportunity for the application of the available methods; i.e., they have had as a minimum both a course of instruction on the changing of behavior in the life situation and a proper initiation of a course of relaxation-desensitization. This minimum takes up to about 15 interviews, including anamnestic interviews and *no patient who has had 15 or more interviews has been omitted from the series* [emphasis added].

We may conclude from this that some patients (how many we do not know) having up to 14 interviews have been excluded from the sample—a procedure highly favorable to the success of the method but which violates the simplest canons of sampling. Wolpe's final sample of 122 consists of those patients most likely to show improvement, since both they and he were satisfied enough with the first 14 (or less) interviews to warrant proceeding further. Those patients least likely to improve are those most likely to drop out early (14 sessions or less) and not be included in the computation of success rate. The fact that a large number of poor-prognosis patients would very likely be eliminated during these early sessions is supported by a variety of research findings (Strickland and Crowne, 1963), which show that most dropping-out of untreatable or unsuccessful cases occurs during the first 10 sessions. This serious sampling bias would be expected to spuriously inflate the percent showing improvement.

When we add this to whatever unknown factors operate to delimit the original population (presumably there is some self-selection of patients who seek out this form of treatment), it becomes apparent that little confidence can be given to the reports of success.

Observer Bias. Psychologists have long been aware that human beings are fallible observers, particularly when they have predispositions or vested interests to protect. In controlled studies, we try to protect judges from their own biases by not acquainting them with the hypotheses, or with the nature of the groups they are judging, or by using blind and double-blind designs. This problem is particularly acute with regard to psychotherapy because both therapist and patient have investments of time, involvement, competence, and reputation to protect. For these reasons, workers in the area have become extremely skeptical of claims put forth for any method which rests on the uncontrolled observation of the person administering the treatment. At a minimum we expect some sort of external evidence. Beyond this minimum we hope for an independent judge who can compare differentially treated groups without knowing which is which.

In addition, there is the problem of the patient's freedom to report effects which may be seriously curtailed when all his reports go directly to the person who has treated him. It seems reasonable to assume that some patients are prevented from expressing dissatisfaction with treatment when they must report directly to the therapist, either because they do not want to hurt his feelings, or are afraid, or are just saying what they think is being demanded of them, or are being polite, or for some other reason. Again, it would be highly appropriate to provide the patients with the opportunity of reporting results in a situation as free from such pressure as possible.

Examination of the 26 studies reviewed by Bandura reveals a surprising lack of concern with these problems. Of the 26 studies sampled, only 12 report evaluation of results by persons other than the treating therapist; four of these use ratings of the hospital staff (who may be acquainted with the treatment), four use mothers or parents reporting on their children to the treating therapist, one is a wife reporting on her husband to the therapist, and three use a second observer. Obviously, whatever factors enter in to cause observer and reporter biases are allowed full reign in most of these cases. While we cannot conclude from this that the reported results are *due to* observer and reporter biases (as is clearly indicated with the sampling biases), it is impossible to rule them out. Furthermore, a great deal of evidence from many areas of psychology leads us to be very skeptical of claims in which biases of this sort go uncontrolled.

Experimental Control. While control of sampling and observer effects are basic to a wide variety of research activities, including field and clinical research, more exacting control over experimental conditions has long been the *sine qua non* of the laboratory methods of experimental psychology. The power of the experimental method stems, in part, from keeping careful control over all but a few conditions, which are experimentally varied, with the subsequent effects of these variations being observed. Since psychotherapy is not a controlled experiment, it is probably unfair to expect this type of control. However, there are more and less accurate descriptions of what goes on during any form of therapy, and we can demand as accurate a description as possible in lieu of experimental control. Thus, while we are led to believe that methods, such as counterconditioning, extinction of maladaptive responses, methods of reward, and the like, are applied in a manner analogous to their laboratory counterparts, examination of what is *actually done* reveals that the application of the learning techniques is embedded in a wide variety of activities (including many of the traditional therapy and interview techniques) which make any attribution of effect to the specific learning techniques impossible. Let us consider a few examples. From Wolpe (1960):

Case 4. The patient had 65 therapeutic interviews, unevenly distributed over 27 months. The greater part of the time was devoted to discussions of how to gain control of her interpersonal relationships and stand up for herself. She had considerable difficulty with this at first, even though it had early become emotionally important to her to please the therapist. But she gradually mastered the assertive behavior required of her, overcame her anxieties and became exceedingly self-reliant in all interpersonal dealings, including those with her mother-in-law.

From Lazarus and Rachman (1957) on systematic desensitization:

Case 1. The patient was instructed in the use of assertive responses and deep (non-hypnotic) relaxation. The first anxiety hierarchy dealt with was that of dull weather. Starting from "a bright sunny day" it was possible for the subject to visualize "damp overcast weather" without anxiety after 21 desensitization sessions, and 10 days after the completion of this hierarchy, she was able to report that, "the weather is much better, it doesn't even bother me to look at the weather when I wake up in the morning" (previously depressing). . . . During the course of therapy, part of the reason for the development of the anxiety state in this patient was unearthed. When she was 17 years old she had become involved in a love affair with a married man 12 years her senior. This affair had been conducted in an extremely discreet manner for 4 years, during which time she had suffered from recurrent guilt feelings and shame—so much so, that on one occasion she had attempted suicide by throwing herself into a river. It was her custom to meet her lover after work *in the late afternoon*. The dull weather can be accounted for, as this affair took place in London.

From Rachman (1959):

Interview No. 12. The patient having received a jolt in her love relationship, this session was restricted to a sort of nondirective, cathartic discussion. No desensitizing was undertaken because of A.G.'s depressed mood and obvious desire to "just talk."

These excerpts have been presented because they seem representative of the practices of the behavioral therapists. As can be seen, the number and variety of activities that go on during these treatment sessions is great, including, in these few examples, discussions, explanations of techniques and principles, explanations of the unadaptiveness of anxiety and symptoms, hypnosis of various sorts, relaxation practice and training with and without hypnosis, "nondirective cathartic discussions," "obtaining an understanding of the patient's personality and background," and the "unearthing" of a 17-year-old memory of an illicit affair. The case reports are brief and presented anecdotically so that it is really impossible to know what else went on in addition to those things described. What should be abundantly clear from these examples is that there is no attempt to restrict what goes on to learning techniques. Since it seems clear that a great variety of things do go on, any attribution of behavior change to specific learning techniques is entirely unwarranted.

In summary, there are several important issues that must be differentiated. First, a review of both learning theory and of the empirical results of behavior therapy demonstrates that they can claim no special scientific status for their work on either ground. Second, there are important differences of opinion concerning the type of patient likely to be affected by behavior therapy. Grossberg (1964), for example, states: "Behavior therapies have been most successful when applied to neurotic disorders with specific behavioral manifestations" (p. 81). He goes on to point out that the results with alcoholism and sexual disorders have been disappointing and that the best results are achieved with phobias and enuresis. He later states that "desensitization only alleviates those phobias that are being treated, but other coexisting phobias remain at high strength, indicating a specific treatment effect" (p. 83). Wolpe et al. (1964), on the other hand, argues: "The conditioning therapist differs from his colleagues in that he *seeks out* the precise stimuli to anxiety, and finds himself able to break down almost every neurosis into what are essentially *phobic systems*" (p. 11). The best controlled study (Lang and Lazovik, 1963) indicates that "desensitization is very effective in reducing the intense fear of snakes held by normal subjects, though it can be questioned whether this is a phobia in the clinical sense."

Thus, there seems to be some evidence that these *techniques* (as techniques and not as learning theory) are effective with certain conditions.* We feel that this bears stressing because psychotherapy has come to be narrowly defined in terms of dynamic, evocative, and nondirective methods, placing unnecessary limitations on the kind of patient suitable for psychotherapy. First, we must note that behavior techniques are not new (as Murray, 1964, points out in a recent article). Freud and Breuer used similar techniques prior to the development of psychoanalysis, Bagby described a number of these methods in 1928, and therapy based on techniques designed to eliminate undesirable responses was used for many years by Stevenson Smith at the University of Washington Clinic. While most of these techniques have been superseded by the various

*Just how many neurotics fit the phobia and/or specific symptom model is a complicated question, the answer to which depends in part on what one's own point of view leads one to look for. For example, an informal census of the first 81 admissions to the University of Oregon Psychology Clinic in 1964 revealed only 2 patients who could be so classified.

forms of dynamic psychotherapy, recent work (Frank, 1961) suggests that the time may be ripe for taking a fresh look at a variety of methods such as hypnosis, suggestion, relaxation, and other approaches of a more *structured nature* in which the therapist takes a *more active role*. Needless to say, this fresh look would best proceed unencumbered by an inadequate learning theory and with some minimal concern for control. As an example of a nondynamic approach to patient management, we refer to the work of Fairweather (1964) and his colleagues.

REFORMULATION

Up to this point our analysis has been primarily critical. We have tried to show that many of the so-called principles of learning employed by workers with a behaviorist orientation are inadequate and are not likely to provide useful explanations for clinical phenomena. In this section we will examine the potential value of ideas from different learning conceptions. Before proceeding, however, we would like to discuss briefly the issue of the application of "laws," principles, and findings from one area (such as animal experimentation) to another (such as neurosis and psychotherapy). The behaviorists have traditionally assumed that principles established under highly controlled conditions, usually with animal subjects, form a scientific foundation for a psychology of learning. Yet when they come to apply these principles to human learning situations, the transition is typically bridged by rather flimsy analogies which ignore crucial differences between the situations, the species, etc. Recently, Underwood (1964) has made the following comments concerning this problem:

> Learning theories as developed in the animal-learning laboratory, have never seemed . . . to have relevance to the behavior of a subject in learning a list of paired associates. The emphasis upon the role of a pellet of food or a sip of water in the white rat's acquiring a response somehow never seemed to make contact with the human S learning to say VXK when the stimulus DOF was presented. (p. 74)

We would add that the relevance is at least equally obscure in applications of traditional S-R reinforcement theory to clinical phenomena.

We do *not* wish, however, to damn any and all attempts to conceptualize clinical phenomena in terms of principles of learning developed outside the clinic. On the contrary, recent work in learning may suggest certain theoretical models which may prove useful in conceptualizing the learning processes involved in psychotherapy and the development of neuroses. Whether these notions can form the basis for a useful learning conceptualization of clinical phenomena will depend upon the ingenuity with which they are subsequently developed and upon their adequacy in encompassing the facts of neurosis and psychotherapy. Further, we would like to stress that their association with experimental work in the field of learning does not give them any *a priori* scientific status. Their status as explanatory principles in the clinical area must be empirically established within that area. In what follows, then, we will outline some ideas about learning and make some suggestions concerning their relevance to clinical problems.

Our view of learning centers around the concepts of information storage and retrieval. Learning is viewed as the process by which information about the environment is acquired, stored, and categorized. This cognitive view is, of course, quite contrary to the view that learning consists of the acquisition of specific responses; responses, according to our view, are mediated by the nature of the stored information, which may consist of facts or of strategies or programs analogous to the grammar that is acquired in the learning of a language. Thus, "what is learned" may be a system for generating responses as a consequence of the specific information that is stored. This general point of view has been emphasized by Lashley (see Beach et al., 1960), by Miller, Galenter, and Pribram (1960), in the form of the TOTE hypothesis, and by a number of workers in the cognitive learning tradition (Tolman, 1951; Woodworth, 1958). Recently it has even been suggested as a necessary formulation for dealing with that eminently S-R area, motor skills (Adams, 1964; Fitts, 1964).

This conception of learning may be useful in the clinical area in two ways: one, in formulating a theoretical explanation for the acquisition or development of neurosis, symptoms, behavior pathology, and the like, and, two, in conceptualizing psychotherapy as a learning process, and suggesting new methods stemming from this learning model.

A conceptualization of the problem of neurosis in terms of information storage and retrieval is based on the fundamental idea that what is learned in a neurosis is a set of central strategies (or a program) which guide the individual's adaptation to his environment. Neuroses are not symptoms (responses) but are strategies of a particular kind which lead to certain observable (tics, compulsive acts, etc.) and certain other less observable phenomena (fears, feelings of depression, etc.). The whole problem of symptom substitution is thus seen as an instance of response substitution or response equipotentiality, concepts which are supported by abundant laboratory evidence.

Similarly, the problem of a learning conceptualization of unconscious phenomena may be reopened. Traditional S-R approaches have equated the unconscious with some kind of avoidance of a verbalization response. From our point of view, there is no reason to assume that people can give accurate descriptions of the central strategies mediating much of their behavior any more than a child can give a description of the grammatical rules which govern the understanding and production of his language. As a matter of fact, consciousness may very well be a special or extraordinary case—the rule being "unawareness" of the mediating strategies—which is in need of special explanation, rather than the reverse. This view avoids the cumbersome necessity of having to postulate specific fear experiences or the persistence of anxiety-motivated behavior, as has typically been done by S-R theorists with regard to unconscious phenomena. It also avoids equating the unconscious with the neurotic, which is a virtue since there is so much that goes on within "normal" individuals that they are unaware of. It further avoids the trap of attributing especially persistent and maladaptive consequences to painful experiences. As Solomon (1964) points out, the existing evidence does not support the view that punishment and pain lead unequivocally to anxiety and maladaptive consequences.

The view of learning we have outlined does not supply a set of ready-made answers to clinical problems that can be applied from the laboratory, but it indicates what sort of questions will have to be answered to achieve a meaningful learning conceptualization of neurosis and symptoms. Questions such as "What are the conditions under which strategies are acquired or developed?" stress the fact that these conditions may be quite different from the final observed behavior. That is to say, a particular symptom is not necessarily acquired because of some learning experience in which its stimulus components were associated with pain or fear-producing stimuli. Rather, a symptom may function as an equipotential response, mediated by a central strategy acquired under different circumstances. As an example, consider Harlow's (1958, 1962) monkeys, who developed a number of symptoms, the most striking being sexual impotence (a much better animal analogue of human neurosis than those typically cited as experimental neuroses [Liddell, 1944]). Their longitudinal record, or "learning history," indicates that the development of this abnormal "affectional system," as Harlow terms it, is dependent on a variety of nonisomorphic experiences, including the lack of a mother-infant relationship and the lack of a variety of peer-play experiences.

These brief examples are only meant to give a flavor of where a learning conception of neurosis which stresses the acquisition of strategies will lead. A chief advantage of this view is that it has *generality* built in at the core, rather than imported secondarily, as is the case with S-R concepts of stimulus and response generalization.

Let us now turn our attention to the very difficult problem of applying learning concepts to psychotherapy. Basically, we would argue that the development of methods and techniques is largely a function of the empirical skill and ingenuity of the individual-craftsman-therapist. Even a carefully worked-out and well-established set of learning principles (which we do not have at this time) would not necessarily tell us how to modify acquired strategies in the individual case—just as the generally agreed-upon idea that rewards affect performance does not tell us what will be an effective reward in any specific instance.

Bearing these cautions in mind, we might still address ourselves to the question of what applications are suggested by the learning approach we have presented. As a first suggestion, we might consider the analogy of learning a new language. Here we see a process that parallels psychotherapy insofar as it involves modifying or developing a new set of strategies of a pervasive nature. A careful study of the most effective techniques for the learning of a new language might yield some interesting suggestions for psychotherapy. Learning a new language involves the development of a new set of strategies for responding—new syntax as well as new vocabulary. Language learning *may or may not* be facilitated by an intensive attempt to make the individual *aware* of the strategies used, as is done in traditional language instruction which teaches old-fashioned grammar, and as is done, analogously, in those psychotherapies which stress insight. Alternatively, language learning sometimes seems most rapid when the individual is immersed in surroundings (such as a foreign country) where he hears nothing but the new language and where his old strategies and responses are totally ineffective.

Using this as a model for psychotherapy, we might suggest something like the following process: First, a careful study should be done to delineate the "neurotic language," both its vocabulary and its grammar, of the individual. Then a situation might be constructed (e.g., a group therapy situation) in which the individual's existing neurotic language is not understood and in which the individual must develop a new "language," a new set of central strategies, in order to be understood. The detailed working out of such a procedure might very well utilize a number of the techniques that have been found effective in existing therapies, both group and individual, and in addition draw on some new techniques from the fields of psycholinguistics and language learning.

These are, of course, but initial fragmentary guesses, and they may be wrong ones. But we believe that the conceptions on which these guesses are based are sufficiently supported by recent learning research to warrant serious attention. Although this reconceptualization may not lead immediately to the development of effective psychotherapeutic techniques, it may at least provide a first step in that direction.

References

Adams, J. A. Motor skills. In P. R. Farnsworth (Ed.), *Annual Review of Psychology*, 1964, *15*, 181-202.

Bagby, E. *The Psychology of Personality*. New York: Holt, 1928.

Bandura, A. Psychotherapy as a learning process. *Psychological Bulletin*, 1961, *58*, 143-159.

Beach, F. A., Hebb, D. O., Morgan, C. T., and Nissen, H. W. *The Neuropsychology of Lashley*. New York: McGraw-Hill, 1960.

Berlyne, D. E. *Conflict, Arousal, and Curiosity*. New York: McGraw-Hill, 1960.

Blodgett, H. C. The effect of introduction of reward upon the maze performance of rats. *University of California Publications in Psychology*, 1929, *4*, 113-134.

Breland, K., & Breland, M. The misbehavior of organisms. *American Psychologist*, 1961, *16*, 681-684.

Brogden, W. J. Sensory preconditioning. *Journal of Experimental Psychology*, 1939, *25*, 323-332.

Bugelski, B. R. *The Psychology of Learning*. New York: Holt, 1956.

Chomsky, N. Review of B. F. Skinner, *Verbal Behavior*. *Language*, 1959, *35*, 26-58.

Deutsch, J. A. The inadequacy of Hullian derivations of reasoning and latent learning. *Psychological Review*, 1956, *63*, 389-399.

Dollard, J., & Miller, N. E. *Personality and Psychotherapy*. New York: McGraw-Hill, 1950.

Eriksen, C. W. (Ed.) *Behavior and Awareness*. Durham, N. C.: Duke Univer. Press, 1962.

Eysenck, H. J. (Ed.) *Behaviour Therapy and the Neuroses*. New York: Pergamon Press, 1960.

Fairweather, G. W. *Social Psychology in Treating Mental Illness: An Experimental Approach*. New York: Wiley, 1964.

Ferster, C. B., and Skinner, B. F. *Schedules of Reinforcement*. New York: Appleton-Century-Crofts, 1957.

Fitts, P. M. Perceptual-motor skill learning. In A. W. Melton (Ed.), *Categories of Human Learning*. New York: Academic Press, 1964. Pp. 244-285.

Frank, J. D. Problems of controls in psychotherapy as exemplified by the psychotherapy research project of the Phipps Psychiatric Clinic. In E. A. Rubenstein and M. B. Parloff (Eds.), *Research in Psychotherapy*. Washington, D. C.: American Psychological Association, 1959.

Frank, J. D. *Persuasion and Healing: A Comparative Study of Psychotherapy*. Baltimore: Johns Hopkins Press, 1961.

Fromm-Reichmann, Frieda. *Principles of Intensive Psychotherapy*. Chicago: Univer. Chicago Press, 1950.

Gibson, J. J. *The Perception of the Visual World*. Boston: Houghton Mifflin, 1950.

Gonzales, R. C., and Diamond, L. A test of Spence's theory of incentive motivation. *American Journal of Psychology*. 1960, *73*, 396-403.

Goodwin, W. R., and Lawrence, D.H. The functional independence of two discrimination habits associated with a constant stimulus situation. *Journal of Comparative and Psysiological Psychology*, 1955, *48*, 437-443.

Grossberg, J. M. Behavior therapy: A review. *Psychological Bulletin*, 1964, *62*, 73-88.

Guthrie, E. R. *The Psychology of Learning*. New York: Harper, 1935.

Guttman, N. Laws of behavior and facts of perception. In S. Koch (Ed.), *Psychology: A Study of a Science*. Vol. 5. New York: McGraw-Hill, 1963. Pp. 114-179.

Harlow, H. F. The nature of love. *American Psychologist*, 1958, *13*, 673-685.

Harlow, H. F. The heterosexual affectional system in monkeys. *American Psychologist*, 1962, *17*, 1-9.

Hebb, D. O. *The Organization of Behavior: A Neurophysiological Theory*. New York: Wiley, 1949.

Herbert, M. J., and Harsh, C. M. Observational learning by cats. *Journal of Comparative Psychology*, 1944, *37*, 81-95.

Hilgard, E. R. *Theories of Learning*. New York: Appleton-Century-Crofts, 1956.

Hull, C. L. *Essentials of Behavior*. New Haven: Yale Univer. Press, 1951.

Knight, R. P. Evaluation of the results of psychoanalytic therapy. *American Journal of Psychiatry*, 1941, *98*, 434.

Köhler, W. *Gestalt Psychology*. New York: Liveright, 1929.

Krasner, L. Studies of the conditioning of verbal behavior, *Psychological Bulletin*, 1958, *55*, 148-170.

Krasner, L. The therapist as a social reinforcement machine. In H. H. Strupp (Ed.), *Second Research Conference on Psychotherapy*. Chapel Hill, N.C.: American Psychological Association, 1961.

Krechevsky, I. The genesis of "hypotheses" in rats. *University of California Publications in Psychology*, 1932, *6*, 45-64.

Lang, P. J., and Lazovik, A. D. Experimental desensitization of a phobia. *Journal of Abnormal and Social Psychology*, 1963, *66*, 519-525.

Lawrence, D. H. The nature of a stimulus: Some relationships between learning and perception. In S. Koch (Ed.), *Psychology: A Study of a Science*. Vol. 5. New York: McGraw-Hill, 1963. Pp. 179-212.

Lawrence, D. H., and DeRivera, J. Evidence for relational transposition. *Journal of Comparative and Physiological Psychology*, 1954, *47*, 465-471.

Lazarus, A. A. The results of behaviour therapy in 126 cases of severe neurosis. *Behaviour Research and Therapy*, 1963, *1*, 69-80.

Lazarus, A. A., and Rachman, S. The use of systematic desensitization in psychotherapy. *South African Medical Journal*, 1957, *32*, 934-937.

Leeper, R. L. Learning and the fields of perception, motivation, and personality. In S. Koch (Ed.), *Psychology: A Study of a Science*. Vol. 5. New York: McGraw-Hill, 1963. Pp. 365-487.

Lewin, K. *Field Theory in Social Science*. New York: Harper, 1951. Ch. 4, pp. 60-86.

Liddell, H. S. Conditioned reflex method and experimental neurosis. In J. McV. Hunt (Ed.), *Personality and the Behavior Disorders*. New York: Ronald Press, 1944. Ch. 12.

Lundin, R. W. *Personality: An Experimental Approach*. New York: Macmillan, 1961.

Mackintosh, N. J. Extinction of a discrimination habit as a function of overtraining. *Journal of Comparative and Physiological Psychology*, 1963, *56*, 842-847.

Miller, G. A., Galanter, E. H., and Pribram, K. H. *Plans and the Structure of Behavior*. New York: Holt, Rhinehart & Winston, 1960.

Miller, N. E. Liberalization of basic S-R concepts: Extension to conflict behavior, motivation, and social learning. In S. Koch (Ed.), *Psychology: A Study of a Science*. Vol. 2. New York: McGraw-Hill, 1959. Pp. 196-292.

Moltz, H. Imprinting, empirical basis, and theoretical significance. *Psychological Bulletin*, 1960, *57*, 291-314.

Murray, E. J. Sociotropic learning approach to psychotherapy. In P. Worchel and D. Byrne (Eds.), *Personality Change*. New York: Wiley, 1964. Pp. 249-288.

Olds, J., and Milner, P. Positive reinforcement produced by electrical stimulation of septal area and other regions of rat brain. *Journal of Comparative and Physiological Psychology*, 1954, *47*, 419-427.

Osgood, C. E. *Method and Theory in Experimental Psychology.* New York: Oxford Univer. Press, 1953.

Postman, L. Perception and learning. In S. Koch (Ed.), *Psychology: A Study of a Science.* Vol. 5. New York: McGraw-Hill, 1963. Pp. 30-113.

Rachman, S. The treatment of anxiety and phobic reactions by systematic desensitization psychotherapy. *Journal of Abnormal and Social Psychology,* 1959, *58*, 259-263.

Riley, D. A. The nature of the effective stimulus in animal discrimination learning: Transposition reconsidered. *Psychological Review,* 1958, *65*, 1-7.

Ritchie, B. F., Aeschliman, B., and Peirce, P. Studies in spatial learning. VIII. Place performance and the acquisition of place dispositions. *Journal of Comparative and Physiological Psychology,* 1950, *43*, 73-85.

Rotter, J. B. *Social Learning and Clinical Psychology.* New York: Prentice-Hall, 1954.

Scott, J. P. Critical periods in behavioral development. *Science,* 1962, *138*, 949-958.

Skinner, B. F. *The Behavior of Organisms: An Experimental Analysis.* New York: Appleton-Century-Crofts, 1938.

Skinner, B. F. *Verbal Behavior.* New York: Appleton-Century-Crofts, 1957.

Solomon, R. L. Punishment. *American Psychologist,* 1964, *19*, 239-253.

Spence, K. W. The differential response in animals to stimuli varying within a single dimension. *Psychological Review,* 1937, *44*, 430-440.

Strickland, Bonnie R., and Crowne, D. P. The need for approval and the premature termination of psychotherapy. *Journal of Consulting Psychology,* 1963, *27*, 95-101.

Thistlethwaite, D. A critical review of latent learning and related experiments. *Psychological Bulletin,* 1951, *48*, 97-129.

Tolman, E. C. *Purposive Behavior in Animals and Men.* New York: Appleton-Century, 1932.

Tolman, E. C. Sign gestalt or conditioned reflex? *Psychological Review,* 1933, *40*, 391-411.

Tolman, E. C. *Collected Papers in Psychology.* Berkeley: Univer. California Press, 1951.

Tolman, E. C., and Honzik, C. H. Introduction and removal of reward and maze performance in rats. *University of California Publications in Psychology,* 1930, *4*, 257-275.

Underwood, B. J. The representativeness of rote verbal learning. In A. W. Melton (Ed.), *Categories of Human Learning.* New York: Academic Press, 1964. Pp. 47-78.

Watson, A. J. The place of reinforcement in the explanation of behavior. In W. H. Thorpe and O. L. Zangwill, *Current Problems in Animal Behavior.* Cambridge: Cambridge Univer. Press, 1961.

Wolpe, J. *Psychotherapy by Reciprocal Inhibition.* Palo Alto: Stanford Univer. Press, 1958.

Wolpe, J. Reciprocal inhibition as the main basis of psychotherapeutic effects. In H. J. Eysenck (Ed.), *Behaviour Therapy and the Neuroses.* New York: Pergamon Press, 1960. Pp. 88-113.

Wolpe, J., Salter, A., and Reyna, L. J. (Eds.) *The Conditioning Therapies.* New York: Holt, Rinehart and Winston, 1964.

Woodworth, R. S. *Dynamics of Behavior.* New York: Holt, 1958.

Yates, A. J. Symptoms and symptom substitution. *Psychological Review,* 1958, *65*, 371-374.

Zener, K. The significance of behavior accompanying conditioned salivary secretion for theories of the conditioned response. *American Journal of Psychology,* 1937, *50*, 384-403.

5

A Dynamic Synthesis of Analytic and Behavioral Approaches to Symptoms

MICHAEL E. MURRAY, PH.D.

This is a remarkable paper for its simple and straightforward review of both the behavioral and psychoanalytic conceptions of symptom formation and maintenance, followed by an integration of the theory such as to provide a rationale for the selection of treatment in a given patient.

Dr. Murray points out that symptomatic behavior may be a lacuna in a basically healthy personality for which faulty learning is the most significant etiological factor, and therefore a behavioral approach to the most efficient intervention. Other symptoms, arising as symbolic expressions of past or current intrapsychic conflict, may be maintained and habituated by behavioral reinforcement even once the initial conflict is resolved. He points out that when diagnostic evaluation includes a careful assessment of both dynamic issues and learning in the etiology and maintenance of symptomatic behavior, it is possible to make a reasoned judgment as to whether to initiate a purely psychodynamic, a purely behavioral, or a combined approach to treatment.

1 SUNDAY

	INBOUND			OUTBOUND	
Leave Watertown Square	Arrive Mt. Auburn Bridge	Arrive Harvard Station	Leave Harvard Station	Arrive Mt. Auburn Bridge	Arrive Watertown Square
6:32A	6:39A	6:50A	7:10A	7:21A	7:28A
7:32	7:39	7:50	8:10	8:21	8:28
8:32	8:39	8:50	9:06	9:19	9:27
9:29	9:37	9:49	10:10	10:23	10:31
10:35	10:43	10:55	11:00	11:13	11:21
11:25	11:33	11:45	11:50	12:03P	12:11P
2:15P	12:23P	12:35P	12:40P	12:53P	1:01P
1:05	1:13	1:25	1:30	1:44	1:52
1:55	2:03	2:15	2:20	2:34	2:42
2:45	2:53	3:05	3:10	3:24	3:32
3:35	3:43	3:55	4:00	4:14	4:22
4:25	4:33	4:45	4:50	5:04	5:12
5:15	5:23	5:35	5:40	5:54	6:02
6:05	6:13	6:24	6:30	6:43	6:51
6:55	7:03	7:14	7:20	7:33	7:41
7:45	7:53	8:04	8:10	8:23	8:31
8:35	8:43	8:54	9:00	9:13	9:21
9:25	9:33	9:44	9:50	10:03	10:11
10:15	10:23	10:34	10:40	10:51	10:58
11:05	11:12	11:23	11:30	11:41	11:48
11:55	12:02A	12:13A	12:20A	12:31A	12:38A
12:45A	12:52	1:03	1:04	1:15	1:22

FARE 60¢

Seniors 65+ w/MBTA Senior ID Card	15¢
Persons w/Disabilities w/Transportation Access Pass (TAP) (Medicare Card holders are automatically eligible for TAP)	15¢
Blind Persons w/Mass. Comm. for Blind ID Card	FREE
Children Ages 11 and under	30¢
Children under 5 yrs.(limit of two, when with adult)	FREE
Students w/MBTA Pupil ID Badge	30¢

EXACT CHANGE REQUIRED

VALID PASSES

Local Bus ($0.60)	$20.00/mo.
Combo ($1.50)	$46.00/mo.
Combo _Plus_ ($1.70)	$48.00/mo.
Zone - 1 ($2.00)	$64.00/mo.
Zone - 2 ($2.25)	$72.00/mo.

1998 HOLIDAYS:
April 20 - See Sat.
May 25 - See Sun.
June 17 - See Wkdy
July 4 - See Sun.
Sept. 7 - See Sun.
Oct. 12 - See Sat.
Nov. 11 - See Sat.
Nov. 26 - See Sun.
Dec. 25 - See Sun.

Route 71
Watertown Square - Harvard Station via

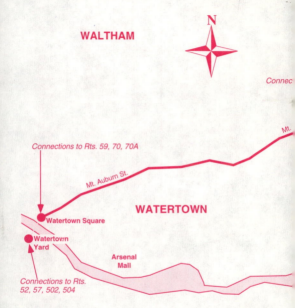

WALTHAM

N

Connec

Mt.

Connections to Rts. 59, 70, 70A

Mt. Auburn St.

WATERTOWN

● Watertown Square

● Watertown Yard

Arsenal Mall

Connections to Rts.
52, 57, 502, 504

5

A Dynamic Synthesis of Analytic and Behavioral Approaches to Symptoms

MICHAEL E. MURRAY, PH.D.

The treatment of psychologic and behavioral problems can be largely divided into theoretical and mythological camps.[1-4] These two groups include the psychodynamic, insight-oriented therapists, whose largest constituency embraces psychoanalytic, theoretical principles, and the behavior therapists, who adhere to operant and respondent conditioning models. The two orientations have some techniques in common, but each school is based upon entirely different models of man, and they have in general remained separated, alienated, and antagonistic toward one another.[5,6]

A number of attempts have been made to synthesize psychoanalytic and behavioral theories beginning as early as 1916.[7] Unfortunately, no real synthesis has been forthcoming as most papers either reinterpret behavior techniques in psychodynamic terms[8-12] or reformulate psychoanalytic theory from a learning framework.[13,14] The most hopeful efforts have been reports on a number of practical therapeutic approaches designed to combine psychodynamic and behavioral techniques in the actual treatment of patients.[15-20] However, the majority of the literature still finds two well-defined camps with behaviorists sharply criticizing psychodynamic therapists for their lack of scientific methodology[21-23] and dynamic therapists attacking the behaviorists for their failure to appreciate the quality of mind and the complexity of psychopathology.[24-27] The general theme is that the therapist must make a choice as to which treatment orientation he will choose.[28]

Such a situation places the conscientious, pragmatic therapist at a disadvantage as he seeks the most appropriate and powerful treatment modalities for his patients. In actual clinical work the therapists must make treatment decisions which can have major impact on the patient's life, and esoteric theoretical issues must give way to practical clinical

Reprinted by permission from *American Journal of Psychotherapy, 30*:561-569, 1976.

considerations. The confusing claims and accusations which the behaviorists and psychoanalytic theorists make can result in narrow-focus
treatment prejudices which rob the patient of optimal therapeutic opportunities. Following a brief summary of both positions, my discussion
will present a theoretical synthesis of the dynamic and behavioral approaches to symptoms and outline a practical guide to clinical treatment
considerations with regard to symptoms.

BEHAVIORAL VIEW OF SYMPTOMS

The behaviorists approach symptom behaviors from a learning-theory perspective. Inappropriate, unconstructive behavior patterns are not
seen as symbolic manifestations of an underlying psychologic disorder,
but rather the behaviors themselves are this disorder. No mentalistic,
theoretical framework or interpretation is employed to explain neurotic
or psychotic behaviors. The patients' responses are simply behavior
habits that are initiated and maintained by contingent reinforcement,
either primary or secondary. The etiology of the disruptive behaviors is
to be found in the patient's reinforcement history, though such information is not necessary for effective treatment. Removal or modification of
inappropriate behaviors is accomplished by changing the antecedent
stimuli that cue the particular behaviors and by rearranging contingent
reinforcement consequences.

In general, behaviors may be modified by the application of punishing consequences following disruptive behaviors or by withdrawing the
contingent positive reinforcement which maintains the response, a process called extinction. Positive behavior patterns are then developed,
again through proper use of contingent reinforcement. The behavioral
emphasis is upon the effects of external stimuli, the reinforcing and
punishing consequences of specific responses, and the complex interaction between subject and environment.[29] The behaviorists have made an
important contribution in specifying the conditions under which behaviors are brought about and maintained. In addition, the emphasis on
behavior has resulted in a systematic and thorough description of the
specific responses and larger behavior problems which create hardships
and interpersonal isolation in psychiatric patients. This basic behavioral
approach has brought forth a variety of innovative techniques which
have shown themselves highly effective in treating a number of behavioral disorders.

PSYCHODYNAMIC VIEW OF SYMPTOMS

The psychodynamic approach is based upon an inferential, mentalistic scheme which employs a psychologic explanation of behavior

symptoms. The emphasis is upon the structure and workings of mind and primary considerations are given to the internal, intrapsychic processes of the individual as he responds to and interacts with his environment.

Symptom formation is essentially a sequential process which arises out of intrapsychic conflict and the elaboration of ego mechanisms to bring about psychic equilibrium.[30] The first step in symptomatic behavior is an increase in anxiety and tension which results from an increase in instinctional, unacceptable drives, from the cathecting of unconscious conflicts, or from an incident in life which causes unusual trauma, threat, danger, frustration, or the loss of a significant other.

If the increased anxiety cannot be handled by normal coping mechanisms, it impinges upon the ego's integrity and executive functioning capabilities. The threat of ego disintegration results in a partial regression of the ego to a main level of fixation and infantile conflicts. These conflicts become intensified and the ego is confronted with the possible eruption of unconscious, repressed material. To combat the upsurge of repressed conflicts and drives, the ego processes bring a number of defensive maneuvers into play, which neutralize and transform the unacceptable materials into a form which is ego syntonic. What emerges is a symptom which may be behavioral, physiologic, or psychologic.

The symptom is a compromise which allows for the reduction of tension and anxiety and establishes a neurotic yet adaptive equilibrium between the conscious and unconscious. This represents the primary gain of the symptom formation. In addition, the psychologic symptom may allow for a secondary gain which involves direct reinforcement from the environment for the symptomatic behavior. If a symptom is removed by changing behavioral contingencies without dealing with the underlying conflict, it will become necessary for the individual to create new symptoms to maintain his intrapsychic balance. This process is called symptom substitution.

A PRACTICAL SYNTHESIS

Those behaviors, thoughts, and feelings which are generally referred to as psychologic symptoms are the main impetus which brings patients to the psychologists and psychiatrists. No matter what his theoretical orientation, the mental health specialist must make a serious study and evaluation of the symptom behavior pattern in diagnostic, dispositional, or treatment preparations. Any psychotherapy attempt which fails to acknowledge and deal practically with the frustrating and disabling manifest symptoms is at best an intellectual exercise and is destined for failure. The therapist must deal with the patient and his symptoms with an appreciation for the complexity of the individual human condition. A failure to consider either the external variables of organism-environment interaction, or the intrapsychic functions of needs, structure, and economy will limit treatment effectiveness.

Symptom formation involves a complex interaction between internal symbolic expression and secondary reinforcing consequences in the patient's environment. Basic needs, impulses, and fantasies are shaped, punished, frustrated, and actualized through interaction with other people. Symptoms exist to serve multilevel, adaptational functions, and ultimately the attribution of a primary etiology is in the eye of the beholder. A wide range of interpretations, be they for the chicken or the egg, possess an element of truth. In actual clinical practice, however, a conceptual framework allowing for practical, effective disposition and management is necessary.

Symptoms may be loosely classified under two general headings: those symptoms which are isolated and are apparently a result of faulty learning and those symptoms which appear to have developed as a result of intrapsychic conflict. The first group of symptoms usually presents itself in patients who demonstrate good psychological adjustment and ego functioning. Such patients present behavioral complaints which can be recognized as ego-alien lacunae which are within a basically intact personality structure. Such behaviors may be quite disabling, but often arise from traumatic events, specific familial-behavioral aberrations, or inadequate knowledge and opportunity for training. In such cases, the behaviors do not indicate underlying psychopathology; rather, the presenting problem is the disease. Perhaps the most common problems of this type are phobias and certain specific sexual dysfunctions.[18]

The task of deciding whether the symptom is an isolated lacuna or a part of a more encompassing disturbance of personality function is often made more difficult by the appearance of secondary emotional responses to the primary behavior problem. Feelings of inadequacy, insecurity, shame, and depression are common reactions to social and behavioral deficits. If, upon close examination, the individual has no decrement in functioning other than his reported symptoms and feelings about them, the therapist should consider direct symptomatic-behavioral treatment before prolonged and expensive analytic procedures are · employed.

The second type of symptoms grows out of psychologic conflicts and unresolved personality complexes. The specific symptoms are only one aspect of an underlying personality disorder. Often there are a number of inappropriate symptom behaviors, and the symptom formation may actually invoke styles of thought, feeling, and awareness, as dramatically exemplified in obsessive-compulsive and hysterical personality disorders. Often ego functioning is fragile, threatened, and ineffective.

The patient may complain of generalized and specific anxieties. Interpersonal problems are common and may be manifest in various aspects of life, including business, marriage, or friendship relations. The symptomatic behaviors have more disadvantages than advantages from a practical, adaptive viewpoint; however most of these problem behaviors have resulted in some secondary gain or reinforcement. The primary psychologic gain of reduced anxiety, penitence, and symbolic expression of conflict is usually discernible, given the patient's present situational conditions and family psychiatric history. Evaluation for treatment purposes must also involve a careful consideration of the present environmental reinforcement contingencies operating upon the behavioral and symptom processes.

Earlier concerns regarding symptom substitution in behavioral treatment of patients with more encompassing personality disorders have in large part subsided as a result of subsequent research[29] and the further development of psychoanalytic theory. Marmor states:

> Earlier psychoanalytic assumptions concerning symptom substitution were based on what we now know was an erroneous closed-system theory of personality dynamics. If the conflictual elements involved in neurosis formation are assumed to be part of a closed system, it follows logically that removal of the symptomatic consequences of such an inner conflict without altering the underlying dynamics should result in some other symptom manifestation. If, however personality dynamics are more correctly perceived within the framework of an open system, then such a consequence is not inevitable. Removal of an ego-dystonic symptom may, on the contrary, produce such satisfying feedback from the environment that may result in major constructive shifts within the personality system, thus leading to modification of the original conflictual pattern. Removal of the symptom may also lead to positive changes in the perception of the self, with resultant satisfying internal feedbacks, heightening of self-esteem, and a consequent restructuring of the internal psychodynamic system.[8]

The majority of the conflicts and psychic traumas which the individual has during his lifetime are resolved and subsequently decathected without psychotherapy. The work may be done at a conscious or unconscious level but the complex is neutralized and no longer provides an impetus for behavior. In some cases, an unconscious conflict may produce symptomatic behavior which becomes habituated in the person's behavioral repertoire by external reinforcement. Through the natural healing process of mind or through the termination of the conflict-producing situation, the underlying complex may become decathected, but the symptomatic behavior remains.

These behaviors may be destructive, yet they provide a secondary reinforcing gain. Thus, the symptom itself has become the pathology. If the symptomatic behaviors are severe enough, they may result in more global personality disturbances, including loss of self-esteem, insecurity, fears and anxieties, and diminished capacity for interpersonal relationships. At this point the primary treatment concern is the removal of the symptom by the shortest and most effective means possible. When the pathologic behavior ceases, a broad range of constructive changes may take place in the form of improved self-confidence and feelings of self-worth.

Thus, symptomatic behavior can be of two types depending upon its etiology and extent. The behavior may be a lacuna in a basically healthy personality which results from faulty learning, trauma, or cultural or familial aberrations. Symptomatic behaviors can also rise as symbolic expressions of intrapsychic conflicts and fixations. The conflict may be an ongoing concern which provides the impetus for the symptom and will produce other responses such as anxiety, confusion, fear, or other acting-out behaviors, if the behavior is removed without dealing with the underlying conflict. However, even in such cases, secondary gain which helps maintain the symptom should be carefully investigated. If the symptoms are very disturbing, their direct removal can provide the patient with increased hope and confidence and aid in the process of the dynamic, reconstructive psychotherapy.

Finally, many maladaptive behaviors which originally arose out of underlying internal conflicts may become habituated through contingent, external reinforcement and be retained even if the initial conflict is resolved. The symptom now becomes the primary concern since the impetus for the behavior has an external rather than an internal focus.

CLINICAL IMPLICATIONS

This broader theoretical construct of symptom formation and maintenance has several clinical implications for diagnosis, disposition, and treatment. As new techniques and methodology become available, the clinician is able to select the treatment of choice, be it behavioral, psychodynamic, supportive, interpersonal, or some combination of therapies. The proper disposition of the patient follows from adequate assessment of the person's symptom-behavior pattern with respect to his history and total personality functioning. Treatment considerations are then based upon the individual's unique problems. The type of symptoms and severity or destructiveness of the symptoms is of primary concern.

An initial behavioral approach aimed at direct symptom removal is indicated in two types of symptoms. The first includes those symptoms and behavioral maladjustments which are the result of faulty and inadequate learning experiences and are often associated with cultural and experiential deprivation. The patient's general personality and interpersonal functioning are good. Second, behavior therapy is the initial choice with individuals whose symptoms were originally created as a response to intrapsychic conflict, but who now continue to engage in the disturbing behaviors even after the initial complex has been decathected by a change of the life situation, psychotherapeutic intervention, or personal growth and healing. The response patterns have become habituated and are now maintained by contingent external reinforcement. As the symptomatic behaviors are given up, the patient may require more traditional psychotherapy in order to resolve existential concerns and stresses as well as to aid in the establishment of new goals, behaviors, and interests. Even in cases where symptomatic behavior bears little relationship to total personality dynamics, the symptomatic treatment should not preclude other therapeutic needs which may arise from the ongoing processes of therapy and life.

Psychodynamic and analytic psychotherapy approaches are indicated when symptomatic behaviors represent only one aspect of a more encompassing personality or interpersonal disturbance. In such cases, the symptomatic behaviors serve the individual adjustment at a number of psychosocial levels and attitudinal and internal gains must be dealt with as well as the current reinforcement contingencies. Therapeutic intervention is often required at an intrapersonal level, an interpersonal level, and even a family-systemic level.

Even in the patient whose primary treatment need is analytic psychotherapy, the therapist may wish to institute or seek out behavioral treatment for specific symptoms. This is especially true in cases where the symptoms are particularly dangerous or disruptive to the patient's life. The patient who engages in illegal behavior such as exhibitionism, child molesting, or overtly aggressive actions often requires behavioral therapy in addition to dynamic psychotherapy. The inclusion of desensitization procedures in the ongoing therapy is quite helpful in the treatment of phobic patients. In addition, when the therapist feels that the existence of a specific symptom is causing personality disruption far beyond its severity in terms of poor self-image, despair, or fear, he may augment therapy with behavioral techniques. The positive feedback and relief from anxiety and fear which accompanies the symptom removal may reduce resistance and speed up the analytic therapy process.

Finally, behavioral intervention should follow intrapersonal and interpersonal therapy in treating couples with sexual dysfunctions. Elimination of sexual problems requires the teaching of specific behavior techniques and sexual information as well as work with communication patterns, interpersonal dynamics, and individual history, attitudes, fears, and expectations.

In conclusion, the responsible clinician can no longer afford the luxury of rigid theoretical frameworks and must consider what techniques and methods constitute the optimal treatment strategy for his individual patients. In his assessment of symptoms he must consider intrapsychic dynamics, external reinforcement contingencies, and the current life situation. The examination of behavioral symptoms with regard to type, severity, and secondary personality reactions is important in determining the disposition of the patient and in aiding in the selection of the treatment techniques employed in the ongoing psychotherapy process.

SUMMARY

Symptoms are considered from a practical clinical perspective and the implications for diagnosis, disposition, and treatment are outlined. The symptom-formation process involves a complex interaction between internal symbolic expression and secondary reinforcing consequences in the patient's environment. Basic needs, impulses, and fantasies are shaped, punished, frustrated, and actualized through interaction with other people. Symptoms may be roughly classified as follows: symptoms which are isolated and are apparently a result of faulty learning; symptoms which appear to have developed as a result of intrapsychic conflict. Depending upon the characteristic and extent of the symptom formation, either a traditional or behavioral therapy approach may be indicated. In certain cases a combination of therapeutic approaches is necessary.

REFERENCES

1. Lazarus, A. A. *Behavior Therapy and Beyond.* McGraw-Hill, New York, 1971.
2. Rimm, P. C. and Masters, J. C. *Behavior Therapy: Techniques and Empirical Findings.* Academic Press, New York, 1974.
3. Bandura, A. *Principles of Behavior Modification.* Holt, New York, 1969.
4. Marmor, J. Psychoanalytic therapy and theories of learning. In *Science and Psychoanalysis.* Masserman, J., Ed. Grune and Stratton, New York, 1964. [See also Chapter 3, this volume.]
5. Lazarus, A. A. Some reactions to Castello's paper on depression. *Behavior Therapy,* 3:248, 1972.
6. Shectman, F. A. Operant conditioning and psychoanalysis: contrasts, similarities, and some thoughts about integration. *Am. J. of Psychother.,* 29:72, 1975. [See also Chapter 6, this volume.]
7. Watson, J. B. Behavior and the concept of mental disease. *Journal of Philosophical Psychology and Scientific Method,* 33:589, 1916.

8. Marmor, J. Dynamic psychotherapy and behavior therapy: are they irreconcilable? *Arch. of Gen. Psychiatry, 24*:22, 1971.[See also Chapter 2, this volume.]

9. Alexander, F. The dynamics of psychotherapy in the light of learning theory. *Am J. Psychiatry, 120*:440-448, 1963. [See also Chapter 1, this volume.]

10. Marmor, J. Psychoanalytic Therapy as an educational process. In *Modern Concepts of Psychoanalysis.* Masserman, J. & Salzman, L., Eds. Philosophical Library, New York, 1962.

11. Klein, M. H., Dittmann, A. T. and Parloff, M. B. *et al.* Behavior therapy: observations and reflections. *J. Consult. Clin. Psychol., 33*:259, 1969. [See also Chapter 14, this volume.]

12. Kubie, L. S. Relation of the conditioned reflex to psychoanalytic technique. *Arch. Neurol. Psychiatry, 32*:1137, 1934.

13. Kimble, G. A. *Hilgard and Marquis' Conditioning and Learning.* Appleton, New York, 1961.

14. Dollard, J. and Miller, N. E. *Personality and Psychotherapy.* McGraw-Hill, New York, 1950.

15. Susskind, D. J. The idealized self image (ISI): a new technique in confidence training. *Behavior Therapy, 1*:538, 1970.

16. Marks, I. M. and Gelder, M. G. Common grounds between behavior therapy and psychodynamic methods. *Br. J. Med. Psychol., 39*:11, 1966. [See also Chapter 10, this volume.]

17. Brady, J. P. Psychotherapy by a combined behavioral and dynamic approach. *Contemporary Psychiatry, 9*:536, 1968. [See also Chapter 15, this volume.]

18. Masters, W. H. and Johnson, V. E. *Human Sexual Inadequacy.* Little, Brown & Co., Boston, 1970.

19. Kaplan, H. S. *The New Sex Therapy.* Brunner/Mazel, New York, 1974. [See also Chapter 25, this volume.]

20. Woody, R. H. *Psychobehavioral Counseling and Therapy: Integrating Behavior and Insight Techniques.* Appleton-Century-Crofts, New York, 1971.

21. Eysenck, H. J., Ed. *Behavior Therapy and the Neuroses.* Pergamon Press, New York, 1960.

22. Wolpe, J. *Psychotherapy by Reciprocal Inhibition.* Stanford University Press, Stanford, California, 1958.

23. Ullmann, L. P. and Krasner, L., Eds. *Case Studies in Behavior Modification.* Holt, Rhinehart & Winston, New York, 1965.

24. Murray, M. E. The treatment of autism: a human protest. *J. Humanistic Psychol., 14*:57, 1974.

25. Breger, L. and McGaugh, J. L. Critique and reformulation of "learning-theory" approaches to psychotherapy and neurosis. *Psychol. Bull., 63*:338, 1965. [See also Chapter 4, this volume.]

26. Locke, E. A. Is "behavior therapy" behavioristic? *Psychol. Bull., 76*:318, 1971.

27. Weitzman, B. Behavior therapy and psychotherapy. *Psychol. Rev., 74*:300, 1967. [See also Chapter 7, this volume.]

28. Eysenck, H. J. and Rachman, S. *The Causes and Cures of Neurosis.* Routledge, London, 1965.

29. Mahoney, M. J., Kazdin, A. E. and Lesswing, N. J. Behavior modification: delusion or deliverance. In *Behavior Therapy and Practice.* Franks, C. M. and Wilson, G. T., Eds. Brunner/Mazel, New York, 1974.

30. Cameron, N. *Personality Development and Psychotherapy.* Houghton Mifflin, Boston, 1963.

Operant Conditioning and Psychoanalysis

Contrasts, Similarities, and Some Thoughts about Integration

FREDERICK A. SHECTMAN, PH.D.

This short paper by Shectman goes over much that has been covered in the previous papers, but it presents a useful organization of the contrasts and similarities between an operant conditioning approach and psychoanalysis in terms of the data employed, the use of theory, the balance between idiographic and nomothetic factors, the role of continuity, views of etiology, and technique. An important additional point that Shectman makes is about the different conceptions of man involved in the two orientations, i.e., one that sees man as being guided, regulated, and molded entirely by outside forces, and one that puts more emphasis on internalized regulatory controls. Like the preceding authors, Shectman asserts that each approach enriches the other and pleads for efforts to achieve integration between them.

Operant Conditioning and Psychoanalysis

Contrasts, Similarities, and Some Thoughts about Integration

FREDERICK A. SHECTMAN, PH.D.

CONTRASTS

Data

The differences between an operant conditioning orientation and a psychoanalytic one are readily apparent, for example, the former focusing on what is outside and observable and the latter on what is inside and less evident; the first stressing behavior and the second emphasizing overall personality organization. Thus, an analytic approach does not exclude the data of operant conditioning (what is outside-observable), but an operant conditioning orientation does exclude the data of psychoanalysis (internal processes) because of its tie to what is palpable and hence measurable. It does not attend to inferred constructs which are at the heart of the psychoanalytic framework and provide it with what its adherents regard as its richness and explanatory power to make understandable what otherwise appears incomprehensible. (Nothing pejorative about operant conditioning nor complimentary to psychoanalysis is implied here. Rather, these are just differences which flow from the dissimilar data bases.)

Unlike psychoanalysis, a reinforcement approach does not commit one to any particular theory of personality disturbance because it stresses observable behavior rather than theoretical constructs. As Lindsley[1] has submitted:

> To a behaviorist a psychotic is a person in a mental hospital. If psychosis is what makes, or has made this person psychotic, then psychosis is the behavioral deviation that caused the person to be hospitalized, or that is keeping him hospitalized.

Reprinted by permission from *American Journal of Psychotherapy*, 29:72-78, January 1975.

Use of Theory

While psychoanalysis has a theoretical framework which can dictate the therapeutic interventions of its practitioners, operant conditioning therapy provides no such theoretical guidelines. It is not a theory but is instead a set of procedures based on experimentally founded principles. As such, a reinforcement approach is inclined to use social acceptability as a criterion for guiding the action of its practitioners, as Lindsley implied above (cf. Portes[2]).

SIMILARITIES

Idiographic-Nomothetic

It has been noted:

> Psychoanalysis was initially a method of therapy which later attempted to become a science; behaviorism was initially a scientific theory which only recently has tried its hand at therapy. The beginnings of psychoanalysis were idiographic, those of behaviorism nomothetic. From here derives the "badness" of psychoanalysis as scientific theory.[2]

And, presumably, the "goodness" of behaviorism stems from its elegant neatness, straightforwardness of its learning principles, and anchorings in laboratory research. But is this really the case? For has not psychoanalysis sought to develop general scientific principles which grow out of the intensive and systematic study of the individual? And, on the other hand, it is evident from journal reports that the application of reinforcement techniques is very much geared to individual differences and not used globally in an impersonal fashion. Both approaches agree, then, in concentrating on a single person but understanding the person's behavior in broad terms which transcend that individual, that is, both orientations work idiographically but conceptualize nomothetically. Lindsley[1] makes this case clear for behaviorists in stating:

> Since the behavioral properties of psychosis are highly individual, each experiment must be conducted in such a fashion that each patient serves as his own control . . . intensive investigation of single psychotics is the only way that a number of different behavioral deficits may be catalogued with respect to individual psychotics in attempts to locate and define syndromes of behavioral deficits which could define subtypes of psychosis.

Within this framework it would appear that Lindsley is also talking very much about nosology and diagnosis, issues of great importance to psychoanalysis but generally avoided by behaviorists. Lindsley's assertion thus reflects more of a similarity between the two approaches than is usually seen to be the case.

Continuity

Psychoanalysis tends to assume a continuity between different forms of psychopathology—so that neuroses, psychoses, and character disorders can be understood by the same fundamental psychologic principles. Operant conditioning practitioners also tend to regard abnormal behavior as part of a continuum stretching from normality to abnormality:

> Abnormal behaviors and normal behaviors can be viewed as reciprocally related, and those with disturbed behavior as exhibiting considerable abnormal behavior, or little normal behavior. Normal behavior probability can be increased by decreasing probability of abnormal behavior, or abnormal behavior can be decreased by the controlled increase of normal behavior.[3]

Etiology

While psychoanalysis carefully examines the past history of the patient, particularly his childhood, operant conditioning has been charged with not considering historical antecedents but focusing only on present conditions. However, operant conditioning does look at the past, but in terms of prior reinforcement schedules. Ferster[4] suggests that "it is possible that many of the symptoms which bring the patient to therapy are largely a by-product of inadequate positively reinforced repertoires." Thus, the therapeutic "assumption [is] that a patient's behavior, whatever historical factors may have been responsible for its present state, is manipulatable through variations in the concurrent controlling environment."[5]

SIMILARITY OF TECHNIQUES

Psychotic Verbalizations

Allyon and Haughton[6] have shown how the frequency of psychotic statements by hospital patients can be manipulated, depending upon the floor personnel's reactions to the patient's verbalizations. For example, positive reinforcement (cigarettes or candy, or demonstrating interest by showing careful attention) and negative reinforcement (looking away, acting busy, appearing distracted or bored) had differential effects upon the ratio of psychotic to neutral verbalization.

A psychoanalytic approach can embody similar principles, for example, telling a patient who speaks in metaphor or cryptic language to speak plain English because otherwise he is just not understandable. The attempts to suppress the incomprehensible and to have it translated into what is understandable can be regarded in effect as negative reinforcement of one form of behavior and positive reinforcement of another form. At other times, though, a staff member may try to enter into the metaphoric communication with the idea of understanding leading toward lessening psychotic talk, for example, a diminishing need by the patient to keep distance via his private language. Communication with the other person may become more rewarding (positively reinforcing) as the patient feels less threatened and allows himself to be more understood, with a concomitant decrease in psychotic talk. Is this not similar to the operant conditioners' practice of successive approximation, when each response is reinforced which more closely approximates the desired behavior than did the preceding reinforced response?

Superego Deficiency

A reinforcement program has been used in Achievement Place, a community living setting designed to modify the behavior of "predelinquent" boys.[7] In dealing with what psychoanalysis would regard as superego deficiency, this program uses tokens to reward desired superego behavior (for example, washing hands before meals and doing homework) and to punish antisuperego behavior (for instance, back talk and fighting). In the psychoanalytically oriented C. F. Menninger Memorial Hospital, there is a strong belief in confronting and interpreting pathologic defensive operations which in themselves bring about ego weakness (for example, lack of superego integration) and whose undoing may actually strengthen the ego.[8] Such efforts may be viewed, *in part*, as negative reinforcement—especially since the use of defensive maneuvers like "splitting" often lead to a curtailment of activities and ever closer observation of what the patient does and not what he says.

Improvement (diminution of pathologic defensive behavior) leads to increased privileges and responsibilities—positive reinforcement of desired behavior. However, while the behavior modification approach would stop here with the cessation of the undesirable behavior, the psychoanalytic one would continue on—regarding that behavior as but a symptom which, when reduced, means that conflicts are being internalized and therefore more accessible to further understanding, rather than being lived out by making the hospital team into a policeman or watchdog.

The Need for Integration

The behaviorist would account for the success of the adolescent who leaves Achievement Place and does not resort to antisocial behavior by talking in terms of behavior generalizing from the token rewards to social reinforcers like approval and esteem. In view of the behavior modification therapist's refusal to take into account what goes on internally—and particularly to do without a concept of "self"—an analytically oriented clinician could ask, "How can social reinforcement work if the individual is not aware of himself and, consequently, cannot value his own image?"[2] But if such a question might prove awkward for a behaviorist, what would an analyst say to a behaviorist who charges him with tautology in accounting for the differential outcomes for youths who leave Achievement Place; that is, the psychoanalyst might suggest that the adolescents who slip back to their antisocial behavior failed to internalize and integrate superego components, while those who maintain behaviors rewarded in Achievement Place do internalize and integrate. But here the dependent variable (failure or success in internalization) is not clearly differentiated at all from the independent variable (those conditions which make for failure or success in internalization).

Indeed, psychoanalysis needs a way of answering questions about internalization, for major alterations in behavior and a substantial impact on personality differentiation and structure formation is presumed to occur as a consequence of "identification." Whereas the behaviorist can talk in terms of reinforced responses based on contingencies which result in behavioral repertoires, psychoanalysts have little to rely on to account theoretically for how crucial identifications happen. Writing on this topic, Schafer[9] notes:

> Learning is so closely related to internalization that one finds it difficult to disentangle the two concepts. The psychological and psychoanalytic literature is not much help in this regard . . . learning on the one hand and processes of introjection and identification on the other hand cannot be regarded as mutually exclusive; nor do they constitute alternative explanations.

And yet the need for integration of learning theory and psychoanalytic concepts has been seen before. Rapaport[10] took psychoanalysis to task because of its failure to produce a dynamic learning theory of its own, and Piers and Piers[11] have sought to bridge the gap between more traditional modes of learning (conditioning and insight) and that mode critically important for psychoanalysis (identification). What is it, then, that stands in the way of such a needed rapprochement?

DIFFERENT IMAGES OF MAN

Perhaps one obstacle is the divergent conception of Man which each of the two orientations under discussion implicitly (if not explicitly) embraces. For the behaviorist, even when the individual's behavior is desirably "shaped up," the emphasis is still on externals, for example, social reinforcers and correctional feedback systems. Methodological values (what is observable and hence measurable) dictate an implicit view of Man as being guided and regulated by outside agents which ever need to be maintained in one form or another. To the psychoanalyst, such a view is reserved for people who suffer from characterological disturbances in their ability to internalize values and controls. For the behaviorist to accept such a view as characteristic of Man and not simply as one form of psychopathology leaves the psychoanalyst cold. For him, it is a repugnant framework which conceptualizes Man as an aggregation of habits or group of behaviors to be shaped and manipulated.

This conception violates the psychoanalyst's belief in the complexity and humanism of the individual—especially doing injustice to the rich internal life of Man which psychoanalysis has sought to illuminate. For the behaviorist, on the other hand, such views smack more of values than science and leave him impatient in wanting to further his understanding via experimentally rooted investigation.

In their dismay, however, at the exclusion by the other of much that is held dear, both parties would do well not to perpetuate what has occurred before; that is, the polarization into camps which ignore each other and overlook the kind of commonalities discussed above, and thereby fail to enrich their respective approaches by discarding elements of the other's framework rather than integrating such concepts into their own. A case in point is the failure of psychoanalysis to use the contributions of the behaviorists to work toward a better psychoanalytic theory of learning. In short, both sides need to overcome the "splitting" of the separate systems of behavior modification and psychoanalysis in order to achieve a more integrated and comprehensive view of personality development and organization.

Summary

Contrasts and similarities between an operant conditioning approach and a psychoanalytic one are discussed in terms of the data employed, use of theory, the place of what is idiographic and nomothetic, the role of continuity, views of etiology, and types of techniques utilized. The need for integration of these two viewpoints is elaborated, especially the need of psychoanalysis for a dynamic learning theory. Such a theory could draw upon what the behaviorists have contributed. A major obstacle to this rapprochement is seen in the divergent conceptions of Man which each orientation embraces and which make for unnecessary polarizations which need to be overcome.

References

1. Lindsley, O. R. Characteristics of the behavior of chronic psychotics as revealed by free-operant conditioning methods. *Dis. Nerv. Sys.*, 21 (Suppl.): 66, 1960.
2. Portes, A. On the emergence of behavior therapy in modern society. *J. Consult. Clin. Psychol.*, 36:303, 1971.

3. Isaacs, W., Thomas, J., and Goldiamond, I. Application of operant conditioning to reinstate verbal behavior in psychotics. *J. Speech Hear. Disord.*, 25:8, 1960.
4. Ferster, C. B. Reinforcement and punishment in the control of human behavior by social agencies. *Psychiat. Res. Rep.*, 10:101, 1958.
5. Sidman, M. Operant techniques. In *Experimental Foundations of Clinical Psychology*, Bachrach, A. J., Ed. Basic Books, New York, 1962, pp. 170-210.
6. Allyon, T., and Haughton, M. The modification of symptomatic verbal behavior of mental patients. *Behav. Res. Ther.*, 2:87, 1964.
7. Phillips, E. L., Phillips, Elaine A., Fixsen, D. L., and Wolf, M. M. Achievement place: modification of the behaviors of pre-delinquent boys within a token economy. *J. Appl. Behav. Anal.*, 4:45, 1971.
8. Kernberg, O. The treatment of patients with borderline personality organization. *Int. J. Psychoanal.*, 49:600, 1968.
9. Schafer, R. *Aspects of Internalization*. International Universities Press, New York, 1968.
10. Rapaport, D. The structure of psychoanalytic theory: a systematizing attempt. In *Psychology: A Study of a Science*, Vol. 3, Koch, S., Ed. McGraw-Hill, New York, 1959, pp. 55-183.
11. Piers, G., and Piers, M. W. Modes of learning and the analytic process. Paper presented at the meeting of the VIth International Congress of Psychotherapy, London, 1964.

7

Behavior Therapy and Psychotherapy

BERNARD WEITZMAN, PH.D.

Weitzman's article is notable because it represents an early effort on the part of a sophisticated psychologist to reconcile the therapeutic results of systematic desensitization not only with classical psychoanalytic theory, but also with Jungian theory, interpersonal theory, and cognitive decision theory. After effectively demolishing Eysenck's tendency to talk of "learning theory" as though there were a single theory of learning, when in fact there are many—a point previously made by Estes et al. in 1954 and by Breger and McGaugh in 1965—Weitzman goes on to demonstrate how much more complex Wolpe's technique of systematic desensitization actually is as compared with the rather simplistic explanation that is usually given (i.e., reduction of anxiety by reciprocal inhibition due to muscular relaxation). In actuality, "a wealth of dynamically rich" fantasy material that has been essentially ignored is conjured up by patients during the silent periods of "relaxation." Weitzman appropriately insists that the existence of these central processes in behavior therapy must not be ignored, and should be incorporated into a comprehensive theory of the behavioral therapeutic process. He chides dynamic psychotherapists for ignoring this challenge and offers some ingenious explanations of how such a theory might be formulated within the framework of a number of diverse theories. He also presents some tentative examples of how systematic desensitization can be utilized within a framework of dynamic understanding in psychotherapy—techniques that subsequent authors have been able to carry further (see Section III of this volume).

Behavior Therapy
and Psychotherapy

7

Bernard Weitzman, Ph.D.

A number of procedures which would, a decade ago, have claimed the status of "psychotherapies" (cf., e.g., Wolpe, 1958) have in the recent past characterized themselves as "behavior therapies." It is intended by its users that this nomenclature shall be pregnant with meaning (cf. Eysenck, 1960). Properly understood, it reflects the long-resisted penetration of clinical practice by that form of "scientism" which, earlier, had a hand in leading academic "psychologists" to their sea change into "behavioral scientists." While attempts to articulate the historical factors which underlie such transformations are always speculative, there seems little doubt that, in the case of clinical practice, the publication of Wolpe's psychotherapeutic manual is one causal nexus. The apparent effectiveness of the techniques devised by Wolpe, in particular the procedure called "systematic desensitization" (cf. Grossberg, 1964), has won him a following, and has invited the use of an argument of virtue by association in a bid to legitimize the host of procedures calling themselves "behavior therapies."

Many psychologists in clinical practice have found quite irresistible the promise of quick and effective results which Wolpe's procedure holds forth, despite a host of objections to it which arise from the various "dynamic" orientations. Others, feeling tempted, have resisted the demons of mechanization and dehumanization, and the danger of "loss of soul" which is understood to be implicit in the *Weltanschauung* of behaviorism. This resistance is buttressed by theoretical allegiances and made to seem necessary by a variety of therapeutic rubrics, for example, the expectation of symptom substitution, a problem which will be treated in some detail later.

The rejection, on grounds of principle, of behavior therapy by the

Reprinted by permission from *Psychological Review*, 74:300-317, 1967. Copyright 1967 by the American Psychological Association.

clinical community, and the derogatory treatment of dynamic therapies by behavior therapists, have had the inevitable consequence of generating premature crystallizations of positions in both camps. The lines of battle have been most sharply and articulately drawn in the writings of Eysenck (1960), who asserts:

> . . . behavior therapy is an *alternative* type of treatment to psychotherapy [i.e., it is not ancillary], . . . it is a *superior* type of treatment, both from the point of view of theoretical background and practical effectiveness; . . . in so far as psychotherapy is at all effective, it is so in virtue of certain principles which can be *derived from learning theory* . . . psychotherapy itself, when shorn of its inessential and irrelevant parts, can usefully be considered as a minor part of behavior therapy. (p. ix)

While the position taken by Eysenck is more extreme than other behavior therapists might prefer, its clarity makes it a useful target for analysis. Some comments on the contents of Eysenck's statement will clear the way for the major substance of this essay, that is, an examination of the grounds upon which clinicians have based their rejection of behavior therapy.

THE THEORETICAL BACKGROUND OF BEHAVIOR THERAPY

The evidence of the practical effectiveness of behavior therapy, while not conclusive, is indeed impressive. However, if one notes (as Eysenck does) that the term *behavior therapy* refers to a large and diverse group of treatment methods, clarity requires that the question of effectiveness must be put to each method. If one extracts from the mass of data the results of systematic desensitization therapy, one is left with an impression which is rather different from that intended by Eysenck. The residue, that is, the evidence of the practical effectiveness of behavior therapies other than systematic desensitization, while interesting, would excite the enthusiasm of few clinicians (cf. Grossberg, 1964). As a first step then, the accuracy of Eysenck's statement might be increased by appropriately reading "systematic desensitization" where he has written "behavior therapy." This sharpening of focus permits a more cogent appraisal of the evidence, and a more lucid analysis of the problems.

An issue of considerable importance is raised by Eysenck's claim of theoretical superiority for behavior therapy. It has been pointed out, from both camps, that analytic theory requires that symptom substitution or recurrence must attend a symptomatic treatment which, by definition, does not affect the dynamic sources of the symptoms. The evidence is rather impressive that neither substitution nor recurrence typically follows treatment by systematic desensitization. When occasional recurrences are reported, they are described as being of low intensity and, apparently, never catastrophic. Wolpe and Eysenck have both explicitly contended that this evidence constitutes a decisive empirical argument against psychoanalysis. A detailed analysis of the theoretical grounds upon which this contention is based will be undertaken later in this discussion. At this point, however, it must be noted that a crucial logical alternative, that is, that systematic desensitization does, as a technique, in some way affect the total psychological matrix, has not been given due theoretical consideration by behavior therapists or by psychotherapists. Attempts have been made to demonstrate, *empirically*, the specificity of the effects of systematic desensitization, that is, to demonstrate that desensitization is confined, in the locus of its effects, to the undoing of specific conditioned associations. The evidence, however, is not altogether convincing and certainly not conclusive. As long as the issue is empirically open, the *logical* analysis must be allowed.

When this analysis is undertaken it appears that there are implications of the data for Eysenck's theoretical model which have not been examined, and which seem to indicate that the Eysenckian position is vulnerable to criticisms similar to those leveled at psychoanalysis. Eysenck (1957) views neuroticism as a genetically determined constitutional predisposition. That is, all else being equal, there is a genetic determination of the likelihood that one individual will develop neurotic symptoms more readily than will another individual. Obviously, behavior therapy, in removing symptoms, cannot be expected to alter this genetic base. Thus, the likelihood of developing symptoms, insofar as this is genetically given, will remain constant. It would seem reasonable to assume that, in statistical mass, the number of patients treated as neurotics in any therapeutic setting will contain a disproportionately large number of individuals high in genetically determined neuroticism. If this reasoning is correct, Eysenck's model would seem to predict a high incidence of new symptom formations in patients who have already been treated for neurotic symptoms. Indeed, if one takes seriously the reports of almost total absence of new symptoms in patients treated by systematic desensitization, a problem of some difficulty arises for the Eysenckian model. On the one hand, there are difficulties in attempting to solve the problem by entertaining the speculation that a lasting transformation of learning processes has been achieved by this technique if one is determined to deny that there are any nonspecific characterological consequences attending its application. (An analysis of some of the conceptual difficulties of S-R theories in "explaining how *generality* of behavior results from specific learning experiences" has been presented by Breger and McGaugh, 1965, p. 348.) On the other hand, if it is granted that there are such nonspecific consequences, the genetic hypothesis must be formulated in a manner which makes such consequences intelligible. The alternatives for Eysenck would seem to entail a surrender, both of the current conception of genetically determined neuroticism and of the insistence upon the specificity of the effects of desensitization.

Eysenck's intention, however, is not to burden his own theory with the support of his claim to theoretical superiority for behavior therapy. Rather, the burden falls more broadly on something called "learning theory." An issue which exists for many clinicians seems to pivot about the intrinsic relation which is claimed to exist between behavior therapy and this "learning theory." The clinician is asked to agree that if he accepts the method as therapeutically valid and gives credence to the data which support assertions of its effectiveness, he must "buy" some "S-R" model of man. But what model of man is, in fact, required? A number of comments on this relationship may be helpful.

In the foreword to a volume reporting the outcome of a summer symposium on learning theory (Estes, Koch, MacCorquodale, Meehl, Mueller, Schoenfeld, and Verplanck, 1954), the editor writes:

> It might be supposed that there would crystallize out from such a critical and unbiased analysis of theories and the experimental evidence on which they rest, some one basic theory of the learning process which all reasonable persons could accept. If there were any such expectations among the members of the group, they were soon dissipated. Each theory appeared to exist within its own closed system and to defy direct comparison and the pooling of data. Concepts, techniques, apparatus, units of measurement, and definitions of terms were peculiar to a given theory and could not safely be lifted out of their own frame of reference. Each theory, then, had to be examined and analyzed separately for internal consistency and the degree to which it satisfied the logic of science. (p. vii)

In the context of a discussion similar to the present one Breger and McGaugh (1965, p. 341) conclude: "The claim to scientific respectability by reference back to established laws of learning is . . . illusory." In light of these reports it seems somewhat misleading to speak as if there were a monolithic system properly called "learning theory." Indeed, Eysenck (1960) concedes this point. To the objection that "learning theorists are not always in agreement with each other," he answers:

> . . . those points about which argument rages are usually of academic [theoretical] interest rather than of practical importance. Thus, reinforcement theorists and contiguity theorists have strong differences of view about the necessity of reinforcement during learning and different reinforcement theorists have different theories about the nature of reinforcement. Yet there would be general agreement in any particular case about the optimum methods of achieving a quick rate of conditioning. . . . (p. 15)

In fact, only an eclectic learning theory which systematically avoids examination of the relations between its own assumptions—that is, a nontheoretical amalgamation of pragmatic principles—can hope to derive the effects of a behavioral setting as complex as the therapeutic interview. Whether or not the methodological consensus which Eysenck assumes really exists (the reader is referred once more to the quotation from Estes et al., 1954), the theoretical limitation which is acknowledged must be as constraining for those procedures called "behavior therapy" as for psychotherapy. That is, if there is no "learning theory" competent to handle the data of behavior therapy, there is no "learning theory" competent to handle the data of psychotherapy. If, then, one accepts the data of behavior therapy, one is faced, not with a set of necessary theoretical conclusions, but with a set of theoretical problems.

THE METHOD OF SYSTEMATIC DESENSITIZATION: AN INQUIRY

Since the most impressive data have been produced by Wolpe's method, it will be worthwhile to turn now to a more detailed consideration of systematic desensitization, and the relation of its practical methodology to Wolpe's conception of it.

Wolpe (1962) has described the genesis of systematic desensitization in discussing his replication of Masserman's (1943) study. Masserman produced "neurotic" behavior in cats by directing blasts of air at the animals as they began to eat. Wolpe, in his replication, demonstrated that the confrontation of appetitive and avoidant drive states is not a necessary condition for eliciting this symptomatology; that is, he obtained apparently the same form of neurotic behavior by shocking cats in the absence of food. (It is worth noting, en passant, that Wolpe has claimed that this demonstration undermines the psychoanalytic theory of the relation of symptom and conflict. While his study does seem to provide evidence concerning necessary conditions, it is not relevant to the premise that drive conflict is a *sufficient* condition for symptom formation.)

Wolpe then "deconditioned" the fear reaction by a procedure in which a gradual, stepwise approach was made to the feared stimuli (the experimental cage and room), each step accompanied by feedings. Feedings, sometimes repeated at a given step, led to extinction of the fear response at that level of approach and permitted feeding to be initiated at the next step. The animals were, finally, free of any signs of neurotic behavior. This result was rationalized by the assumption that the eating response inhibits the occurrence of anxiety and leads to the extinction of the anxiety response to the stimuli which are present at a given step.

Wolpe reasoned that eating is only one of a variety of behaviors which may be used to inhibit anxiety. This thinking led to the application of the procedure to human subjects. Relaxation was substituted for eating as the anxiety-inhibiting response, and the resulting method was called "systematic desensitization."

A description of this method sounds strikingly like the method used by Wolpe to cure his cats: The human subject is trained, by a short form of the Jacobson (1938) method, to develop high-strength relaxation responses. He is then, while in a relaxed condition, presented, one at a time, with preselected stimuli, known to produce anxiety and arranged in a series of intensity or approach steps. When, after one or a number of presentations, a given step elicits no anxiety response, the next stimulus in the intensity hierarchy is presented, until the most intense stimulus produces no anxiety.

In this description, however, is hidden a form of analogy-making which gives comfort to the behavior therapist but which obscures differences of profound significance between the systematic desensitizations of cats and men. The reaction of the clinician, that "they are treating patients the way they treat cats," fails to penetrate the flaws of the analogy. (It is not entirely beside the point to note that this reaction implicitly grants the legitimacy of the behavioristic interpretation of cat behavior. The necessity of that interpretation is, of course, open to question.) It is crucial that the above, stylized description of systematic desensitization be concretized and given a more detailed procedural analysis.

The human subject is trained in voluntary relaxation. The training directs the subject to careful observation of certain internal states, to the discrimination of tensions in the major muscle groups of the body, and to the voluntary cessation of muscular responding. When this highly complex "response" has been acquired, a stimulus is presented. That is to say, the patient is directed by the therapist to *imagine a stimulus* which he has previously described to the therapist and which he has placed, for the use of the therapist, among other anxiety-producing stimuli in a given hierarchical position. The patient is, in fact, required to produce a vivid visualization of a scene. It is this visualization which is the "stimulus" bandied about in discussions of systematic desensitization. As Breger and McGaugh (1965, p. 340) have put it, "the use of the terms stimulus and response are only remotely allegorical to the traditional use of these terms in psychology." The importance of this characterization of the stimulus is underlined by the fact that *inability to produce such visualizations is grounds for rejecting a patient for treatment by this method.* Having "presented a stimulus," the therapist lapses into silence for periods of up to 1 minute. *Any stimulus present in this situation is produced by the patient's internal processes.*

The therapeutic effect of systematic desensitization thus seems to be produced in periods of silence. That is, the therapist describes a scene which, presumably, sets a process in motion. So long as this process continues neither therapist nor patient speaks, and neither acts. There is, thus, for the content of the therapeutic process itself, no response of record. In other words, the question of what transpires during these silences is not, and has not been, asked. In reaction to the formulation of this question, and to frequent spontaneous reports from patients who were concerned that their inability to maintain static visualizations of the scene described by the therapist might hamper therapy, the author undertook regular inquiry into the contents of these silences. Six patients being treated by the method of systematic desensitization were interviewed. An interview was conducted at the end of each session of desensitization, providing a sample of approximately 200 interviews. Without exception, when closely questioned, patients reported a flow of visual imagery. The initiating scene, once visualized, shifted and changed its form. Moreoever, these transformations took place continuously and, when the imagining was terminated by the therapist, had produced images which were quite removed in their content from the intended stimulus. These contents, and the transformations they exhibit, compel a characterization as a form of spontaneous and apparently autonomous fantasy familiar to many dynamically oriented therapists and, in fact, a therapeutic focus for those analysts who use Jung's (1959) method of active imagination. (While there is one report in the literature—Weinberg and Zaslove, 1963—of " 'involuntary' manipulations of the imaginal process," during treatment by systematic desensitization, the observed shifts in the intended stimulus are understood by the authors as a form of "resistance" to the treatment.)

What emerges from this inquiry is the information that the initiating scene presented by the therapist undergoes a series of transformations and elaborations which are under the control of the patient's internal, psychological processes. With this information in hand, it is not surprising, to a dynamically oriented therapist, to find that a wealth of dynamically rich and exciting material results from desensitizations obtained with Wolpe's method. For example, in one case, immediately upon conclusion of a desensitization series dealing with the patient's fears about the eventual death of his mother, he spontaneously reported:

> It was as if my feelings about my mother were transformed. Whenever I thought about her dying what I really felt was a fear of my being deserted by her. Now if I think of her dying I feel sorry for *her* [patient's emphasis]. For the first time I feel sorry for her instead of for myself.

Such a reminder of the fact that one is engaging processes of profound depth and complexity is hardly unique in the writer's experience. Opportunities for similar observations will probably present themselves to any behavior therapist who is willing to listen, and might be expected to serve as a caution against the simplistic view that only a stimulus-response connection is being affected by the therapy.

To note that the stimulus of record in this procedure is a self-produced visualization, and then to observe that the period in which the therapeutic effect is produced is characterized by a flow of images and symbolic materials, stretches the analogy to Wolpe's procedure with the cats rather thin. The grounding of behavior therapy in the history of the past decade of experimental psychology, which behavior therapists hope has elevated them above the analytic schools and made a science of therapy, is placed in jeopardy by this finding. I am not aware of the existence, in the literature of experimental psychology generated by learning theories, of anything more than an unpaid promissory note in regard to conceptualizations of this form of cognitive activity.

When one notes, in addition, that in this procedure an internally produced, imagined representation of a stimulus has a reality, in terms of its observable and specifiable behavioral consequences, equal to what one might expect of an externally produced stimulus, it is clear that the current conceptual horizons of S-R learning theories have been passed. What in fact seems to be demanded by these data is a conceptualization geared to understanding man as a cognitive being.

In all fairness to behavior therapists it should be noted that Wolpe has offered demonstrations of effectiveness for other procedures, including the vivo presentations of actual stimuli, based on his general principle of reciprocal inhibition, and using responses other than relaxation for the inhibition of anxiety. In addition, other behavior therapies have used therapeutic analogues which are, at least without closer scrutiny, better approximations of laboratory procedures with animals. The present critique, however is justified by the status of systematic desensitization therapy, and does not require modification if its applicability to behavior therapies is not universal. In other words, the writer is not willing to prejudge the question of whether a single set of processes is responsible for the successes reported by every therapeutic school.

Defense of Psychotherapy

Neither cognitive psychologists nor psychoanalysts have yet seized upon the data of systematic desensitization as providing an opportunity for theoretical growth. Nor have dynamically oriented therapists fulfilled their professional responsibility, which, or so it appears to me, requires the most careful investigation of a method which makes and supports claims to therapeutic efficacy. Here I am in full agreement with Eysenck (1960) when he says:

> . . . I have noted with some surprise that many psychotherapists have refused to use such methods [behavior therapies] . . . on *a priori* grounds, claiming that such mechanical methods simply could not work, and disregarding the large body of evidence available . . . only actual use can show the value of one method of treatment as opposed to another. (p. 14)

An attempt to weaken the claims of behavior therapists of the theoretical superiority of their position by a critical attack may be welcomed by analytically oriented psychologists but is not likely to prove constructive. It is, rather, necessary to turn attention to the attacks made upon psychotherapy and to seek out the legitimate sources of its defense. While this examination is cast in a theoretical context, it should be noted that there is also at issue, waiting offstage but providing a background of urgency, a question of therapeutic responsibility; that is, what degree of theoretical certainty justifies withholding an available therapeutic method from a client?

The Therapy-Theory Distinction

There are two issues, typically confounded in the literature, which need to be separated before an intelligible analysis can proceed. It is claimed by behavior therapists that the clinical successes of behavior therapy invalidate psychoanalysis. Statistics on rates of "cure" are adduced in support of the claim that behavior therapy is more effective than psychoanalysis. Whatever the persuasiveness of these statistics, final judgment is a complex matter. Definitions of therapeutic practice and diagnostic criteria remain inadequate. The uses of the word *cure* by behavior therapists and psychotherapists are often incommensurable. Regardless, however, of history's verdict on the value of psychoanalytic therapy as it is practiced today, the problem will remain that psychoanalysis as a theory requires evaluation by criteria different from those by which therapy is evaluated.

There appears in many places in the analytic literature the articulation of an awareness of Freud's intention to consider analytic theory and therapy as distinct endeavors. The metapsychology incorporates analytically derived data but goes, with full comprehension of this step, far beyond the data. On the other hand, the metapsychology requires, if it is to be properly implemented in practice, procedures which have not yet been invented. Thus Reich (1949) wrote:

> All problems of techniques converge in the one basic question whether and how an unequivocal technique of analytic therapy can be derived from the theory of the neuroses. . . . Ample experience[s] . . . have shown that we have hardly made a beginning at this task. (p. 3)

A responsible critique of psychoanalysis by behavior therapists would need to make this distinction clear. The adequate response from psychoanalysts would also make this distinction. If behavior therapy is indeed the more effective instrumentality, this fact should instigate a reexamination of the untapped technical resources of analytic theory. One cannot expect progress to follow from defensive denials.

The Problem of Symptom Substitution

On other fronts, genuinely theoretical attacks have been leveled at psychoanalysis. The most potent of these is the claim that, according to analytic theory, symptom substitution or recurrence *must* follow a course of treatment which removes a symptom by treating it directly, that is, without altering the underlying source of the symptom. In fact, analysts have tended to the belief that symptomatic treatment may be worse than no treatment at all, that is, that it may be dangerous. Both Eysenck and Wolpe have stated that psychoanalytic theory is decisively undermined by the failure of this prediction. The expectation of symptom substitution is a clinical prejudice of long standing, but the data seem to require a reevaluation.

Freud (1936) considered the possibility that a symptom may be a behaviorally fixed pattern which has inherited the total cathectic energy of the impulse which existed at its time of origin:

> . . . of the repressed instinctual impulse itself we assumed that it persisted unchanged for an indefinite period in the unconscious. Now our interest shifts to the fate of the repressed, and we begin to feel that this persistence, unchanged and unchanging, is not a matter of course, is perhaps not even the rule. . . . Do there therefore still exist the old desires, of the earlier existence of which analysis informs us? The answer appears obvious and certain. The old repressed desires must still persist in the unconscious, since we find their lineal descendents, the symptoms, still alive. *But this answer is inadequate*; it does not make it possible to distinguish between the two possibilities that, on the one hand, *the old desire now operates only through its descendents*, the symptoms, *to which it has transformed all its cathectic energy, or on the other hand, that the desire itself persists in addition*. . . . There is much in the phenomena of both the morbid and the normal life of the psyche which seems to demand the raising of such questions. In my study of the breakdown of the Oedipus complex, *I became mindful of the distinction between mere repression and the true disappearance of an old desire or impulse*. (p. 83; italics mine)

Successful symptomatic treatment may be taken as evidence for this second alternative, which might be extended and elaborated in ways entirely compatible with analytic theory.

On another level of analysis, Rapaport (1959) has noted that psychoanalysis is, essentially, a postdictive system. It can rationalize events after their occurrence but cannot predict these events. This assertion is, in part, based upon Freud's conception of the energetic relations between the systems of the psychic economy. The originally unitary nature of the psychic structure is conceived as remaining, in certain essential characteristics, unalterable. Thus the energetics of those psychic systems which emerge in the course of the development of personality remain highly interactive. This interactivity makes it extraordinarily difficult to predict the consequences of alterations of energy distributions in one psychic system upon the other systems. Is it possible, then, to state what follows of theoretical necessity from the removal of a symptom? Such an alteration of experience and behavior is, after all, likely to involve a not inconsiderable redistribution of cathectic processes. From this vantage it would appear that predictions of symptom substitution follow from a clinical rubric, and not with strict necessity from the analytic theory of the neuroses.

These considerations can be carried still further. Another line of analysis arises from the consequences of the thesis that the ego depends, for its development, on the greater efficiency of the secondary, as compared to the primary, process. That is, because the operations of the secondary process lead to increasing mastery of the relation of the psychic structure to object reality, exercise of the secondary process results in the binding of libidinal energies to the service of the emerging ego. Among the services to which energy is bound is that termed "repression." If one now considers the consequences for the ego, in its relations with object reality, of the removal of a symptom, the strands of the analysis come together. The removal of a symptom typically involves an increased mastery of object relations; for example, in the case of the person who is freed to express love or hostility, or the person who is able, for the first time in a decade, to climb a flight of stairs without trembling. Such increased mastery must lead to an increment in the bound energy available to ego functioning. Even if one must insist that the dynamic source of an original symptom formation remains unaffected by the removal of that symptom, the consideration that an increase in bound energy may well lead to an increase in the effectiveness of repressive cathexes should prohibit any *certain* prediction that symptom substitution must follow.

A final line of analysis of this problem is stimulated by a consideration of Freud's conception of symptoms in their relation to anxiety. It is useful to compare this conception with Wolpe's behavioristic formulation. Wolpe conceives of anxiety as *the neurosis*. As such, it is simply an acquired, that is, learned, maladaptive response. In this formulation anxiety is not given a functional role in the psychic system. Freud, on the other hand, envisions symptoms, that is, maladaptive responses, as means used by the ego to protect itself from danger. Anxiety, in this context, serves as a signal to the ego that a dangerous instinctual demand is growing in strength. In response to this impending danger a symptomatic action is engaged which binds a portion of the energy available to the instinctual demand. This binding reduces the imperiousness of the instinctual demand and permits the ego to avoid engaging it. Thus conceived, the symptom is a behavior substituted for the behavior demanded by the instinctual arousal. It is a maladaptive substitute because the danger to the ego, which may, at the time of symptom formation, have been actual, no longer exists. The ego never discovers that the danger is past because every arousal of the instinct produces a signal of anxiety, which in turn produces a discharge of the instinctual energy through the substitutive action, that is, the symptom. Of immediate relevance to the problem in hand is that in order to bind, successfully, the energy of the instinct, the substitute formation must bear a certain meaningful relation to the original object of the instinct. That is, the symptom formation is governed by the same principles which govern every displacement from an original instinctual object. This is another way of saying that the symptom must contain, in some measure, a symbolically adequate representation of the original object. Thus, for example, an external, phobic stimulus must symbolically represent the meaning of the internal danger.

This analysis leads to another formulation of the belief that symptom substitution must follow symptom removal, but also contains a suggestion of the possible error of this belief. If a symptom is removed, it is argued, the instinctual demand is unaltered, but now the ego has been deprived of its safety valve, that is, of its means of binding the instinctual energy. Without a means of discharge available the urgency of the impulse will increase, anxiety signals will come more and more frequently, and in the end the ego will either be inundated or a new substitute formation, that is, a new symptom, will appear to bind the energy which is pressing forward.

Among the many assumptions, both explicit and implicit, in the above argument, the postulated relation between an instinctual demand and its object underpins both psychoanalytic method and theory. Every displacement of cathexis from an existing object is determined by, and participates in, a system of associative and symbolic meaningfulness. It is this fact which permits the reading of dynamic messages in the overt behaviors of people. It is this premise which permits psychoanalytic theory a solution of the problem of joining an apparently limitless field of variations in human behavior to a limited number of motivational sources. Thus, when a therapist confronts a symptom as a substitute formation he is, by definition, confronting the inner dynamic as well, albeit at a remove. Insight is, after all, conceived as the grasping of this relationship in a particular instance. To speak analytically of treating a symptom is theoretically inexact, unless one envisions the psychic equivalent of a scalpel which can enter a body of tissue, excise a desired portion, and leave lower tissue layers unaffected.

The treatment of a symptom by the method of systematic desensitization has no sensible analogy to such an idealized surgical procedure. On the contrary, the entire ego system is engaged in an eidetic and introspective task. The patient confronts his fear and inhibits his flight reflex. His fear, then, decreases. This fact should not upset the analytic theorist. If, in treating a symptom, we are treating the symbolic carrier of a feared instinctual demand, it satisfies the "logic" of our understanding of unconscious processes to expect far-reaching effects. To the degree to which a substitute formation is an adequate binder of cathectic energy, we may expect that a reduction in the strength of the signal anxiety which sustains this formation will represent an increase in ego tolerance of the instinctual demand. Freedom from fear, theory leads us to expect, is characteristic of increased ego strength, and may signal the possibility of creating more adequate binding behaviors. Why then predict symptom substitution?

It would neither surprise nor distress the author if psychoanalytic theorists should find fault with the above arguments. If a critique leads to a more convincing and elegant penetration of the proper relationship between the data of behavior therapy and analytic theory, the intention of the present analysis will have been realized. What is of importance is that this relationship be examined. The considerations already outlined suggest the futility of the position taken by Wolpe and Eysenck. To maintain that the failure of symptom substitution to occur with any regularity following symptom removal by the interventions of behavioral therapists constitutes a decisive argument against the validity of psychoanalysis is to seriously underestimate its theoretical resources. Similarly, the unexamined prediction that symptom substitution must occur, as the grounds for a refusal by clinicians to give the use of the technique of systematic desensitization due consideration, must be rejected.

Some Interactions of Desensitization with Psychotherapy

The consequences, for a psychotherapist, of acknowledging the possible utility of systematic desensitization, bear illustration. One may tentatively accept the data which report the effectiveness of this technique and which deny contraindicating consequences. One may use the technique to give relief to one's patients. When the use of this technique is allowed, and when its implications are permitted to interact with an existing analytic, or other, orientation, possibilities occur which, while quite foreign to the behavior therapists, may lead to technical and theoretical growth.

For example, the occurrence of resistance in analytic work lends itself to an analysis which suggests the use of systematic desensitization. Resistance, in general, is assumed to occur when a train of associative production approaches forbidden unconscious material. This approach produces anxiety signals which excite the defenses of the ego and which lead to renewed efforts at repression of the material in question. What would follow if a patient were presented with the associative content which energizes repressive cathexes as a stimulus for desensitization?

In order to explore this question, two patients in analytic therapy were given brief training in the relaxation method (Jacobson, 1938) used in preparation for systematic desensitization. (The author is aware of the concern which many therapists will feel in regard to the effects of this procedure upon the transference. While this is a problem of great theoretical importance, an adequate treatment would require at least as much space as is taken by the present article.) When these patients reported dreams for which they were able to produce only sparse associative material, the systematic desensitization procedure was used. Specifically, the patient was asked to relax and was then asked to imagine either the last image of the dream, or another image in the dream which seemed particularly significant or disturbing to him. (The procedure may be described as a marriage of the methods of active imagination as developed by Jung, and systematic desensitization.) When a scene produced no further anxiety reaction, the patient was again asked for associations to the dream. On the 12 occasions (10 with one patient and two with the other) when this procedure was attempted, the outcome was the production of a flood of associative material. Both patients developed spontaneous interpretations of their dreams in the course of this process during six of the sessions in which the method was used. A control for this observation is suggested by a history of unsuccessful efforts by these patients to engage the images in their dreams by the method of active imagination prior to relaxation training. Other explorations suggest themselves, in abundance, upon consideration of the possibilities involved.

A promising area of research which has been opened in the literature is the application of systematic desensitization to the treatment of the psychosomatic complaints. Insofar as a conception is entertained in which the breakdown of an organ system is envisioned as a consequence of the repression of impulses to express significant affect, systematic desensitization offers the possibility of direct hypothesis testing. Among the most interesting desensitizations, from a dynamic point of view, are those which free a patient to express his feelings. For example, in two cases which the author has not yet reported in the literature, the desensitization of anxiety produced by impulses to express hostility led to the disappearance of migraine syndromes of extended duration. The time and energy which would be involved in a full-scale, controlled investigation of psychosomatic illness, using the method of systematic desensitization to test the hypothesis of its relation to affect suppression, seems to this writer a small price to pay for the potential gains in understanding and therapeutic power. Applications to general medicine may also be envisioned in areas in which psychosomatic effects are apparent, for example, the postulated relations between preoperative emotional stress and postoperative prognoses. What gains would there be in desensitizing a patient's unrealistic fears about his impending surgery?

An Empirical Critique of Systematic Desensitization and a New Method of Treatment

Dynamic points of view also suggest possible technical innovations in the desensitization procedure itself which are not likely to present themselves to a behavior therapist of a learning theory persuasion. One such suggestion arises from the ground-breaking investigations of Gendlin (1962) undertaken from his Rogerian orientation. Gendlin has described the consequences of attending to internal, felt body-states associated with affective arousal. It is his observation that the decision to remain verbally quiet and passive while directing attention to feelings in the body results in the experience of an increase in the richness and complexity of these feelings and a sequence of transformations of the felt "meaning" of the sensations. There is typically reported a brief, sharp rise in the intensity of the feeling, followed by a decline in the intensity as the associative richness connected with the feeling is directly experienced.

Explorations of Gendlin's procedure, both by this writer and in the reports of patients who were asked to observe themselves in this way, produced descriptions bearing a marked resemblance to the reports of content flow which were obtained from the investigations of imagining during systematic desensitization which were reported earlier in this paper. The possibility presented itself that during systematic desensitization visualizations, time limitations placed on the imagining of a given scene do not permit the patient's feeling to pass the peak of anxiety. It thus appeared possible that the necessity of multiple, hierarchical presentations was an artifact of the technique itself.

Four patients were involved in an investigation of this possibility. Each of two of the patients who were already being treated by systematic desensitization was given a new set of instructions. The patient was told to relax as usual and to imagine the scene presented by the therapist; but as soon as a feeling arose he was to direct his attention to the way his body felt. He was to focus attention on the strongest locus of feeling and to keep watching it no matter what distracting thoughts or images came to mind, and no matter how intense the feeling might become. The patient was presented with scenes from his prepared hierarchies. The first presentation to each patient was made at the beginning of a session in which a new hierarchy was scheduled for treatment, and consisted of the most intensely disturbing scene in that series. A single presentation was limited to 15 minutes. The therapist repeated, every minute, one or another paraphrase of the following: "Attend to the way you feel. Don't talk! Don't think! If thoughts come, let them pass through your mind. Don't attach yourself to them. Keep watching your feelings." Each session consisted of two such presentations followed by half an hour of discussion of the contents which had been experienced. Both of the patients reported intensifications of anxiety, floods of associations, changes in their understanding of what they were feeling, and, finally, complete disappearance of any affect they were willing to call anxiety in regard to the contents treated. (The interested reader is referred to Gendlin, since my description of the experienced process would add nothing to what he has already described in detail.) Both patients felt that, *in contrast to their experience with systematic desensitization*, they "made sense to themselves," felt good about themselves and "in touch with themselves" (cf. Gendlin, 1962) after each session. In addition, while the *effects* of desensitization were experienced as "real," the procedure seemed magical and mysterious. By contrast, in this new procedure, the patients felt that *they* had healed themselves.

Four such sessions were conducted with each patient. Each of the "Gendlin-like" sessions was followed by one session devoted to the standard systematic desensitization procedure in order to determine whether desensitization had, in fact, occurred. The first scene presented was, in each case, the same scene which had been treated by the "Gendlin-like" procedure. In the case of one of the patients, the systematic desensitization presentations of the scenes in *descending* hierarchical order produced no anxiety reactions whatever. In vivo behavior gave strong evidence that desensitization had taken place. In the case of the other patient, two of the four hierarchies followed the above pattern. The other two hierarchies showed an anxiety residue, although the patient felt that the anxiety was considerably less than he had anticipated when preparing the hierarchies. For each of these hierarchies, a second "Gendlin" session produced apparently complete desensitization.

Two additional patients were treated by the "Gendlin" procedure. In both cases the treatment was begun without prior relaxation training and, consequently, without experience of systematic desensitization. Each of these patients went through a standardized series of diagnostic sessions used in cases intended for treatment by systematic desensitization, which included the preparation of anxiety hierarchies. At the beginning of the first treatment session the patient was instructed to relax as well as he could and to attend to the way his body felt, that is, sensations of his clothing on his body, the chair against his back, the feeling in his "gut," etc. He was then given the instructions which have been described above and was presented with the most intense scene of his lowest hierarchy. One patient was flooded with anxiety and could not bear to continue on this first and two subsequent attempts. The procedure was, therefore, temporarily abandoned. The results with the second patient were identical with those which have been described for patients experienced with systematic desensitization. In this case, however, the "Gendlin sessions" were not alternated with systematic desensitization sessions. The evidence that desensitization occurred is, therefore, confined to self-reports and in vivo behavioral evidence.

The patient with whom the procedure had failed was subsequently trained in relaxation. Treatment by the "Gendlin procedure" was then resumed and, on this attempt, replicated the three cases which have been described. Relaxation training seemed to have had a striking effect. On the occasions of the initial attempts the patient reported poor visualization of the scenes described to him by the therapist. After relaxation training visualizations were vivid and feelings during sessions were sharp and distinct. The patient reported the, to him, fascinating observation that, while the anxiety was as strong during sessions following relaxation training as he remembered it having been before, he felt more in touch with his body and better able to tolerate the feeling. Relaxation training of the Jacobsen type may prove to be a means of bringing patients into contact with their internal processes. Rather than fostering repression under the guise of relaxation, as one analyst has expressed his concern (Hillman, 1960), relaxation training may tend to induce an increased receptivity to unconscious contents.

It hardly seems necessary to point out the urgency of attempts to replicate these findings. These results, should they prove replicable, suggest that the use of intensity gradients and other means of controlling anxiety arousal may be unncessary for desensitization, and call into question a crucial procedural and theoretical emphasis in systematic desensitization. Wolpe came upon this treatment procedure, in part, by analogy to his successful desensitization of conditioned phobic reactions in cats. It does not detract from the impressiveness of the successes this analogy has generated in the treatment of human subjects to suggest a modification and indeed a radical revision of his method. It may be that with human subjects a method which encourages an engagement of the dynamics of the anxiety reaction with a subject's cognitive processes will also produce desensitization.

In spite of the very preliminary nature of the data which have been described, they would seem to offer reason for optimism. Attempts to produce confrontations of the data and method of systematic desensitization with other perspectives and frames of reference may prove to be a source of enrichment of therapeutic practice and theory.

ANALYTIC INTERPRETATIONS OF BEHAVIOR THERAPY

Earlier in this discussion a challenge was made of Eysenck's assertion that the effects of psychotherapy can be understood in terms of principles derived from "learning theory." It remains, for the purposes of this paper, to show that the effects of behavior therapy (systematic desensitization) can be understood in terms of principles derived from analytic theories. In other words, it seems desirable to offer a preliminary demonstration that confrontations of analytic theories with the method of systematic desensitization may be undertaken with some degree of plausibility on theoretical grounds. In what follows an attempt will be made to show that psychotherapists can derive, from their theoretical perspective, means of understanding the effects of the technique of systematic desensitization. That is, some of the resources of analytic theories will be tapped in an effort to frame interpretations of the way in which the specific therapeutic interventions of this form of behavior therapy produce their effects. These interpretations should *not* do violence to dynamic points of view, and *should* lead to a rational expectation that desirable results will follow.

A Psychoanalytic Interpretation of Systematic Desensitization

A number of suggestions have already been made, for example, in the discussion of symptom substitution, which could lead to a rational derivation of the effects of systematic desensitization by psychoanalytic theory. There are, however, in the body of Freud's writings a number of formulations which lend themselves even more precisely to this purpose. For example, Freud (1936) considers that an analysis of anxiety yields three attributes: "(1) a specific unpleasurable quality, (2) efferent or discharge phenomena, and (3) the perception of these" (p. 70). This is true for symptomatic anxiety as well as for signal anxiety which leads to a mobilization of ego defenses and symptom formation. Were it possible to confront the ego with impulses which generate the signals of anxiety, by, for example, asking the patient to imagine himself engaged in the expression of an impulse from which he normally flees, and, were it possible, at the same time, to prevent or inhibit the occurrence of anxiety signals by, for example, inducing deep relaxation and raising the threshold of the discharge phenomena, reality-oriented binding of cathexes might be expected to follow. While aware of the oversimplifications in this analysis, the writer fails to see any urgent reason why the suggestions which it makes available should not be explored by the technique of systematic desensitization.

An Interpretation by Complex Psychology of Systematic Desensitization

Within the writings of Jung, as well, is contained abundant conceptual material for analyses similar to that which has been outlined for Freud. Strikingly suggestive parallels may be found in Jung's (1960) monograph on paranoid dementia. The terms of definition of the complex theory as they are presented in that paper lend themselves to our present purpose.

The psyche is conceived as consisting, in part, of an indefinite number of clusters of relatively autonomous associative complexes. Each complex is organized around an emotionally toned content which draws to it materials bearing similarities of meaning and materials which occur as stimulus input during periods of time in which that particular complex is behaviorally dominant. In ordinary circumstances the complex of greatest strength, stability, and clarity is called the "ego." The ego depends, for its stability, on the fact that it includes in its associative cluster the range of proprioceptive stimulation produced by normal bodily tone. Most stimuli which occur in the presence of this normal proprioceptive state are drawn into association with the ego complex and share its clarity and stability. When a stimulus, by its associative properties, excites a complex other than the ego, it also excites an alteration in body tone. This altered body tone is part of the ego-alien complex, and induces an alteration of proprioception. It is in such altered states of proprioception that we have emotions. The emotional state is characterized by a weakening to the ego complex, that is, a loss of its usual behavioral dominance, and a change of consciousness best described as a loss of apperceptive clarity. (For an extended theoretical discussion of the far-reaching conclusions as to the nature of consciousness to which Jung was led by these germinal considerations, the reader is referred to Jung, 1954.)

It seems to follow that if a content which ordinarily disturbs the ego complex could be made to occur without producing an alteration in proprioception, that is, without an emotional excitement, the consequence should be an integration of this content to the ego complex. The therapeutic gains would be considerable. If systematic desensitization produces effects which can be understood in this way, many interesting avenues of exploration will be opened to Jungian theorists.

An Interpretation of Systematic Desensitization from the Viewpoint of Interpersonal Psychiatry

From the vantage point of interpersonal psychiatry a relatively straightforward interpretation can be formulated. Anxiety, in Sullivanian thinking, has a clearly articulated function in determining personality structure. Anxiety generates and is involved in maintaining a set of defensive processes, primary among which is the "self." Insofar as the habitual responses of the self are designed to avoid anxiety, they tend to have the character of parataxic thinking, that is, thought processes in which association by contiguity rather than connection by rational structure is the guiding principle. An adult who is capable of syntactic or rational thought may, nonetheless, exhibit parataxic habits in the presence of anxiety. Anxiety typically produces this weakening of rational processes. While this set of concepts is already suggestive in the present context, its relationship to systematic desensitization is clarified by a further consideration. Sullivan (1940) supposed that the necessary precondition for emotional states is an increase in skeletal-muscular tension. This increase in tension, when it passes a threshold value, produces that clouding of consciousness which, when we perceive it, we call anxiety. It is this clouding of consciousness which results in the failure of rational thought mentioned above.

It follows that if the adequate stimulus for an increase in skeletal-muscular tension could be presented in such a fashion as to limit, or avoid, the increase in tension which is ordinarily contingent upon it, a clouding of consciousness might be avoided. The stimulus in question should, in these circumstances, come under the scrutiny of the syntactic process and might be expected to undergo rational integration. Systematic desensitization is "tailor-made" for testing this hypothesis, which should it be validated, provides a possible rationale for the use of this technique by analysts of the interpersonal school.

An Interpretation of Desensitization Therapy by Decision Theory

Psychotherapists who are oriented toward decision-making models of cognitive functioning, and who prefer to avoid dynamic formulations of the analytic variety, should also find little difficulty in rationalizing the use of systematic desensitization. A single example, very loosely based upon the theory of signal detection and focused on the anxiety hysteric, will serve to illustrate this contention. (Another approach, from the point of view of "cognitive" learning theory, is outlined by Breger and McGaugh, 1965.)

Anxiety may be conceived as the adequate stimulus for an avoidance or flight response (signal anxiety in the Freudian sense). Anxiety thus reflects an organization of the utilities matrix which controls the decision-making process by which responses to certain stimulus classes are selected. Existing utilities may require that a stimulus class which has the demonstrated power of evoking the anxiety signal be avoided, so that no signal is generated. The situation will now be such that for a given class of stimuli, the threshold of the avoidance response has been lowered. In order to insure a high percentage of successes in the avoidance of danger the person is willing to make avoidance responses to a range of contents which include many innocuous stimuli. At the same time, avoidance of the anxiety signal will require that avoidance responses be initiated at the first signs of such proprioceptive alterations as might imply possible anxiety. Given a base level of proprioceptive stimuli which are not perceptually articulate, any given increase (as determined by the utilities) in the intensity of proprioceptive feedback, such as that produced by increased skeletal-muscular tension, may be an anxiety signal. We thus have a person who responds as if there were reason to be anxious to a wide range of stimuli, both external and proprioceptive. We say that such a person has unadaptive anxiety. If, in the therapeutic setting, we alter the a priori possibilities of stimulus input by decreasing the intensity of proprioceptive feedback, we decrease the "false alarm" rate and raise the threshold of avoidance responses to signals of anxiety. This can be accomplished by inducing a state of skeletal-muscular relaxation. If, at the same time, we decrease the chaos of perceptual inputs by directing a patient to close his eyes and, further, by asking that he produce a vivid visualization of particular stimuli, we once again reduce the a priori possibilities of "false alarms." The experience of specific stimuli which have, in the past, been the occasion for anxiety signals, in the presence of reduced intensity of proprioceptive feedback, might be expected to produce "therapeutic" alternations of utilities matrices. The task of rationalizing the effects of systematic desensitization should not present formidable difficulties for other cognitive theories.

CONCLUSION

This paper has attempted a form of relatively systematic desensitization, in regard to the use of a therapeutic technique, upon the dynamically oriented clinical-academic community. It must, however, be noted that many objections to the use of systematic desensitization which may be raised on analytic grounds have only been lightly touched upon in this paper, or not mentioned at all. The interpretation of the transference relationship, to select only one example, will require a formidable theoretical effort. It would miss the point, quite decisively, to proceed as if no problems remained.

On the other hand, exploratory arguments have been drawn with the intent of persuading psychotherapists of the urgency of examining the grounds of their resistance to the use of systematic desensitization and of reevaluating the theoretical necessity of these grounds. The primary motivation of this attempt is the conviction of the writer (qualified by the obvious need for better controls and further investigation) that systematic desensitization works, that is, that it produces behavioral change, reliably, sometimes dramatically, and therapeutically. Within the areas to which it has been applied it has demonstrated impressive effectiveness. It remains to determine the best theoretical formulation of the processes involved in producing its effects. The limit of its applicability and the best form for its application are empirical questions. However, as a source of data and as a source of therapeutic power, it demands exploitation.

The question of the form this exploitation *should* take has led to the theoretical exercises in this paper, and to the empirical investigations described. What shall be the field of investigation, and the theoretical attitude with which this tool will be applied? The stakes seem too high to settle for a battle between behavior therapists and psychoanalysts. That there is danger of this happening has been pointed out by Andrews (1966) in his appeal for more open scientific communication. Everyone, including the patient, is likely to lose in such warfare. There is room for each persuasion to increase its technical and theoretical sophistication. Preliminary considerations have been presented with the intention of demonstrating that proprietary rights to this technique cannot be established on theoretical grounds. In other words, there is nothing to fear, in the technique or in the data it generates, for psychoanalytic or cognitive theorists, provided they actively engage the problem. There is no reason to fear that the engagement will force them to "throw the psyche out of psychology." There is reason to think they may emerge from the combat with new strength. Freud (1936) put the alternative succinctly: "When the wayfarer whistles in the dark, he may be disavowing his timidity, but he does not see any the more clearly for doing so" (p. 23). There are theoretical grounds for the use of systematic desensitization, for hypothesis generation, and for experimental tests of its consequences from a variety of points of view.

So long as the relationship of theory to its data is sufficiently loose that logical arguments can take precedence over empirical arguments, and empirical decisions seem out of reach, we can, perhaps, justify uncritical loyalty to our preconceptions. When, however, a means presents itself of bringing our therapeutic concepts to an empirical confrontation we are obligated to do so. None of us can assume that we possess enough foresight to envision the theoretical consequences, the model of man which the data will require. Perhaps it helps to remember the words of the prophet, that the better is always the enemy of the good, and that the good must give way if the better is to be. In any case, whatever the outcome, to collect the data and to construct the model seem to this author to be our professional obligation.

REFERENCES

Andrews, J. D. W. Psychotherapy of phobias. *Psychological Bulletin*, 1966, *66*, 455-480.

Breger, L., and McGaugh, J. L. Critique and reformulation of "learning theory" approaches to psychotherapy and neurosis. *Psychological Bulletin*, 1965, *63*, 338-358. [See also Chapter 4, this volume.]

Estes, W. K., Koch, S., MacCorquodale, K., Meehl, P. E., Mueller, C. G., Jr., Schoenfeld, W. N., and Verplanck, W. S. *Modern Learning Theory*. New York: Appleton-Century-Crofts, 1954.

Eysenck, H. J. *The Dynamics of Anxiety and Hysteria*. New York: Praeger, 1957.

Eysenck, H. J. (Ed.), *Behavior Therapy and the Neurosis*. New York: Pergamon Press, 1960.

Freud, S. *The Problem of Anxiety*. New York: Norton, 1936.

Gendlin, E. T. *Experiencing and the Creation of Meaning*. New York: Free Press of Glencoe, 1962.

Grossberg, J. M. Behavior therapy: A review. *Psychological Bulletin*, 1964, 62, 73-88.

Hillman, J. *Emotion*. London: Routledge and Kegan Paul, 1960.

Jacobson, E. *Progressive Relaxation*. Chicago: University of Chicago Press, 1938.

Jung, C. G. The spirit of psychology. In J. Campbell (Ed.), *Spirit and Nature*. New York: Pantheon, 1954. Pp. 371-444.

Jung, C. G. *The Archetypes and the Collective Unconscious*. New York: Pantheon, 1959.

Jung, C. G. *The Psychogenesis of Mental Disease*. New York: Pantheon, 1960.

Masserman, J. H. *Behavior and Neurosis*. Chicago: University of Chicago Press, 1943.

Rapaport, D. The structure of psychoanalytic theory: A systematizing attempt. In S. Koch (Ed.), *Psychology: A Study of a Science*. Vol. 1. New York: McGraw-Hill, 1959. Pp. 55-183.

Reich, W. *Character-Analysis*. New York: Noonday, 1949.

Sullivan, H. S. *Conceptions of Modern Psychiatry*. New York: Norton, 1940.

Weinberg, N. H., and Zaslove, M. "Resistance" to systematic desensitization of phobias. *Journal of Clinical Psychology*, 1963, 19, 179-181.

Wolpe, J. *Psychotherapy by Reciprocal Inhibition*. Stanford: Stanford University Press, 1958.

Wolpe, J. The experimental foundations of some new psychotherapeutic methods. In A. J. Bachrach (Ed.), *Experimental Foundations of Clinical Psychology*. New York: Basic Books, 1962. Pp. 554-575.

Learning Theory and Psychoanalysis

EUGENE WOLF, M.D., D.P.M., F.R.C. PSYCH.

In this eloquent and persuasive paper, Wolf explicates the differences between the classical conditioning theory of Pavlov and the operant conditioning concepts of Skinner, and their applications to psychodynamic theory and practice. He makes the telling point that for many people the traumatic life situations into which they are inextricably bound renders them just as immobilized, for all practical purposes, as dogs in a Pavlovian frame, and that this may explain why, like Pavlov's dogs, they persist in their neurotic responses despite the fact that these responses are maladaptive. He suggests that transference and countertransference reactions can be seen as learned responses based on earlier stimuli, which then become generalized to similar ones in later life. He then comes to a formulation, essentially similar to Alexander's concept of the corrective emotional experience, that stresses the therapist's capacity to respond differently to the patient from the way previous human figures have done. Like Alexander and Marmor in the previous two papers, he stresses the mutual benefit that both psychoanalytic and behavioral psychiatrists can derive from an integration of both models.

Learning Theory and Psychoanalysis

Eugene Wolf, M.D., D.P.M., F.R.C. Psych.

At a time when cybernetics has come to relate the behavior of man to that of lifeless machines, we cannot possibly turn our backs on the model of something as close to man as is another mammal. The animal model is, however, a potentially double-edged weapon. It can be a blessing to the extent to which we succeed in establishing all that man and animal have in common, but it can also prove to be a hindrance to the extent to which we fail to establish the relevant features in which the two differ at the same time.

Persistence of Maladaptive Behavior

It is a characteristic feature of ontogenetic and even of phylogenetic learning that responses, or systems of responses, which are no longer adaptive and enhancing the needs of the organism tend to be shed and discarded. In the absence of constancy of living conditions, the maintenance of life of individuals as well as species is dependent on their flexible adaptivity, which consists as much in their capacity to extinguish and abandon patterns of behavior that are no longer appropriate to the changed conditions, as in their capacity to acquire and retain new appropriate ones. All this is in full keeping with the reward-punishment model of learning: adaptive behavior being reinforced by its own rewarding outcome is retained, whereas unadaptive behavior which cannot be reinforced by its own harmful outcome is cast off and extinguished.

In applying this "instrumental" ("operant") model of learning to human psychopathology, we come up against the disconcerting paradox that maladaptive patterns in man, once acquired, may be retained for years in spite of their repeatedly *unrewarding and even incapacitating out-*

Reprinted from *British Journal of Medical Psychology,* 39:1-10, 1966, by permission of Cambridge University Press.

come. Learning theorists have put forward a number of attempts to explain this contradiction. One way of accounting for the persistence of a pathological pattern, such as a phobia, is that it is essentially an avoidance response to a feared stimulus or situation. Even though it is not appropriate or no longer appropriate, by avoiding the stimulus the organism deprives itself also of further opportunities to unlearn what may be, or may have already become, an inappropriate response (Eysenck, 1960). But if avoidance behavior is designed to avoid suffering, how can this apply to mental patients? Is a psychogenic disorder designed to avoid suffering, or is it suffering itself? If the disorder really protects the patient from suffering, why call any kind of procedure that deprives him of such protection "therapeutic"?

In the avoidance hypothesis the persistence of the morbid pattern is ascribed to absence of reexposure, i.e., absent opportunities not only for further reinforcements but also for extinction through nonreinforcement. A more commonly put forward explanation is that maladaptive patterns persist because they *are* being constantly reinforced by their own rewarding outcomes. The reinforcing reward may be a negative one, such as repeatedly experienced relief from fear, but the rewarding outcome may also be a positively pleasurable one. But in either case is this not a contradiction in terms? Why call a pattern that is rewarding to the organism "maladaptive"? And why cure patients of patterns that are beneficial to them?

All forms of mental and bodily sickness may be to some extent compensated for by the various allowances made by society for the temporarily or permanently disabled. It is also an indisputable clinical fact that under certain circumstances a psychogenic illness may prove to be the lesser of two or more alternative evils available to the patient. But by being a lesser evil, *illness as a whole never ceases to be an evil* in its consequences for the patient. Whatever the secondary and partial gains accruing from illness may be, it would be scientifically untenable to argue that mental ill-health, with the concomitant suffering and limitations to effective living, can ever *outweigh motivationally* mental health in the *totality* of satisfactions. If this were the case, patients would never ask to be relieved of their illness and it would become altogether debatable how far pathological behavior is at all maladaptive.

From the point of view of learning and motivation, what else can the rationale underlying "aversion therapy" imply but that the illness to be erased by it is either pleasurable to the patient, or at least less unpleasurable than is a series of induced vomiting or some other disagreeable procedure? Treatment by punishment is, of course, no novelty in the history of our discipline. Though in former ages it was not meted out with methodological precision, some may think that the demonological rationale was perhaps more logical.

INSTRUMENTAL AND CLASSICAL MODELS OF LEARNING

Hull (1943) does not distinguish between "classical" and "instrumental" conditioning as being two essentially different modes of learning. Though he utilizes classical Pavlovian concepts, his monistic single-factor theory is in fact built up on the Thorndikean reward-punishment model of behavior. Unlike Hull, Skinner (1938) is theoretically more consistent, in that he admits at least in principle the existence of classical as distinct from instrumental conditioning, and even gives it the separate term of *respondent* behavior to distinguish it from the *operant* variety. However, Skinner presents his two-factor view of learning rather by way of introduction, whereas in his actual work he has concerned himself with the operant variety of learning. An outspoken two-factor theorist has been Mowrer (1953), but his contributions are not directly relevant to the present discussion.

There can be no doubt that classical and instrumental conditioning have numerous features in common. In the case of *rewarding* outcomes that follow a particular response, it is extremely hard to say whether there is any essentially different principle involved. Whether the attainment of food following a particular response by an *unimmobilized* animal in a maze is the rewarding outcome of its *own behavior*, or whether the attainment of such food following the salivary response by an *immobilized* animal in a Pavlovian frame is the rewarding outcome of the *experimenter's behavior*, may, indeed, be no more than a difference in experimental technique, but not in the learning process itself.

There is, however, a fundamental difference between the two varieties of learning when a particular response is followed not by reward, but by *punishment*. In the case of a mobile animal opportunities to repeat a particular punishment are restricted, for the simple reason that further approach responses are inhibited and replaced by a defensive avoidance response. In Hullian theory it is not the punishment that reinforces the avoidance response, but the rewarding relief from pain, or even from fear of such pain. In the instrumental model of learning only rewards can act as a reinforcer of behavior: it cannot reinforce approach responses, it can only inhibit them; nor can punishment reinforce avoidance responses which are designed precisely to avoid its further repetition. In Hullian theory punishment cannot function as a reinforcer because it possesses no need-reducing or drive-reducing property.

Punishment, however, does have a reinforcing capacity in the classical model of the immobilized animal. An experimental animal can effectively avoid a traumatic stimulus or situation only if it is free to move about in space, as is the case in the instrumental variety of learning. Liddell (1944), for instance, placed his experimental goat in a Pavlovian frame with loops under its limbs to prevent locomotion and with electrodes attached to one of its forelegs. Following the clicking of a telegraph sounder, Liddell continued to apply electric shocks to the foreleg until the goat was trained to produce the defensive flexion of the foreleg to the mere acoustic stimulus. In this case the *punishing unconditioned stimulus* itself was the *repeatedly administrable reinforcer* of the acquired response to the conditioned acoustic stimulus. This model of learning can, of course, only apply if the organism has no option of escaping from the traumatic situation.

True, our human patients are not tied up in Pavlovian frames, but is this at all relevant? After all, they do not move about in mazes or Skinner boxes either. What is crucial, surely, is whether a patient can or cannot escape from his traumatic life situation. Is it so simple even for a physically or mentally flogged child to run away and keep away from its mother for good? Is it at all easy for a human adult to escape from a distressing marital or employment situation, even if the distress imported into such a relationship of dependence is largely or entirely of his own making? For if his life situation is in fact inescapable, and the learning model that applies to his illness is the classical one, then it is not at all paradoxical that his illness should persist "despite" the repeatedly punishing outcome of his maladaptive behavior. In such a case the repeated punishments themselves would constitute the reinforcing and perpetuating factors of his disorder. And conversely, if psychogenic disorders were governed by the principles of the operant model of learning, the maladaptive patterns would, as a result of their own disabling consequences, be self-obliterating, and there would be in this world no need or place for either psychotherapists or behavior therapists.

METHODOLOGICAL ISSUES

Psychodynamics cannot afford for long to ignore the gravity of the methodological challenge, nor does it have to concede that the value of an investigation lies in its formalistic perfections, and not in its contribution to the understanding and alleviation of mental ill-health. *It is not at all unscientific if in their choice of data to be investigated clinical workers are not guided by the best available method, but if, instead, in their choice of the best available method they are guided by such understanding of the issues involved as has emerged from the pooled experience of generations of practitioners to be relevant to the disorders they are concerned with.*

There are grounds to believe that whatever the theoretical banner under which a therapeutic procedure is carried out and whatever the rituals employed in the course of it, what really matters is not what the therapist *subjectively* thinks he does to the patient, but what, directly or indirectly, consciously or unconsciously, he does to the patient *in fact*. Yet in recent years some behaviorists have confined their scientific misgivings to such therapeutic procedures as have been traditionally referred to under the general term of psychotherapy (Eysenck, 1965). As far as their demand is concerned that the therapeutic process be stripped of all artistic status and be placed on a scientific footing instead, it is a welcome challenge to the conceptual looseness and complacency of some psychotherapists, and deserves unqualified support.

Until such time as the hypothesis that the stimuli that are ever operative in the learning and unlearning of psychogenic disorders are social ones is adequately confirmed by stringent methods of verification, there is admittedly room left for disagreements. But if, by way of contrast, the scientific weight claimed for behavior therapy hypotheses is to be conceded, clear evidence is required to show that the *social stimuli*, considered by many as paramount determinants of human behavior, were an *adequately controlled variable* in their own investigations and therapies. The work of Crisp (1964) carried out in collaboration with V. Meyer is a pioneering attempt to bring under control the social variable which the *impact of the behavior therapist* on the patient constitutes. Until such time as this crucial control is satisfactorily established, behavior therapy can claim to excel psychotherapy in hardly more than the appearance of a scientifically validated theory.

The Validation of Psychoanalytic Hypotheses

Although current psychodynamic theories are by now fairly saturated with clinically significant hypotheses, it has not been possible to test them in their original form by more rigorous quantitative methods because of their very conceptual framework. Freud was not, and could not have been, a behaviorist, and psychoanalytic theory is couched in the language of traditional subjective psychology. However, behaviorists have by no means discarded all contributions made by their predecessors or even by contemporary nonbehaviorists. For what was characterized of the transformation of traditional academic psychology into a behavioral science was not so much discovery of fundamentally new facts as the development of a fundamentally *new approach* to the same psychological phenomena and processes. Although behaviorism grew almost concurrently with psychoanalysis, the two disciplines have developed for several decades in virtual isolation from each other. Especially since the last war, however, there has been among psychoanalytically oriented workers a growing awareness that the behavioral approach, with its experimental and methodological advantages, is destined to open new insights into psychopathology.

Early attempts by Luria (1932) or Sears (1944) to verify experimentally psychoanalytic concepts in their original form encountered serious methodological difficulties. However, the growth of behaviorist psychology has stimulated a number of leading clinicians and learning theorists to relate psychodynamics to *maladaptive behavior* (Alexander, 1946; Masserman, 1946; Mowrer, 1953; Dollard and Miller, 1950; Cameron and Magaret, 1951; Leary, 1957; Rotter, 1954). Their attempts have proved successful to the extent to which psychodynamics was not merely "translated" into the language of learning theory, but actually *integrated* with it.

It is a known fact that psychoanalysis operates with terms, and refers to psychological phenomena, which are all too often unobservable and operationally undefinable. Moreover, its hypotheses are not sufficiently explicit to preclude ambiguity; nor can many of them be considered definitive and final, if for no other reason than that they are still controversial. It can be meaningful to formulate in behavioral terms only those psychodynamic principles which are more or less generally accepted by most writers and workers of psychoanalytic derivation.

A PSYCHODYNAMIC MODEL OF LEARNING

The psychodynamic model of learning presented in this discussion leans in its general outlines on Sullivan's (1955) interpersonal theory of psychopathology, on Alexander's (1946) formulation of the transference in terms of generalization and on his concept of the "corrective emotional experience" to which the patient is exposed in the therapeutic relationship, and on Masserman's (1946) concept of conflict behavior.

In the model put forward here it is assumed that underlying the mental and bodily symptomatology of a psychogenic disorder is a breakdown in adaptive *interpersonal behavior*. An individual's characteristic patterns of behavior to other people, as much as to objects, are learned principally during the formative years of childhood in the course of interactions with significant members of the nuclear family. The interpersonal patterns thus acquired are, with greater or lesser modifications, transferred by way of social generalization into relationships with comparable, equivalent, or derivative human figures. Maladaptive patterns acquired in earlier traumatic relationships may continue manifestly into adulthood in the form of personality anomalies, or may, in the course of subsequent corrective experiences, undergo repair. Such repair may be from a clinical point of view more or less complete or only superficial and tenuous. A precariously integrated system of interpersonal behavior constitutes a latently predisposed personality structure that may break down and decompensate under precipitating stress in later life, and the individual may, as a result, revert (regress) to earlier patterns of immature behavior.

The survival and persistence of typical interpersonal patterns and their carry-over into successive relationships of the same category (intimacy, authority, peers) is the recurrent theme of psychiatric case histories, and has been referred to by Freud under such terms as *repetition-compulsion* or *neurosis of destiny*. Pathological patterns of interpersonal behavior are maladaptive to the extent to which they come to be transferred rigidly into new relationships which are only similar but in which they are *no longer appropriate*. The morbidly *extended gradient of social generalization*, whereby patterns of behavior are prcmptly and indiscriminately elicited in the patient by human figures only remotely resembling earlier ones, is a measure of the severity of the traumatic interpersonal experiences to which he was previously exposed and in the course of which the patterns were originally acquired. That the gradient of stimulus generalization is a function of the severity of the previous trauma has been experimentally demonstrated in both animal and man (Hilgard and Marquis, 1961), and its primary function is apparently defensive. The greater the risk to the organism, the more widespread are the precautions taken against the danger of repetition: as if the organism were "once bitten—twice shy" not only with identical stimuli, but also with *similar stimuli*. Pathological social generalization by a child or adult, affecting certain interpersonal relationships, may be thought of in psychological terms as a form of impelling "prejudice" against human figures of a certain category. Patterns of response acquired in relation to an excessively authoritarian father, for instance, are maladaptive when they are compulsively and indiscriminately elicited by other subsequent figures in authority, irrespective of how closely the new figures resemble the father's own personality in fact. Patterns of this sort, when displayed by the patient toward the therapist, Freud called "transference."

From his first observations of transference phenomena in the early nineties of the last century, it took Freud (1964*a*) nearly twenty years to discover and describe the " 'countertransference' which arises in the physician as a result of the patient's influence," requiring him to recognize it in himself and to overcome it if the patient is to be changed at all. According to Freud (1964*b*): "It must not be supposed, however, that the transference is created by analysis and does not occur apart from it. Transference is merely uncovered and isolated by analysis. It is a universal phenomenon . . . and in fact dominates the whole of each person's relations to his human environment." This universality of the transference he was able to establish from his patients' own accounts of their repetitive life stories. However, the phenomenon of the countertransference he was only able to identify in himself, for the simple reason that the therapeutic situation was his only available opportunity to investigate *both ends* of a relationship of the patient. Had the rules of psychoanalytic technique not precluded Freud's access to independent environmental data, it would not have taken him long to note that the countertransference was no less ubiquitous than the transference itself. Countertransferences roused by the individual in the lay environment tend to be equally spontaneous and ununderstood, and to have no modifying impact on the transferential patterns. Lay countertransferences are of no theoretical or practical consequence as far as the psychoanalytic model itself is concerned, but in the model of psychodynamic learning submitted in this discussion it constitutes an indispensable link of interaction and interpersonal feedback.

PERSISTENCE OF INTERPERSONAL PATTERNS

With the exception of early life, no new human relationship is ever initiated at the moment of encounter right from scratch. Into newly opened relationships man always carries over experiences and modes of conduct acquired in previous similar relationships, and this represents his own share in the common undertaking. We could never benefit from previous life experiences if we did not ubiquitously indulge in a normal degree of interpersonal generalization. Even when a patient comes to see us for the first time his initial behavior is less determined by our own conduct than by that of our colleagues whom he had seen before us. If *they* happened to be unduly impatient with him, we should not be surprised to find him distrustful and unconfiding with us too. Since the examination of an uncommunicative patient, especially when the available time is limited, may be a severe test of endurance even for a trained psychiatrist, we should not be surprised if our oversensitive patient does not fail to note *our* inner sighs of despair also. This will naturally only comfirm his preconceived assumption that we and our colleagues are much the same kind of people. Having thus failed our patient's test means, unfortunately, that we too have, in our turn, succeeded in perpetuating his uncommunicativeness. What is more, our own responses have, at the same time, predetermined the despair of the psychiatrist who is destined to examine him after us. If we may find a patient to be rather exasperating in one single interview, how much nonreinforcing tolerance can be expected from lay associates who work or even live with him day in and day out?

If a hysterical, psychopathic, or paranoid patient is today still like he was yesterday, this is due to the fact that once again he has succeeded in compelling his environment to "repay him in kind." If the environment is mentally "normal" in that it responds *appropriately*, once again it will drive him hysterical, psychopathic, or paranoid, as the case may be. It is extremely difficult even to refrain from the patronizing responses which the emotionally immature and dependent patient is consistently drawing from his environment. The element of reinforcing condescension usually implicit in such protective responses will, of course, only continue to bar him from rising to maturity and independence.

Relatives and associates will readily provide us with vivid accounts of how very difficult and trying it is to respond to a patient differently from what is appropriate to his own conduct. And this is precisely what we are supposed to do in psychotherapy: unlike the natural environment of the patient we are to behave and respond *inappropriately* and, therefore, "abnormally." Ours is the arduous task of behaving and responding to the patient not according to what he actually is, but what he is not, that is to say, according to what we would like him to be. For as long as the surrounding world of the functional psychotic continues to treat him as a madman, psychotic is he doomed to remain. The same, of course, goes not only for antisocial criminals and neurotics, but for all of us. We all persist in being whatever we are as a result of the fact that we continually succeed in compelling our environments to respond to each one of us in the very particular way in which they actually do.

It is a measure of Freud's genius to have discovered that the extent to which we can at all prove helpful to a patient is a function of our capacity to control our own responses to him. We are often unaware of subtle metacommunications whereby we give away to our patients the reactions which they compulsively rouse in us. Parents, even if they know that they should strive to behave to their disturbed child not according to what he actually is, but according to what they would like him to be, find it very difficult to observe this rule consistently. Yet this, fortunately, is only a general tendency, not a rigid law. We are all familiar with the abrupt and sometimes dramatic changes that may take place in the attitude of the environment to a person who has suffered a breakdown. The homeostatic effect of the various allowances made by the human environment following his admission to hospital, or even mere acceptance into outpatient medical care, is fairly well known. Even the law, and society in general, take a different view of crimes committed by the mentally ill offender, and waive the usual rule of making the punishing response fit the crime.

Investigations of *both ends* of a patient's extratherapeutic relationships show that, once afflicted by maladaptive patterns, the patient becomes himself an indirect source and a carrier of repeated self-injury mediated by the retaliatory properties of the equally sensitive human environment. He tends to contaminate each new and as yet unbiased relationship with a carry-over of morbid patterns acquired in comparable former relationships. By compulsively recreating his earlier interpersonal relationships and situations, *he also tends to reproduce the traumatizing features of his previous environments* only to keep him confirmed in his illness. It may even be illusory to imagine that when we fail to cure a patient, we merely fail to do him any good by way of omission. Are we really justified in assuming that there is no appreciable difference between a psychogenic illness which remains unchanged in the absence of any treatment and an illness which remains unchanged following unsuccessful therapeutic intervention? Could it not be argued that in his relationship to us we have inevitably confirmed the patient's problems, making our next colleague's task one grade more difficult?

The Psychotherapeutic Process

To say that interpersonal dynamics are at play in the persistence of maladaptive behavior does not imply that the disorder could spontaneously fade away following a period of social seclusion and protection from reinforcing environmental traumata. Extinction of a response to a certain stimulus is not the same as forgetting the stimulus altogether. On the contrary, extinction implies the obliteration of the response in any further encounter with the same stimulus. If an impotent patient keeps away from women, true, his difficulties may not be clearly manifest. But treatment means to abolish this inhibitory response whenever he is reexposed to the same, or the same kind of, erotic relationship. The concepts of reinforcement and nonreinforcement are meaningless unless they coincide with reexposure to the conditioned stimulus or situation. An experimentally established salivary response cannot be extinguished by failing to sound the bell altogether, but by repeatedly sounding the bell and yet failing to reinforce the exhibited response.

Nonreinforcement in psychogenic disorders, too, can prove therapeutic only if it is coupled with reexposure to certain interpersonal situations. However, reexposure to the original traumatic relationship is no more essential for abolishing the patterns than it is for perpetuating them. A comparable interpersonal situation with analogous significance, such as the therapeutic relationship, may prove sufficiently effective and corrective for this purpose. It goes without saying that the almost instantaneous reexposure of the experimental animal to *physical* stimuli can bear no comparison in complexity with the laborious psychological reexposure of the patient in the therapeutic situation.

The patient's interpersonal generalizations are bound to envelop also the therapist, and from him, too, the patient will tend to draw and extract countertransferential responses. As Freud says, it is only to the extent to which the therapist will prove capable of differentiating himself in the patient's own experience from previous human figures, that the inappropriate and disabling patterns can be surrendered and no longer exhibited in further interpersonal encounters.

FIRSTHAND AND SECONDHAND LEARNING

We can benefit from experimental psychology only if the relevant dissimilarities as well as the similarities between animal and human learning are borne in mind. There is no valid reason why the behavior of a person in response to the verbal and nonverbal stimuli emitted by another person could not be fitted into a behavioral stimulus-response scheme, with the interposed central processes constituting a Tolmanian intervening variable. The obvious advantage of such a behavioral scheme lies in the fact that, quite independently of intrapsychic processes, the testing of psychodynamic hypotheses can be confined to observable data. In principle, interpersonal behavior in dyadic relationships is not only observable, but also measurable (Wolf et al., 1964). It is perfectly feasible that with the aid of adequate methods it should be possible to investigate, in both longitudinal and transverse studies, not only the relationship of psychogenic symptoms to maladaptive interpersonal behavior, but also such processes as the development and vicissitudes of interpersonal patterns or the universality of transference phenomena (Wolf, 1966).

It would be fallacious to expect that the methodological approach evolved in the investigation of animal behavior is equally adequate to all aspects of human behavior. The behavior of a laboratory animal may be a subject of direct observation by nonparticipant observers. It does not follow, however, that a laboratory setting which even in the human adult has proved suitable for investigating his characteristic responses to *objects and tests* is equally suitable for investigating his characteristic responses to *other people*. Unlike the prompt responses that may be elicited in animals and infants to pleasant and unpleasant stimuli, an interpersonal response may take days, months, or even years to materialize, as may be the case in acts of retaliation. However, the *prolonged latencies* with which man often responds, especially to people he significantly depends upon, are not the only reason why interpersonal behavior is unsuited for observation within the confines of limited time and space. Another reason is that one could not possibly accept, say, the behavior of a parent to his child as observed in the setting of a clinic to be a *representative sample* of his overall behavior to the child at home.

The sole function of learning is to benefit from previous relevant experience, and this much is undoubtedly common to both man and animal. That is why man, when not impulsive and whether inves-

tigators like it or not, is a thinking creature who before finally deciding
how to respond to a significant person's act, often prefers to take his
time and weigh such an act in the light of his previous interpersonal
experiences. But this is not the most fundamental difference between
human and infrahuman learning. For, unlike the animal which is only
capable of profiting from *its own experiences* which it has itself been exposed to, man, by virtue of his capacities to communicate verbally, can,
in addition, also profit from the personal *experiences of other people*, such
as parents or friends. He may decide to consult the latter before finally
responding to the other person whom he, say, contemplates divorcing.
But this is by no means all, for he may, as an alternative or additional
intermediary response consult a book on this particular subject or perhaps
a psychiatrist, with the aim of profiting from the *combined and pooled experiences of many more contemporaries and even past generations*, registered in
both the book and the psychiatrist's erudition not as verbatim accounts
of innumerable life histories, but in a generalized and abstracted form of
perhaps some psychodynamic theory of marital problems.

That there is a fundamental difference between the therapeutic benefit derived from firsthand experiences and secondhand ones, was empirically established by Freud. Not being behaviorally orientated he
could only conceptualize the contrast between them in the traditional
language of subjective psychology as "emotional" versus "rational"
reeducation. In his latest formulation of the therapeutic process Freud
laid all the emphasis on the "emotional" experience attained with the
aid of concrete interpretations, as against the inefficacy of abstract "intellectual" insight imparted to the patient.

Only what a child or adult has learned from secondhand sources is
susceptible to correction or even denial by secondhand as well as
firsthand revelations. However, knowledge or lessons drawn from other
people's experiences have no corrective capacity if they run counter to
the patient's own firsthand experiences. A psychogenic disorder that
has grown out of his own interpersonal experiences can be unlearned
only by exposing him to *new disconfirming firsthand experiences*. By sheer
force of logical argument we could not possibly convince an antisocial
psychopath, who was not only a subject of parental hostility but also of
repeated imprisonments and social ostracism, that society or some
people are really well disposed to him and want to help him. For what
he knows from firsthand experience to have been true for certain, in the
course of his therapeutic reeducation he requires to see for himself not
that it was not true, but that it is *no longer* true. He should be offered
experiential opportunities to discover for himself that in the therapeutic
situation his behavior is anachronistic and no longer appropriate. This is
in essence the analysis of the transference.

Maladaptive interpersonal patterns can be unlearned only in the face-to-face situations which the patient has a compulsive need to subject to empirical testing to see if they are any different from previous traumatic ones. Such testing is only feasible if there are opportunities to evoke invalidating social feedback (Wolf, 1957, 1960). Information conveyed by some impersonal route such as a book or a public lecture, through which in the last analysis innumerable anonymous sufferers and ex-sufferers are addressing their pooled and abstracted experiences to the patient, may be highly instructive but not curative. Recognition of this fact is nowadays implicit in every variety of psychotherapeutic procedure in which face-to-face social encounters with therapist, staff members, and fellow patients are considered indispensable.

Conclusion

We should allow ourselves neither to be carried away by the animal model too literally nor to be driven by the complexities of social behavior to the other extreme. What we require is not a *behavioral animal model to copy*, but a *behavioral approach to apply* in psychiatric thinking and practice. In a fruitful cooperative spirit the clinician stands as much to gain from the learning theories based on the animal model as does the learning theorist stand to gain from the empirically established principles of learning and unlearning pathological behavior which only pertain to man but have *no direct counterpart in the animal*.

The learning theory model and the psychoanalytic model are by no means incompatible alternatives. On the contrary, they bear out each other's most important contributions, and interdisciplinary integration of the two models is likely to open up sharper insights into the genesis and treatment of psychogenic disorders. I submit that their integration is sooner or later inevitable, however passionately some or many of us may choose to resist it. Psychoanalysis cannot remain for much longer outside the behavioral sciences, nor can the science of human behavior for much longer ignore the body of knowledge amassed by the psychoanalytic schools of thought.

References

Alexander, F. and French, T. M. (1946). *Psychoanalytic Therapy.* New York: Ronald Press.

Cameron, N. and Magaret, A. (1951). *Behavior Pathology.* Boston: Houghton Mifflin.

Crisp, A. H. (1964). Development and application of a measure of 'transference.' *J. Psychosom. Res.* 8:327-335.

Dollard, J. and Miller, N. E. (1950). *Personality and Psychotherapy.* New York: McGraw-Hill.

Eysenck, H. J. (1960). Personality and behavior therapy. *Proc. R. Soc. Med.* 53:504-508.

Eysenck, H. J. (1965). The effects of psychotherapy. Critical review in *Int. J. Psychiat.* 1:97-178.

Freud, S. (1964a). *Collected Papers,* 4th ed. vol. II, p. 289. London: Hogarth Press.

Freud, S. (1964b). *An Autobiographical Study,* 2nd ed. p. 76. London: Hogarth Press.

Hilgard, E. R. and Marquis, D. G. (1961). *Conditioning and Learning,* rev. ed. pp. 340-342. London: Methuen.

Hull, C. L. (1943). *Principles of Behavior.* New York: Appleton-Century-Crofts.

Leary, T. (1957). *Interpersonal Diagnosis of Personality.* New York: Ronald Press.

Liddell, H. S. (1944). *Personality and the Behavior Disorders,* vol. I, pp. 389-412. Ed. J. McV. Hunt. New York: Ronald Press.

Luria, A. R. (1932). *The Nature of Human Conflicts.* New York: Liveright.

Masserman, J. H. (1946). *Principles of Dynamic Psychiatry.* Philadelphia-London: Saunders.

Mowrer, O. H. (1953). *Psychotherapy — Theory and Research.* New York: Ronald Press.

Rotter, J. B. (1954). *Social Learning and Clinical Psychology.* New York: Prentice-Hall.

Skinner, B. F. (1938). *The Behavior of Organisms.* New York: Appleton-Century-Crofts.

Sears, R. R. (1944). *Personality and the Behavior Disorders,* vol. I, pp. 306-332. Ed. J. McV. Hunt. New York: Ronald Press.

Sullivan, H. S. (1955). *Conceptions of Modern Psychiatry.* London: Tavistock Publications.

Wolf, E. (1957). *Congress Report, 2nd Int. Congr. Psychiatry,* vol. III, pp. 270-277, 284-291. Ed. W. A. Stoll. Zurich: Orell Fuessli.

Wolf, E. (1960). *Progress in Psychotherapy,* vol. V, pp. 51-58. Ed. J. H. Masserman and J. L. Moreno. New York: Grune and Stratton.

Wolf, E., Dytrych, Z., Grof, S., Kubicka, L. and Srnec, J. (1964). A methodological approach to social maladaptation. Mutual social perception inventory. (In Czech.) *Cs. Psychiat.* 60:34-37.

Wolf, E. (1966). Psychogenic disorders and interpersonal behavior. *J. Psychosom. Res.* 10: 119-126.

Psychoanalysis and Behavior Therapy

LEE BIRK, M.D., AND
ANN W. BRINKLEY-BIRK, PH.D.

In this article, two experienced clinicians, trained in both psychoanalytic and behavioral paradigms, present cogent arguments for the advantages of a combined psychodynamic-behavioral approach by a single therapist or (for groups) a single team of cotherapists. They offer a number of clinical vignettes to illustrate their basic theme that the insight-seeking methodology of psychoanalytic psychotherapy and the change-producing techniques of behavior therapy form a complementary system. They assert that a conceptual as well as a clinical integration of the two approaches is not only possible but needed, in order to most fully utilize the data presented in the therapeutic process.

9

Psychoanalysis and Behavior Therapy

LEE BIRK, M.D., AND
ANN W. BRINKLEY-BIRK, PH.D.

Most readers of this journal are already sufficiently familiar with the historical developments of psychoanalysis and behavior therapy to recognize the extent to which the theoretical and methodological divergence of the two traditions is due to the different scientific/epistemological biases of their founders. That psychoanalysis and behavior therapy developed from and were formally determined by separate, seemingly incompatible methodological and metaphysical underpinnings is by now a well-established commonplace in the history of science. But that the two traditions should continue to generate essentially separate and uncooperative clinical schools can no longer be supported by differences in their philosophical/scientific determinants; there *is* a conceptual interface between psychoanalysis and behavior therapy. In this paper, we will be focusing on the prospects for broadening this nascent interface into an effective theoretical synthesis of these two traditions—a synthesis that eventuates clinically in the mutual potentiation of psychoanalytic and behavioral techniques.

Real and widespread synergistic cooperation between advocates of the two schools has been slow in developing[1; 2, pp. vii-ix, 1-6, 38-41]; at present, the integration of behavioral and psychoanalytic techniques* in the treatment repertoire of the single clinician is the result of ad hoc adaptations and is still without a solid conceptual foundation. For about half a

*Following Glover,[3] Cushing,[4] Tabachnick,[5] and Marmor,[6] we see no clearcut criteria (especially conceptually) for differentiating between psychoanalysis and psychoanalytic psychotherapy. In this article we use the term *psychoanalysis* to refer not just to classical psychoanalysis (dyadic, four to five times a week, on the couch) but also to the many variants of psychoanalytic therapy—including group, family, and couple therapy—that are largely derived from psychoanalysis.

From *American Journal of Psychiatry*, 131:499-510, May 1974. Copyright 1974 by the American Psychiatric Association. Reprinted by permission.

147

decade, however, there have been at least a few modest steps toward de facto convergence on a practical, clinical level. The joint session of the American Academy of Psychoanalysis and of the American Psychiatric Association at APA's 1973 annual meeting is typical of this trend. Moreover, it is no longer unusual for psychoanalysts and behavior therapists to refer patients (even including themselves!) to each other or to collaborate in the treatment of difficult cases. Despite this and a series of papers over the past ten years that have emphasized their common features,[7-10] coexistence, [11,12] and even convergence,[13] real conceptual integration has barely begun and it remains true that "on the whole, both behavior therapists and dynamic psychiatrists seem to have been unwilling to inform themselves sufficiently to be able to consider the observations presented by the other approach."[2, p. 6]

There have been a few instances, however, in which writers have gone beyond a merely hortatory approach to this integration. One of the earliest papers illustrating this trend toward true integration and synthesis was a 1966 paper by Crisp[14] that presciently discussed *both* "transference" and effects as in "social repercussion effects" due to successful behavior therapy. A few years ago one of us (L.B.) presented a brief but much-rebutted paper, "Behavior Therapy: Integration with Dynamic Psychiatry,"[15] and in early 1972, Feather and Rhoads published an important paper entitled "Psychodynamic Behavior Therapy."[16] This nascent trend toward true integration reached its fullest development to date with two papers presented in May 1973 at the joint session mentioned above: one by Rhoads and Feather[17] and one by one of us (L.B.).[18] These two papers are noteworthy for the amount of conceptual and practical integration they embody: each describes the work of single clinicians alternately[17] or even simultaneously[18] using both behavioral and psychoanalytic concepts and methods in the treatment of the same patients, the first using relatively short-term individual therapy and the second using intensive five-day-per-week group therapy.

What is really required at this stage, however, is dialogue between clinicians of both schools whose aim is genuine rapprochement, mutual understanding, and the tentative forging of a new clinical learning theory for psychotherapy—a conceptual framework that can embrace and contain the raw data (clinical phenomena) of both psychoanalysis and behavior therapy.

Assumed Differences

The Philosophical Paradigms

Psychoanalytically derived psychotherapies and the behavior therapies are assumed to differ essentially in two ways: in the mechanisms of therapeutic change deemed effective by each school and in the primary areas in which change is assumed to become manifest. These differences are derived from the contrasting sets of assumptions that underlie the theoretical structure of each school. That is, each school was bound to a large extent to the philosophical/scientific parameters that were operating at each stage in its development, since these determined not only what was accepted as workable and true but what were the very standards of truth itself. Insight-oriented psychotherapy, for example, derived its theoretical impetus from the "knowledge-is-power" model underlying post-Newtonian science. That insight should be presumed to be the mark of—and catalyst for—therapeutic change is only a corollary of that model's basic premise. Moreover, the emphasis on insight-mediated change is also perfectly consistent with the primary focus of other scientific models of the time: until the early 1900s, rational reconstruction of the phenomenal world ("making sense of the data") was regarded as the principal concern of the scientific community—more so, that is to say, than mastery or manipulation of the phenomenal world.

The triple-layered (conscious, unconscious, and preconscious) mental structure postulated and accepted by the adherents of Freudian and neo-Freudian psychotherapeutic theory and practice served as a referential base* for the collection of technical explanations and operations that they advocated at the same time that it was assumed to be a second-order source of validation for the choice of therapeutic mechanisms underlying the retrospective-associative methods of psychoanalytically oriented psychotherapists.† For this reason, the primary mechanisms of therapeutic change were believed to serve a dual purpose: on the one hand, to act as signs or indications to the patient and therapist of the current (albeit ameboid) interface between conscious and nonconscious (preconscious or unconscious) and, on the other hand, to be the vehicles for that transit between unconscious and conscious that was assumed to be the major, indeed the necessary, condition for therapeutic change in psychoanalytic psychotherapy.

Slips of the tongue, dreams, and unexpected associations (to name only a few of these mechanisms) are presumed to be interpretable and self-consistent, not primarily within the context of conscious experience but within the expanding framework supplied by the content of con-

---

*This is equally true of the earlier (pre-1920s) "topographical" model of psychoanalysis and of the later "structural" model.

†On reflection, it will be clear that this is circular, in very simple terms, the existence of the unconscious as a receptacle for repressed conflicts and wishes is predicated on the assumption that the content of slips of the tongue, dreams, and so on make indirect reference to unconscious material, but that these mechanisms in turn are believed to be the vehicles of transit between the two mental levels is itself a hypothesis that requires confirmation directly by the above-mentioned existence postulate.

scious and previously unconscious thought together. Indeed, by virtue of this same theoretical ontology, neurotic symptoms are the presumed explicanda of repressed conflicts, wishes, memories, and motivations. The ultimate mark of a successful retrospective probe is not just the recovery of repressed material, therefore, but is also the discovery of subjectively acceptable explanations for the otherwise inexplicable phenomena of ordinary conscious thought and affect, unconscious verbal or motor slips (accidents), and dreams—explanations, that is, that do not so much merely expose the repressed conflicts as make sense of phenomena that appear at first glance to be inconsistent.[19-22]

The emergence of unconscious processes into consciousness—via dreams, slips, associations, affective links, etc., to the hidden conflict or motivation—is mediated by the phenomenon of transference. To recreate the past in the present or react to the present as if it were just like the past is already to have made accessible to interpretation the early learning experiences from which were constructed the matrix of rules operating within the perceptual-interpretive apparatus. It is by means of these "rules" that individuals establish an idiosyncratic pattern in the screening, coding, and storing of experiences.

In working through the transference one might be said to be redetermining the boundary conditions for past and present in the service of both exposing and eliminating the systematic perceptual distortion that the individual brings to his current environment and of shifting or modifying the basic rules by which he typically codes and integrates new experiences. Secondarily and concomitantly, of course, one should expect to change the reality-perception-feeling sequence to the point that cognitive and emotional reactions to external stimuli work with and not against each other. This implies the resolution of conflict, some aspects of which had not previously been fully conscious; in short, it can be said that merely exposing the internal consistency of the items in an individual's psychological inventory is not adequate to the task of bringing into harmony with external reality that individual's emotional and cognitive responses without a corrective emotional experience[23] concurrent with the resolution of the transference neurosis.

In spite of well-specified theoretical and practical differences, behavior therapy and psychoanalytically derived psychotherapy show a marked and similar congruence in the amount of circular reinforcement between operative metaphysical assumptions (or any lack thereof) and the derivation of therapeutic mechanisms. While psychoanalytic psychotherapy can be said to operate within a context in which metaphysical assumptions (i.e., the "mental model" with its triple-layered view of consciousness) both determine and are derived from a carefully chosen set of phenomena that have been granted *a priori* significance, it must be said of behavior therapy that its principles are presumed valid within a context in which, by prescientific decision, *no metaphysical assumptions* are allowed to operate. These are the contexts that validate the choice of treatment mechanisms and that determine the priorities assigned to different outcome criteria.

The Clinical Models

These differences in the two philosophical paradigms are reflected in the dissimilarity in clinical models. Whereas psychoanalysis focuses on learning about previously unconscious motivation and conflicts, emphasizes free association, dream interpretation, and the handling of the interpersonal relationship between the analyst and the patient, and focuses on making the correct cognitive interpretation to the patient,[6, p. 1197] behavior therapy generally has not attempted to deal with unconscious mental processes, nor has it ever really acknowledged their relevance—even, in some quarters, their existence. Moreover, behavior therapy focuses on the patient-therapist relationship only to the extent that this is seen to be important in securing the patient's cooperation with the therapist's treatment plan[2, pp. 27-28] and in enhancing the therapist's effectiveness as a "social reinforcer."[24] With only sparse and limited exceptions, originating mainly from those who have an analytic background[25] or who have otherwise been tainted by analytic apostasies,[26] behavior therapists have not attached therapeutic value to cognitive interpretations, correct or incorrect, nor have they in general even acknowledged the possibility of dealing with cognitive material (what the patient says he thinks or feels) with sufficient scientific objectivity to make this a worthwhile endeavor. This theoretical stance strikes a strangely discordant note* in view of the practical fact that most behavior therapists, especially those more in the tradition of Wolpe than Skinner, *use* self-report data about cognitive matters in carrying out, for example, systematic desensitization and in the construction of hierarchies.[27]

The emphasis by behavioral theorists on observable, objectively

---

*In fact, one of us (L.B.) has pointedly criticized[1] the paradoxical tendency among some behavior therapists to base entire therapeutic strategies wholly on assumed cognitive processes—"covert" imaginal stimuli, "covert" reinforcement, and "covert" punishment—quite without any adequate objective data, even self-report data, to confirm that the therapist's commands to imagine stimulus scenes and to imagine reinforcing and/or punishing events in fact lead to those events within the patient's brain. Psychoanalysis, in contrast, (1) does not attempt to directly manipulate cognitive content, but rather attempts to deal naturalistically with existing cognitive content, and (2) amasses as much self-report data as possible, including data that come from observed verbal slips and associative connections, to support any theories the analyst may have about cognitive content, conscious and unconscious.

manifest data is a consequence of the phenomenological bias inherent in the scientific model that was prominent at the time of the development of behavioral principles. Manipulation of the external environment to effect behavior change is the modus operandi of behavior therapists and is consistent with the parsimony of metaphysical accretions that is characteristic of phenomenologists and others of a behavioral bent who regard observability, objectivity, and repeatability as the hallmark of criteria for existence and truth. In this, clinical behaviorists have taught us much about the importance of extinction in the therapeutic process and about competitive response[28] and behavioral-shaping strategies.[29-34] With their emphasis on the processes of operant conditioning that pervade everyday life, normal, neurotic, and even psychotic, they have opened up self-control and treatment mechanisms that depend on bringing selected behaviors under "stimulus control"[35-40] through the planned use of discriminative stimuli, punishment, and reinforcement. In so doing, they have also added depth, subtlety, and power to the clinician's ability to understand and therapeutically limit what analysts call "secondary gain."[28,41,42]

Both schools have recognized the great importance of what analysts call identification[43,44] and what behaviorists call modeling,[45] although the analysts have been much more alert to the fact that therapeutic (and other) identifications can exert profound, pervasive, and lifelong effects, while the behaviorists have been much more productive in studying modeling experimentally and in manipulating it as a process for the achievement of focused therapeutic goals, such as overcoming specific phobias.

Marmor has recently summed up the "fundamental aspects of Freud's contribution . . . generally accepted by all psychoanalysts."

> On the theoretical side . . . that human behavior is motivated, that our personalities are shaped by the interplay of biological potentials and life experiences, that functional psychiatric disturbances are the result of developmental vicissitudes and contradictory and conflictual inputs and feedbacks, and that early childhood experiences are of special significance in shaping subsequent perceptions and reactions in later life.[6, p. 1197]

And one might say of behavior therapy that it, too, emphatically acknowledges the undeniable role of past learning experiences, recent and remote, in the formation of an individual's adaptive and maladaptive (symptomatic) behavioral repertoire. Thus, in fact, psychoanalytic and behavioral theories are both learning theories; it follows that in effect *psychoanalysis and behavior therapy are both learning therapies*.

In other words, past experience (learning) shapes current behavior and personality, including "neurosis" or "functional psychiatric disturbance," and the role of therapy is to reverse this faulty learning. With this in mind it might really be more accurate to refer to both psychoanalysis and behavior therapy as unlearning and relearning therapies.

Strengths and Limitations of the Two
Therapeutic Methodologies

We have discussed above the theoretical causes for divergence between the psychoanalytic and behavioral traditions. We will turn our attention now to the types of successful therapeutic change and the mechanisms by which those changes are achieved, based on the pure theoretical models of psychoanalytic and behavior therapy, respectively. To this end, we have prepared a series of diagrams to represent the pure models of psychoanalysis and behavior therapy and their combination in schematized form.

Psychoanalysis

In successful psychoanalysis or psychoanalytically oriented psychotherapy, one can predict a necessary and significant change in the patient's level of self-understanding or self-awareness. One mark of successful therapy of this type is the recovery of forgotten or repressed material through the gradual exposure, clarification, interpretation, and extension of associative-affective links between present and past. By means of these emotion-mediated insights, the patient is gradually made aware of his particular psychodynamic inventory—in philosophical terms, of the cognitive assumptions underlying his personal world view. This is the sine qua non of a successful analysis. In addition, the patient would predictably begin to feel better about himself, to experience less guilt and more pleasure, to be freer to work efficiently, and to achieve a greater degree of social integration without concurrent or later self-punishment. In Figure 1, we have indicated this causal nexus by the broad arrow from "insight" to "subjective sense of improvement." This is meant to suggest that if insight occurs—as it must if psychoanalysis is to effect its proper end—subjective confirmation of improvement follows. It goes without saying, however, that objectively manifest behavioral change is not at all a necessary product of insight and insight-based changes in the patient's self-evaluation: "we have learned the difficult lesson that rational understanding alone is not enough, that people can understand only why they behave in certain ways and yet be unable to alter their unsatisfactory patterns."[46]

Case 1. A 25-year-old male graduate student with a 12-year history of a disabling fear of gagging (or actual uncontrolled gagging) in public-speaking situations uncovered the origin of his phobic symptom during group therapy. In a particularly emotional moment, he gained the insight that this problem had to do with his fear of disclosing the guilty secret of his long-practiced habit of playing with his own feces, originally as an imagined substitute for the siblings that he (an only child) lacked. Memory confirmed this insight: the patient's first trouble with gagging (to the point of vomiting) had occurred at age 13 when, during a Sunday-school Bible reading in front of the entire congregation, he was called upon to read the words "and all his bowels spilled out" (at this age he thought

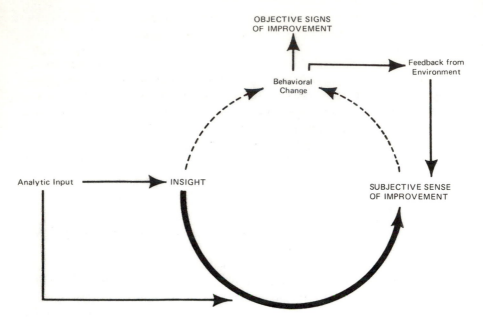

FIGURE 1. The narrow psychoanalytic model.

"bowels" meant feces). In spite of extensive therapeutic efforts to "work through" this insight, he experienced no relief whatever from the symptom. This patient has now been referred for systematic desensitization; he is also continuing in group psychotherapy.

Behavior Therapy

It is now well recognized that discrete behavioral symptoms—for example, specific fears and inhibitions; compulsive habits; obsessive, ritualized, or self-destructive, self-punitive, or self-defeating behaviors; specific behavioral deficits; and certain psychophysiological symptoms[47]—are amenable to modification by a variety of behavioral techniques that do not rely in any way on insight but instead make use of external feedback mechanisms. As Figure 2 indicates, insight and heightened self-awareness are not part of a pure behavior therapy stratagem; instead, the behavior therapist undertakes careful "behavioral analysis" of the leading behaviors in the symptomatic matrix in order to determine what the current sources of reinforcement are that perpetuate these target behaviors. This leads naturally to the design of a specific behavioral program to modify the behaviors that constitute the patient's chief complaints.

Thus, if the behavioral analysis is correctly done, behavioral change and objective signs of improvement will necessarily occur (if they do not, one can legitimately assume an error, omission, or oversimplification in the original behavioral analysis). Both behavioral change per se and its observable or measurable manifestation in objective signs of improvement should elicit greater social rewards, which in turn lead to further shaping of the desired behavioral change, as Figure 2 indicates. According to behavioral theory, maladaptive behavior is defined as just that behavior which routinely elicits punishing responses from the environment and adaptive behavior as that which effects appropriately rewarding social consequences. Although behavioral change and its objective manifestation may be sufficient to cause a subjective sense of improvement, the latter is not a necessary effect.

This happens when the patient's internal reinforcement/punishment system is sufficiently skewed, because of an unanalyzed neurotic distortion in the value system or the perceptual-interpretive apparatus, to permit behavioral change to occur in the absence of the patient's really experiencing subjective improvement. The natural system of rewards and punishments alone may not be effective in modifying maladaptive behavior when there is systematic (neurotic) distortion in the patient's perception or valuation of reward/punishment. In such cases, a systematic amplification of the normal reward/punishment consequences may not be helpful and may even be countertherapeutic.

Case 2. A 45-year-old teacher and mother of four with a 20-year history of multiple severe compulsive habits, manipulative depressive affect, and periodic quasi-suicidal behavior was seen in treatment with her husband by an experienced behavior therapist. She had already had many years of unsuccessful psychotherapy. The therapist noted that the patient's complaints were shifting and migratory following successful work in a given area. Ultimately his efforts with her foundered in the face of his straightforward (noninsight-seeking) efforts to help bring some genuine nonneurotic pleasure into her life. She was then referred to one of the authors (L.B.) for combined behavioral-psychoanalytic work. Previous insight-oriented psychotherapy had failed as well, although the patient had come to recognize the intensity of her guilt over the death of her father. He was an inveterate gambler—in her eyes, an assertive, charming man—with whom she had been incestuously involved as a young woman. His death by suicide followed an argument with her about money. Despite her earlier psychotherapy the patient continued to feel very guilty and to heap punishment on herself and those around her by manipulating and provoking her all-too-compliant and passive husband into low-key but hurtful attacks.

Her previous psychotherapy did not work because, despite considerable insight, it did not interrupt her self-punitive life-style. Her behavior therapy, on the other hand, did not work because it attempted simplistically to eliminate her multiple self-punitive behaviors without altering her basic world view, which provided a cognitive justification for her pervasive need to punish herself. She was in a sense doomed to continue paying off her guilt for her father's suicide until she could achieve sufficient insight into the relationships among her old sexual feelings about her father, her anger at him, and her unconscious wishes for his death. It was the punishment-seeking drive produced by this patient's guilt that distorted her response to what would ordinarily have been reinforcing/punishing events in her environment.

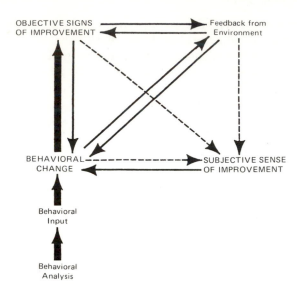

FIGURE 2. The narrow behavior therapy model.

As Figure 2 also indicates, another drawback of pure behavior therapy is that desirable behavioral change can occur either in the absence of a subjective sense of improvement or even in the face of increasingly negative self-report data.

Case 3. A 25-year-old passive-dependent office worker sought behaviorally oriented couple therapy in order to resolve his inhibitions against further involvement with a woman he was otherwise on the verge of marrying. The assignment of graded behavioral tasks accomplished the ostensible goals for which therapy was undertaken, but it resulted in a simultaneous worsening of the patient's chronic success-anxiety to the point that he was experiencing frequent attacks of nausea and vomiting. Insight-oriented probing exposed the patient's previously unconscious fear of his father's retaliatory jealousy. Once exposed, these fears were treated with imaginal desensitization in combination with a flooding and extinction technique of "symptom scheduling." With this combined behavioral-psychoanalytic approach, the patient not only continued to *do* better but also began to *feel* better.

Figure 3 shows the therapeutic power that is gained when, in the treatment of the same patient, there is both an analytic input and a behavioral input. Fundamentally, this is the combined (but not integrated) paradigm that operates when analyst-behavior therapist teams collaborate successfully in the treatment of individual patients.

A Proposed Paradigm for the Clinical and Conceptual Integration of Psychoanalysis and Behavior Therapy

One of the fundamental reasons that psychoanalysis and behavior therapy have such apparently well-entrenched differences in their modi operandi, it seems to us, is that their goals are different. That is to say, successful psychoanalysis is marked by the maximization of self-awareness, "making sense of" increasingly profound levels of psychological data as they become accessible to conscious interpretation. Behavior therapy, on the other hand, is primarily concerned with *modifying* behavior according to external, socially determined standards, by means of the manipulation of environmental contingencies. Both are consistency-oriented therapies in the sense that each attempts to fit together its choice of significant phenomena under an integrating theoretical superstructure but, since these phenomena make up categories that need not be coextensive, the goals and therapeutic results remain essentially disparate. Psychoanalysis works to bring the internal data of consciousness into some sort of harmony mediated by the logic and self-

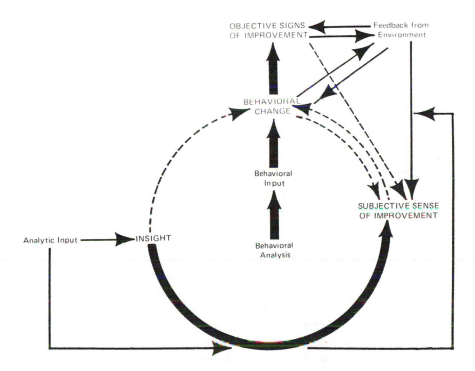

FIGURE 3. The combined model.

consistency of mental events; behavior therapy, on the other hand, works to bring the individual (characterized by the externally manifest phenomena of his behavior) into greater harmony with the physically and socially determined consequences of his own deliberate and idiosyncratic (habitual) actions.

Our proposed model seeks to combine the internal and external aspects of human activity—to regard self-awareness as a potentiator of behavioral change and to view an increasingly realistic assessment of natural social rewards and punishments as a motive for continuing insight-based self-realization. That is, if insight and external feedback systems can be used together to expose, clarify, and change an individual's perceptual and reactive patterns when those have proved ineffective, one has indeed found a way to maximize the fit between an individual, his self-evaluation, his perceptions of external reality, his response to that reality, and his actual existential position.

To be more specific, it is our belief, on the basis of our clinical experience, that psychoanalysis and behavior therapy need no longer represent two warring belief systems or two separate clinical traditions but that, as techniques, each can be used to reinforce the weakest links in the therapeutic input-outcome chain of the other.

For example, even in the specific case of dealing with loss and grieving, usually regarded as an area in which behavioral ideas can contribute little, therapists can learn something of value from both the behavioral and the psychoanalytic traditions. The behavioral literature contains some excellent conceptual contributions to the understanding of the phenomena of acute depression,[42-48] learned helplessness and chronic depression,[49,50] chronic social (maternal and peer) deprivation,[51] and even a few promising studies of the treatment of depression.[42,52,53] Notwithstanding all this, it can still be said that, for obvious ethical reasons, loss and grieving have not been subjects that lend themselves naturally to truly experimental study and, therefore, that those who have pursued the more naturalistic scientific methods, ranging from Freud[54] to van Lawick-Goodall,[55] have made a relatively greater contribution.

Faced with helping a patient to deal with the loss of a child or of a life partner, the therapist may find it useful, to some extent, to conceptualize this in terms of an existentially unhappy state, e.g., an "abrupt loss of available reinforcers," but in our opinion there is no humane and ethical alternative to the therapist's "sharing it, bearing it, and helping the patient to place it in perspective." In this endeavor, we have found this clinical admonition of Semrad's, along with Freud's classic paper "Mourning and Melancholia"[54] and Lindemann's paper on the management of acute grief,[56] to be among the most helpful in the literature and lore of psychotherapy.

Integrated Model

In the integrated model, an insight is regarded not so much as one piece in the puzzle uniquely representative of every individual's psychological identity, but rather as a clue to the developmental origins of a particular emotional/behavioral/cognitive response that is, in the patient's current life, symptomatically overgeneralized from past learning experiences. If it becomes clear to the patient—through insight—what the details of the original situation were and why the response may have been an adaptive one *in that situation*, it becomes increasingly easy for him to learn to discriminate between new experiences that no longer call for the same response/feeling/idea and those that resemble past learning experiences so closely as to be appropriate stimuli for the previously habitual response. Insight, in short, functions as a vehicle for the retraining of an individual's discriminative abilities.[57] One might even say insight *is* discriminative learning, evaluated subjectively.

To reexperience childhood traumata or conflicts as completely as possible is to become convinced of the *particularity* of early learning experiences. Thus, the patient relives past traumatic experiences in order to establish (learn) the particulars of these experiences and in order to minimize the likelihood of continued faulty generalization in later similar situations. Insight based on the exploration and interpretation of transference phenomena is not the only mechanism for promoting recognition of the natural human (and biologic) tendency to recreate past situations in the present* and to respond to them as if universalization of experience were a valid cognitive/emotional induction. In fact, a change in behavior can supply a compelling counterinstance to the prevailing faulty cognitive or emotional set.

All therapists have one objective in common, and that is to help patients respond internally and externally in more adaptive ways, to bring feeling states and behavioral responses into closer alliance. In pursuing this end, psychoanalytic therapists concentrate on improving the patient's perceptual clarity and acuity through the analysis of distortional transference phenomena; behavior therapists direct their efforts toward teaching the patient to stop doing what is maladaptive and begin doing what is situationally adaptive.

Development of Appropriate Responses

With pure analytic therapies a patient may come to see the need for changing his behavior without being able to do so; with pure behavior

---

*Biologically, stimulus generalization is an important learned involuntary component in this process but, in our opinion, there is another demonstrable wish-component in the human situation: a stubborn nostalgic longing for things to be as they were in the "good old days" of comfortable childhood dependence, as well as for the original parental objects of a person's love/hate.[58]

therapy, a patient may change his behavior without learning to see the need for modifying the new learned responses when the subtleties of new situations warrant and demand this modification. A response that is fully adaptive to the nuances of particular new situations depends, therefore, as much on accurate perception of the situation as it does on attention to the natural social feedback consequent to the response. Thus, psychoanalytic psychotherapy and behavior therapy are naturally complementary and resonant[58]; within the psychoanalytic therapies a patient learns to use insight as an incentive for a potentiation of behavior change and within the behavior therapies a patient learns how to change his behavior.

Behavior therapy is not only a technique to modify behavior, because of its emphasis on contingencies of reinforcement/punishment, it is also a profoundly effective technique for teaching people to consider the consequences of their behavior and to reconcile their internal reward/punishment systems with those of the natural social environment (this is especially true of behaviorally oriented group, family, and couple therapies). Even more important is the fact that behavior therapy is an approach capable of teaching patients to be able to provide themselves with effective counterinstances to their own faulty (anachronistic or primitive) views of world and self.

For example, a man in analysis may "know" that his wife is not his mother but if, because of a deficit in his own capacity for effective assertive behavior, she dominates him as his mother did, he will still feel like a little boy with her until this deficit in assertiveness can be remedied. In analytic psychotherapy, in such matters, the patient essentially is left to "work out his own salvation with fear and trembling."* The analyst may repetitively point out that his wife and his mother are quite different, may proddingly question why he did or didn't say X or Y, and may support (and reinforce) him emotionally for nascent efforts at assertiveness, but he *does not teach him how to be assertive*. A behavioral-psychoanalytic therapist would do all of these things and, *if needed*, would also use the behavioral technique of assertive training to teach him how to be assertive with his wife. This would typically include sessions with the wife; such sessions combine the therapeutic advantage of *in vivo* behavioral shaping, enhanced identification/modeling effects, and the systematic undermining of his old "little boy" feelings with his wife.

Not only does the patient learn to change his behavior, but he is also compelled to give up the faulty assumptions, often unconscious or preconscious, about himself and about his wife, that were part of the cognitive/emotional matrix out of which his maladaptive behavior with her

---

*We do not mean here to derogate the didactic advantages, *in classical psychoanalysis*, of the analyst's limiting himself in a disciplined way to the pure task of analysis.

arose, grew, and was neurotically nourished by him in the first place. If uninterrupted, this maladaptive behavior continues to reinforce the erroneous, albeit unconscious, coalescence of wife and mother. When the old behavior is interrupted and replaced by new assertive behavior, however, the new pattern stands in direct contradiction, as a counterinstance, to the chronic unconscious equation of wife and mother. In other words, the patient is behaving as if he no longer believed in this equation. The consequent shift in cognitive set and attendant increase in self-esteem serve as internal reinforcers for the continuance and increasing adaptiveness of the new behavior patterns.

Some of the powerful advantages of such an integrated model are illustrated in Figure 4. This is the paradigm that applies when a single clinician, as in the papers cited earlier by Rhoads and Feather[17] and by one of us,[18] integrates within his own clinical approach behavioral *and* psychoanalytic principles and techniques.

This clinical integration is indicated by the circle labeled "therapist" that contains within it "psychoanalytic understanding and interpreta-

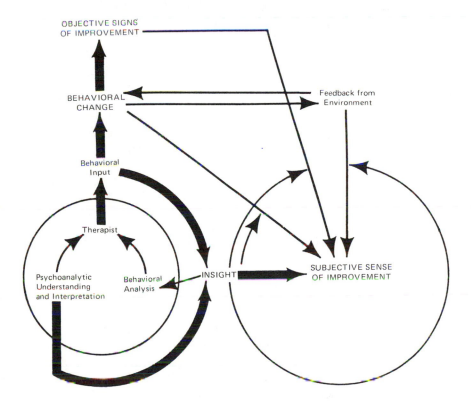

FIGURE 4. The integrated model.

tion" and "behavioral analysis." Insofar as the therapist is able to direct the cognitive content of what he says toward insight while simultaneously managing to keep the behavioral valence (reinforcing/punishing) and timing (contingencies) of his therapeutic interactions consonant with the plan set up during the behavioral analysis, he can effect a significant behavioral change; to that extent he is able to function simultaneously as a behavioral and psychoanalytic therapist. Thus, there is an arrow leading from "therapist" to "behavioral input" as well as an arrow from "behavioral input" to "behavioral change" and one from "behavioral input" to "insight." That is, the therapist may also elect to try to impart cognitive understanding (insight) by means of psychoanalytic comments, questions, and interpretations; although these do not sabotage the behavioral regimen, they are not meant to subserve a particular function in that regimen. This accounts for the arrow leading directly from "psychoanalytic understanding" to "insight."

Another advantage of the integrated single-therapist model is that insight provides the therapist with data about the patient's internal processes, which may serve as internal reinforcers and punishers for behavior that may otherwise consistently defy skillful management of modifications by only external contingencies (for example, a masochistic patient may have a covert guilt-linked need to suffer, so that presumed punishing stimuli are in fact reinforcing). This is indicated by the arrow from "insight" to "behavioral analysis." Finally, as the other three smaller arrows from "insight" indicate, insight can be used to promote movement toward "subjective sense of improvement" from "behavioral change," "objective signs of improvement," and "feedback from the environment." In earlier figures, these were connected only by broken lines: in the absence of the patient's correctly recognizing the value of each of these (because of unanalyzed transference distortions or unresolved self-punitive needs, for example), the three do not *necessarily* lead to a subjective sense of improvement.

Transference and Countertransference

Naturally, considerable skill and experience are required for the therapist to be able to act explicitly as a reinforcer/punisher of certain patient behaviors while also managing to silhouette and interpret transference distortions. Basically, in order to do this the therapist must shift his stance away from the traditionally sought analytic neutrality, against the backdrop of which the transference is first developed and later experienced by the patient as a distortion. Instead, the therapist deliberately and openly attempts to promote the explicit behavioral goals toward which the patient and he together have agreed to work. Within such a therapeutic alliance, intruding transference feelings can be experienced and recognized (with concomitant therapeutic benefit) as a distortion by the patient.

It should be emphasized, however, that the *elicitation of transference phenomena is not a goal* during behavioral-psychoanalytic therapy, although it is certainly a proper and indispensable goal in classical psychoanalysis. The transference phenomena that do occur in the course of behavioral-psychoanalytic therapeutic programs tend to be very strong eruptions of feeling in direct relation to the therapist's interventions. Resolution of transference conflict depends on the patient's being able to see the distinction between the therapist and the early object of his strong and by now overgeneralized feelings. Recognition of the distinction is made considerably easier by the patient's having a real sense of the therapist's individuality—a sense that will, with proper interpretation and help from the therapist, defy further overgeneralized reactions from the patient. The therapist must therefore be a real person to the patient, not only in the sense of being a more effective "social reinforcing machine"[24] but also in order to help correct the faulty cognitive/emotional responses that patients bring from their past learning experiences and incorrectly apply to new individuals and new situations.

Since there need be no concern about impeding the full development of a traditional transference neurosis, transference behavior can be interpreted and managed in a straightforward and open way.

Case 4. A 46-year-old university professor, after almost a year of treatment in intensive behavioral-psychoanalytic group therapy, became quite angry with the therapist (L.B.) when the therapist announced his plan to take a two-week summer vacation. The patient wanted to take a four-week vacation. This discrepancy, he said, would ruin his whole summer. His anger deepened despite the therapist's offer not to charge for the extra two weeks he wanted to be away. Open interpretive group discussion of this led him to an early intellectual acknowledgement of the irrationality of these deep strong feelings—which he continued to struggle with—and of their rootedness in his anger at his wealthy but withholding father over money, at his warmly affectionate but domineering mother over her controllingness, and at both his parents and himself for his still-unresolved dependency needs ("I just wouldn't want to be away on vacation if the group were meeting!").

Countertransference issues are also of course complicated by the decision to use reinforcement or punishment* as part of the therapeutic strategy. The therapist is compelled to examine his choice of behavioral contingencies in the light of his own (perhaps unconscious)† predisposition to reward certain behaviors out of his own needs, rather than be-

---

*The use of punishment may (rarely) include frank aversive procedures; more commonly, however, punishment takes the form of negative interpretations.[18]

†For this reason, we believe that therapists who use behavioral techniques have even more reason than traditional therapists to explore thoroughly their own unconscious processes, ideally within the setting of a classical psychoanalysis.

cause of their social adaptiveness for the patient, or to punish other behaviors as an acting out of his own anger.

For example, a female therapist with unanalyzed castration impulses may unconsciously wish to undermine the assertive traits in her male patients. Thus she may discourage (subtly punish) his assertive responses, while simultaneously overtly reinforcing counteraggressive behaviors in the service of promoting "gentleness" or "sensitivity." Similarly, a therapist with unresolved (perhaps unrecognized) sadistic or angry feelings may choose punishment strategies for personal gratification rather than therapeutic utility.

To sum up, it should be said that the behavioral-psychoanalytic therapist is accepting a great ethical responsibility and should be vigilantly on guard against using learning theory and learning therapies as a way of rationalizing and justifying the acting out of impulses that serve his own needs rather than the patient's.

"SAVING THE PHENOMENA"‡

In the preceding parts of this paper we have tried to highlight the potential therapeutic power that results from broadening the criteria used to determine the set of clinically relevant psychological data and to propose a comprehensive framework into which clinical data of all sorts can be fitted. One of the major features of our proposal is the built-in exhortation neither to overlook phenomena nor to deliberately exclude practical operations merely because they do not conform to preconceived metaphysical or methodological standards of a particular theoretical stance—not to exclude, for example, subjective reports on the grounds that they are not amenable to objective quantification, nor behavior modification by contingency scheduling on the grounds that it does not contribute directly to heightened self-awareness.

We do recognize, however, that the sets of data circumscribed by the strict behavioral and psychoanalytic models constitute categories of differing ontological status. It is a well-acknowledged fact that subjective reports are *about* mental events, feelings, and fantasies but are not the events, feelings, or fantasies themselves. Mental events, sensations, or feelings are private, to the extent that only the individual whose consciousness they shape has privileged access to them. Behaviors, on the other hand, are in a sense their own report and are therefore amenable to scientific description and confirmation by observation, measurement,

‡"Saving the phenomena" (*tithenai ta phainomena*) is a shorthand name for the philosophical argument that originated with the Greek philosophers between those who sought to ignore anomalous "facts" in favor of theoretical purity and those who sought to preserve the facts against an imposed theoretical distortion.

and quantification. And we recognize that these two categories of phenomena require two essentially different approaches, designed to effect two different ends.

Experimental psychologists can employ as a scientific strategy a necessarily restricted view of the "significant phenomena," i.e., of what there is that underlies rigorous scientific theory. But it is not the same for the phenomenological and operational underpinnings of clinical psychiatry; there *are* behaviors and there *are* feelings, dreams, fantasies, fears, ideas, and a collection of techniques for dealing with them that have not yet been conceptually integrated. To exclude any of these in order to preserve intact a favored ideal of methodological rigor is a luxury of scientific strategy that clinical psychiatry cannot properly afford.

* * *

The insight-seeking methodology of psychoanalytic psychotherapy and the change-producing techniques of behavior therapy form a complementary system; the former serves to uncover the early developmental learning experiences that shaped the later maladaptive and overgeneralized emotional/cognitive/behavioral habits, thereby providing therapeutically powerful counterinstances to the patient's prevailing faulty world view and self-evaluation.

REFERENCES

1. Birk L: Psychoanalytic omniscience and behavioral omnipotence: current trends in psychotherapy. *Seminars in Psychiatry* 4:113-120, 1972
2. Birk L, Stolz S, Brady JP, et al: Behavior Therapy in Psychiatry, Task Force Report no 5. Washington, DC, American Psychiatric Association, 1973
3. Glover E: *The Techniques of Psychoanalysis*. New York, International Universities Press, 1955, pp 261-350
4. Cushing JGN: Report of the committee on the evaluation of psychoanalytic therapy. *Bulletin of the American Psychoanalytic Association* 8:44-50, 1952
5. Tabachnick N: Research committee report on psychoanalytic practice. *The Academy* 17(1):3-5, 1973
6. Marmor J: The future of psychoanalytic therapy. *Am J Psychiatry* 130:1197-1202, 1973
7. Alexander F: The dynamics of psychotherapy in the light of learning theory. *Am J Psychiatry* 120:440-448, 1963 [See also Chapter 1, this volume.]
8. Wolf E: Learning theory and psychoanalysis. *Int J Psychiatry* 7:525-535, 1969 [See also Chapter 8, this volume.]
9. Porter R (ed): *The Role of Learning in Psychotherapy*. A Ciba Foundation Symposium. Boston, Little, Brown and Co, 1968
10. Aronson G: Learning theory and psychoanalytic theory. *J Am Psychoanal Assoc* 20:622-637, 1972
11. Marmor J: Dynamic psychotherapy and behavior therapy. *Arch Gen Psychiatry* 24:22-28, 1971 [See also Chapter 2, this volume.]
12. Sloane RB, Staples FR, Cristol AH, et al: *Psychotherapy versus Behavior Therapy*. Cambridge, Harvard University Press, 1975

13. Sloane RB: The converging paths of behavior therapy and psychotherapy. *Int J Psychiatry* 7:493-503, 1969 [See also Chapter 12, this volume.]
14. Crisp AJ: Transference, symptom emergence, and social repercussion in behavior therapy. *Br J Med Psychol* 39:179-196, 1966
15. Birk L: Behavior therapy: integration with dynamic psychiatry. *Behavior Therapy* 1:522-526, 1970 [See also Chapter 19, this volume.]
16. Feather BW, Rhoads JM: Psychodynamic behavior therapy. *Arch Gen Psychiatry* 26:503-511, 1972 [See also Chapter 21, this volume.]
17. Rhoads JM, Feather BW: Application of psychodynamics to behavior therapy. *Am J Psychiatry* 131:17-20, 1974
18. Birk L: Intensive group therapy: an effective behavioral-psychoanalytic method. *Am J Psychiatry* 131:11-16, 1974 [See also Chapter 23, this volume.]
19. Freud S: *An Outline of Psychoanalysis*. Translated by Strachey J. New York, WW Norton & Co, 1949
20. Freud S: The interpretation of dreams (1900), in *Complete Psychological Works*, standard ed, vols 4-5. Translated and edited by Strachey J. London, Hogarth Press, 1953
21. Fenichel O: *The Psychoanalytic Theory of Neurosis*. New York, WW Norton & Co, 1945
22. Nemiah J: Psychodynamic psychotherapy, in *Overview of Psychotherapies*. Edited by Usdin GL. New York, Brunner/Mazel, 1975, pp 36-50
23. Alexander F: *Psychoanalysis and Psychotherapy*. New York, WW Norton & Co, 1956
24. Krasner L: The therapist as a social reinforcement machine, in *Research in Psychotherapy*, vol 2. Edited by Strupp HH, Luborsky L. Washington, DC, American Psychological Association, 1962, pp 61-94
25. Beck A: Cognitive therapy: nature and relation to behavior therapy. *Behavior Therapy* 1:184-200, 1970
26. Stampfl TG, Lewis DJ: Essentials of implosive therapy: a learning-theory-based psychodynamic behavioral therapy. *J Abnorm Psychol* 72:496-503, 1967
27. Locke EA: Is "behavior therapy" behavioristic? (an analysis of Wolpe's psychotherapeutic methods). *Psychol Bull* 76:318-327, 1971
28. Birk L: Social reinforcement in psychotherapy. *Conditional Reflex* 3:116-123, 1968
29. Wolpe J: *Psychotherapy by Reciprocal Inhibition*. Stanford, Calif. Stanford University Press, 1958
30. Skinner BF: *The Behavior of Organisms*. New York, Appleton-Century, 1938
31. Skinner BF: *Science and Human Behavior*. New York, Macmillan Co, 1953
32. Krasner L: Behavior therapy. *Annu Rev Psychol* 22:483-532, 1971
33. Ferster CB: Clinical reinforcement. *Seminars in Psychiatry* 9:101-111, 1972
34. Ayllon T, Azrin NH: *The Token Economy*. New York, Appleton-Century-Crofts, 1968
35. Lindley OR, Skinner BF: A method for the experimental analysis of behavior of psychotic patients. *Am Psychol* 9:419-420, 1954
36. Ferster CB, DeMyer MK: The development of performances in autistic children in an automatically controlled environment. *J Chron Dis* 13:312-345, 1961
37. Harris FR, Johnston MK, Kelley CS, et al: Effects of positive social reinforcement on regressed crawling of a nursery school child. *J Educ Psychol* 55:35-41, 1964
38. Allen KE, Hart BM, Buell JS, et al: Effects of social reinforcement on isolate behavior of a nursery school child. *Child Dev* 35:511-518, 1964
39. Ayllon T, Azrin N: The measurement and reinforcement of behavior of psychotics. *J Exp Anal Behav* 8:357-383, 1965
40. Baer DM, Wolf MM: The reinforcement contingency in pre-school and remedial education, in *Early Education*. Edited by Hess RD, Bear RM. Chicago, Aldine, 1968, pp 119-129
41. Shapiro D, Birk L: Group therapy in experimental perspective. *Int J Group Psychother* 17:211-224, 1967

42. Liberman RP, Raskin DE: Depression: a behavioral formulation. *Arch Gen Psychiatry* 24:515-523, 1971
43. Knight RP: Introjection, projection, and identification. *Psychoanal Q* 9:334-341, 1940
44. Koff RH: A definition of identification: a review of the literature. *Int J Psychoanal* 42:362-370, 1961
45. Bandura A, Walters RH: *Social Learning and Personality Development*. New York, Holt, Rinehart & Winston, 1963
46. Marmor J: *Modern Psychoanalysis: New Directives and Perspectives*. New York, Basic Books, 1968
47. Birk L (ed): *Biofeedback: Behavioral Medicine*. New York, Grune and Stratton, 1973
48. Ferster CB: A functional analysis of depression. *Am Psychol* 28:857-870, 1973
49. Seligman MEP: Depression and learned helplessness, in *The Psychology of Depression*. Edited by Friedman RJ, Katz MM. Washington, DC, Winston-Wiley, 1974, pp 83-113
50. Miller NE: Interactions between learned and physical factors in mental illness, in *Biofeedback and Self-Control*, 1972. Edited by Shapiro D, Barber TX, DiCara LV, et al. Chicago, Aldine, 1973, pp 460-476
51. Suomi SJ, Harlow HF, McKinney WT Jr: Monkey psychiatrists. *Am J Psychiatry* 128:927-932, 1972
52. Lewinsohn PM, Weinstein MS, Shaw DA: Depression: a clinical research approach, in *Advances in Behavior Therapy*, 1968. Edited by Rubin R, Franks C. New York, Academic Press, 1969, pp 231-240
53. Lewinsohn PM: The behavioral study and treatment of depression, in *Progress in Behavior Modification*, vol 1. Edited by Hersen M, Eisler RM, Miller PM. New York, Academic Press, 1975, pp 19-64
54. Freud S: Mourning and melancholia (1917), in *Complete Psychological Works*, standard ed, vol 14. Translated and edited by Strachey J. London, Hogarth Press, 1957, pp 243-259
55. Van Lawick-Goodall J: *In the Shadow of Man*. Boston, Houghton Mifflin Co, 1971
56. Lindemann E: Symptomatology and management of acute grief. *Am J Psychiatry* 101:141-153, 1944
57. Dollard J, Miller NE: *Personality and Psychotherapy*. New York, McGraw-Hill Book Co, 1950
58. Birk L: Psychoanalysis and behavioral analysis: natural resonance and complementarity. *Int J Psychiatry* 11:160-166, 1973

Common Ground between Behavior Therapy and Psychodynamic Methods

10

ISAAC M. MARKS, M.D., D.P.M., F.R.C. PSYCH.,
AND MICHAEL G. GELDER, M.D.

This elegant and classic paper by two nonanalyst psychiatrists was one of the earliest to plead for mutual understanding between the warring camps of behavioral therapy and dynamic psychotherapy. Building their thesis logically and step by step, the authors discuss both the similarities and the differences between the two approaches with clarity and objectivity. They debunk some of the exaggerated claims of many behavioral therapists but, at the same time, point out the comparable limitations of psychodynamic psychotherapy. They correctly point out that for certain types of clinical problems one approach may be superior to the other and that for others a combination of both therapies may be indicated. They illustrate not only how different symptoms can have different meanings, but also how the same symptoms, e.g., anxiety, can result from either limited situational factors or deep-seated personality problems, or even somatic pathology. Similarly, phobias may range from simple, easily desensitized ones to extremely complex ones for which behavioral techniques alone are totally unavailing without benefit of prior or concomitant dynamic psychotherapy. Thus, far from being mutually contradictory, behavior and psychodynamic therapies are seen as complementary.

Common Ground between Behavior Therapy and Psychodynamic Methods

Isaac M. Marks, M.D., D.P.M., F.R.C. Psych., and Michael G. Gelder, M.D.

> *There are numerous parallels between the approach to the problem of personality taken by the learning theorist and that of the psychoanalyst (Kimble, 1961).*

> *Behaviour therapy is derived from the rejection of traditional psychodynamic theories and consists of the application of the principles of modern learning theory to the treatment of behaviour disorders (Grossberg, 1964).*

Introduction

These apparently contradictory quotations exemplify the diverse opinions which are held about psychodynamic and behavior therapies. We shall argue that such differences can be reconciled: common ground does exist, but at other points behavior therapy parts company from psychodynamic therapy. If the points of similarity and difference are examined carefully it becomes clear that each method and theory can contribute to the practice of psychiatry.

Psychological theory should be a pliant servant, not a rigid master. It might be argued that one cannot choose a theory where it fits most economically, and discard it where it does not. This is only true where the theoretical system is a set of tightly dependent constructs, as in some mathematical models. Even in physics the dispute about the wave and particle theories of light was only resolved when both theories were partially vindicated by experiments which showed that under some condi-

Reprinted from *British Journal of Medical Psychology*, 39:11-23, 1966, by permission of Cambridge University Press.

tions light can more usefully be treated as a wave form, but under other conditions it is more useful to regard it as particulate; neither theory alone explained all the relevant phenomena. Psychological and particularly psychoanalytic theories are loosely constructed, and can only be tested adequately part by part, as Farrell (1951) and Kardiner, Karush, and Ovesey (1959) have shown. There is movement now toward reconciling behavioral and psychodynamic theories and methods, though extremists on either side still oppose this.

Throughout this paper we shall mainly emphasize points of similarity between the two methods. There are, however, certain important differences in the aims of the therapists who now use each treatment and these must be recognized at the beginning. Behavior therapists pursue more limited therapeutic aims, being mainly concerned with symptomatic relief, while psychotherapists often attempt a more fundamental reorganization of personality, and concern themselves with the patient's problems in a wide sense. However, we shall argue that behavior therapy can be used in the context of a wider concern with patients' difficulties although this is not always done at present.

When extravagant claims are made for a new method, there is a danger that the good it contains may be lost when its extravagances are uncovered. Mesmerism was a case in point: in 1779 an eminent commission demonstrated the lack of factual basis for Mesmer's theory of animal magnetism; in 1840 another commission pronounced unfavorably on it, but both missed the importance of the hypnotic state as a phenomenon worthy of study. The same caution applies to the assessment of psychological treatments today.

The two methods will now be compared, taking in turn historical antecedents, theory, practical procedures, and claims to success. It will not be possible to cover the whole field; instead the main points of common and disputed ground will be selected, drawing on clinical experience of the two therapies in several neurotic syndromes.

HISTORICAL ANTECEDENTS

Ideas often have mixed pedigrees. It is often difficult to decide whether particular behavioral or psychotherapeutic methods are direct applications of learning or psychodynamic theory, respectively, or whether they originate elsewhere.

Behavior Therapy

This single term covers a wide variety of techniques for which a basis in learning theory is claimed and which attempt to remove symptoms directly or shape new items of behavior by operant conditioning. However, the idea of symptomatic treatment of tics, hysterical paralyses, and other disorders by exercises was much discussed by

French writers at the turn of the century under the name of reeducation (Meige and Feindel, 1907; Janet, 1925) and even earlier attempts to treat writer's cramp in such ways were noted by Poore in 1878. None of these writers was directly influenced by experimental psychology, but the ideas and methods foreshadowed later attempts to manipulate symptoms and were applied to just those conditions for which behavior therapy is now advocated. With the advent of behaviorism, this idea of reeducation gained a theoretical basis and developed more systematically, as in the classical production of a phobia by Watson and Rayner in 1920, and its relief by Cover Jones (1924a,b). Educational writings of the same period were imbued with similar ideas about the treatment of children's fears (Burnham, 1925; Jersild and Holmes, 1935). Freud (1919) himself advocated that phobias should be faced directly as an adjuvant to analytic therapy, though he did not call this reeducation. Pavlov's inquiries into the simplest form of learning—conditioning—caused an enthusiastic extrapolation of his ideas to distantly related phenomena, thus drawing the stricture of McDougall (1923) that "the young student of psychology swears by 'conditioned reflexes,' and is apt to regard the term as the key to most of the riddles of the universe, or at least as the master key of human fate." Both Herzberg (1941) and Leonhard (1963) advocated the use of graduated tasks in treatment without recourse to learning theory. Today's writings on behavior therapy commonly claim a basis in the work of Pavlov and Watson.

Psychodynamic Methods

Psychodynamic methods set out to help patients develop new ways of coping with problems of living in a wide sense. They try to do this by exploring feelings and interpersonal relationships; in so doing they hope to modify presenting symptoms indirectly, but this is often not the primary goal of treatment. These methods are widely known and need not be discussed in detail here. They claim origin in psychodynamic theory which emphasizes motives and drives and most often spring from the work of Freud and other analysts. As with behavior therapy, however, the ancestry can sometimes be seen to be mixed. There have been many methods of psychological healing in different societies through the ages. Toward the end of the nineteenth century interest mounted first in hypnotism and then in other types of psychological healing, as evidenced by the work of Liebault, Bernheim, and Dubois, and the systematic studies of Janet, Freud, Jung, and others. This expanded rapidly with the advent of the various psychoanalytic movements from about 1910. It is perhaps significant that at the same time as McDougall berated uncritical adoption of conditioning as an all-embracing explanatory principle, others made equally sweeping claims for psychodynamic theory and practice.

That both enthusiasms arose about the same time suggests that common elements in the contemporary climate nurtured them, perhaps a desire to repeat the successes of the physical sciences in psychology, · which had then but recently become scientific.

Mutual Influences

As they developed concurrently, both approaches naturally influenced one another, e.g., experimental neuroses were produced in animals and these served as models for certain psychopathological phenomena (Massermann, 1943; Liddell, 1958; Gantt, 1944). Many writers tried to synthesize the languages of conditioning and psychodynamics. One of the earliest attempts at translating psychoanalytic ideas into learning theory was made by Watson (1916): "The central truth that I think Freud has given us is that youthful, outgrown and partly discarded habit and instinctive systems of reaction can and possibly always do influence the functioning of our adult systems of reactions, and influence to a certain extent even the possibility of our forming the new habit systems which we must reasonably be expected to form." Other early attempts at synthesis were made by Schilder (1929), French (1933), and Kubie (1934), while later extensive links were forged by Dollard and Miller (1950), Mowrer (1950), Shoben (1949), and Hilgard and Marquis (1940), all of whom found many phenomena from clinic and laboratory which could be usefully equated. These workers smoothed the path to a fruitful common language. An apparent rivalry only developed in the 1950s when certain writers (Eysenck, 1960, 1964; Wolpe, 1958) propounded therapeutic techniques apparently derived from learning theory and allegedly suitable for all forms of neurosis. The notion that "neuroses are nothing but learned faulty habits" was put forward with the same vigor with which an earlier generation had asserted that neuroses were nothing but the result of repressed conflicts. Simultaneously, these later writers derided psychodynamic treatments in a manner reminiscent of Dubois when he repudiated Bernheim's method of suggestion as being entirely unrelated to his own "moral" treatment, or a little later, of Freud's rejection of Jung and Adler. More recently, however, an increasing volume of opinion (e.g., Kimble, 1961; Piers and Piers, 1964; Abell and Cowan, 1964; Wolf, 1964) again stresses that advocates of both methods often say and do the same thing in a different language, and have given detailed examples.

In the following section we shall examine the theory and practice of each approach separately, and try to define where the two outlooks seem to stand on common ground, and where there are genuine differences.

THEORETICAL CONSIDERATIONS

Introduction

Needless to say, there is no one body of learning or psychodynamic theory; each consists of many streams of thought which mingle and diverge; nevertheless, brevity requires us to write of each as a unity.

The literature on behavior therapy usually stresses the differences between learning and psychodynamic theories. We shall argue that these have been exaggerated, but that one difference is clear: learning theories start with simple phenomena and try to build an explanation of complex behavior from them; psychodynamic theory starts with complex behavior and tries to analyze it into simpler components. It is not surprising, given the present incomplete development of both learning and psychodynamic theory, that learning theories are not always successful in explaining clinical phenomena because these are far removed from the observations on which they were originally based, while psychodynamic theory, which started from clinical observations, is often more useful. Of course, there is always a gap between events inside and outside the laboratory, but experimental models are most useful when this gap is small.

Simple and Complex Learning

How far can complicated neurotic syndromes be explained as the sum total of many conditioned responses, and how far must entirely new principles of learning be invoked? Or does learning per se play only an unimportant part in these disturbances?

Few would doubt the value of laboratory studies of learning. What can be questioned is their relevance to species other than those originally investigated, to learning in a free environment rather than in the laboratory, and to learning complicated as well as simple behavior. These doubts are not restricted to psychiatrists; Kanfer, a clinical psychologist, wrote (1965): "I doubt if much of our rat psychology is applicable even to the field mouse, much less to the adult human . . . the detailed findings simply do not fit the complexity of the uncontrolled everyday environment." Hilgard and Marquis (1940) discuss the same point and conclude that for the time being all that is possible is to attempt the explanation of complex phenomena in simpler terms, knowing that the resulting explanations will be incomplete and imperfect.

This is an important reservation for the psychiatrist who must understand patients' behavior now, and cannot wait for experimentally validated findings to appear, however much he may prefer these in principle. Current learning theories are incomplete and it is often necessary to draw on diverse theories to explain clinical phenomena.

Which Learning Principles?

If it is accepted that it is useful to build complex behavior from simple principles, we must decide which of the many principles of learning to employ. Several attempts have been made to use the laws of simple learning to explain complex behavior. Hull's theory was the basis of an ambitious attempt by Dollard and Miller (1950), but there were wide gaps of knowledge to fill between experimental learning and social behavior. As Metzner (1961) points out, use of the terms *stimulus* and *response* can lend a spurious precision to the description of clinical phenomena because it is seldom possible to define the stimulus and the response in unambiguous terms. To explain complex behavior a more general theory is required which considers how series of stimuli and responses are organized. Skinner's ambitious attempt to explain human language was sharply criticized by Chomsky (1959) because in trying to solve this problem, unsubstantiated assumptions passed for valid generalization from laboratory experiment. A related difficulty is to explain events between stimulus and response in complex behavior. Pavlov adopted the idea of the "second signaling system," Osgood developed the concept of mediating responses, while Skinner simply ignored this problem in his theorizing.

As will be seen, some psychologists have recognized the difficulty of explaining complicated behavior in terms of simple laws of learning and have turned, as psychodynamic investigators did, to a direct analysis of complicated behavior, starting in this case not with neuroses but with the social behavior of children. Bandura's (1946) work on modeling and on the learning of aggression in children exemplifies this. It is intrinsically probable that this kind of approach will yield results more relevant to clinical problems than the results of laboratory experiments with rats.

Explanations of Neurotic Behavior and Psychotherapy

Attempts to use conditioning principles in psychiatry go back at least to Watson's 1916 paper already cited. However, these early attempts too often draw loose analogies between laboratory and clinical events, without forging any convincing detailed links between the two sets of phenomena. Freudian concepts were already in the minds of many early behaviorists when they formulated their theories and some, of course, derive from much earlier philosophical systems, e.g., the terms *pleasure principle* and *positive reinforcement* both express an idea which has origin in the earlier idea of hedonism.

As time went on, more sophisticated language was developed which was capable of describing psychotherapeutic events in greater detail. The contributions of Dollard and Miller, Mowrer, Hilgard and Marquis, and others have been mentioned. It is these which provide the greatest common ground between learning theorists and psychodynamicists, especially in the description of psychotherapeutic transactions. Recent authors go beyond the mere analogizing of the earlier "translators" in that they can describe and predict certain clinical events with more economy and detail. Watson himself recognized that primitive psychological concepts hindered the development of psychodynamics, and laid responsibility for this at the door of the developing psychology of the time. Since then, psychologists have successfully produced better concepts to fit psychotherapeutic data, to the extent that Franz Alexander (1963) wrote that "we are witnessing the beginning of the most promising integration of psychoanalytic theory with learning theory, which may lead to unpredictable advances in the theory and practice of the psychotherapies."

A few examples can be given. Kimble (1961) noted that psychoanalytic and learning theories are similar in several ways: both are historical in orientation, and assume that present behavior is the result of past experience; primary process thinking can be construed as classical conditioning, and secondary process thinking as instrumental conditioning; finally, theoretical concepts such as unconscious motivation, transference, primary and secondary gain, working through past conflicts, could be translated respectively into the language of drives (innate and acquired), stimulus generalization, reward by anxiety reduction, relearning during therapy. Kanfer (1961) viewed change in psychotherapy as a two-stage learning process in which initial change in perceptions is followed by the development of new habits in the proving ground of psychotherapy interviews. He construed that "pushing back the boundaries of the unconscious" described that process in which the range of private experience which became accessible to analysis was extended as important overt responses were reported to the therapist and reinforced directly.

The Two Languages in Practice

Applying such ideas in practice, Abell and Cowan (1964) describe, as an example of instrumental conditioning, the treatment of a woman with social anxiety who felt that people did not like her. When the patient spoke of this the therapist related it to her rejecting behavior which was an anticipation of being rejected herself. As the patient became aware of her own responses first as thoughts (covert behavior) and then in action, verbal labeling helped her to learn to change her maladaptive responses. The patient learned that some responses were inaccurate generalizations from past situations, and could modify them more appropriately to suit present contingencies, a process which can also be called insight. As she made friendly overtures outside therapy and was warmly received, these became reinforced. Abell and Cowan reported that it was possible to predict such changes in a series of patients and to demonstrate them in life situations.

This type of language derived from learning theory is useful to describe certain events in psychotherapy. It could in part be paraphrased into psychoanalytic language by talking of the patient reliving traumatic past experiences during therapy, projecting the derivatives of now unconscious conflicts onto the therapist, who then points out this distortion (transference or parataxis) and enables the patient to develop new modes of conduct freed from these restricting distortions. Either language can be applied to some extent, and there need be no quarrel between them, though they are not completely equivalent. Jones (1964) has shown this, comparing the dynamic concept of repression and the behavioral concept of avoidance learning: in Freudian theory there is an active force which energetically thrusts the idea out of the field of consciousness into which it constantly struggles to return; in behavioral theory repression is merely avoidance of danger signals. Such differences cannot be swept aside; awareness of them can lead in time to testing against clinical data, selection of more accurate and economical concepts, and eventually to greater synthesis. This has been done in limited fashion, for example, with the role of aggression in formation of obsessive symptoms (Marks, 1965).

Sources of Disagreement

There are several sources of disagreement. First, each body of theory explains some events, but not others. Learning theory accounts for the course of some simple phobias more economically than psychodynamic formulations, but it cannot yet usefully explain, say, depressive symptoms. Psychodynamic theory in turn accounts better, for example, for morbid grief reactions. Selected clinical findings can thus be used to support either theory. At their present stage of development both theories have uses, but neither can explain all clinical events; approaches related neither to learning nor to psychodynamic theory must also be used at times.

Secondly, it follows that there are no global tests to decide the better theory; each must be tested against discrete clinical problems. The fact that for a given problem one theory is better does not necessarily mean that the second theory is not superior for other problems.

Thirdly, even with discrete problems, crucial tests are hard to devise because the two theories sometimes make the same predictions. As Berlyne (1964) has pointed out, there is often considerable overlap in the consequences deducible from different psychological theories, and given events may fit several theories equally well; deciding which theory to accept then becomes rather arbitrary.

Theoretical Problems in Relation to Phobias

As we have pointed out, psychodynamic theories arose to explain complex disorders in humans; learning theories focused on simple learning and often derived from animal experiments. This fact makes the results of our own studies of the treatment of phobias more understandable.

Our results (Marks and Gelder, 1965; Cooper, Gelder, and Marks, 1965) show that behavior therapy produces good short-term results in the simplest phobias (e.g., fears of cats, birds, or feathers). Although the group of patients as a whole relapsed partially during follow-up, some individuals remained well even though no conflicts had been dealt with and no transference interpretations had been made. The findings were compatible with the view that these phobias were faulty habits. However, patients with severe agoraphobia who had many other complicated problems and who were treated as inpatients were not helped more by behavior therapy than by control treatments (Gelder and Marks, 1966). Treating these patients' phobias as simple learned habits was not particularly successful. On the other hand, when outpatients with less severe agoraphobia were treated with behavior therapy they improved symptomatically more than matched controls receiving psychodynamic psychotherapy either individually or in a group (Gelder, Marks, Sakinofsky, and Wolff, 1964). Fresh symptoms have not appeared in the symptomatically improved patients any more frequently than in the others. Again, learning theory was useful when the condition was less complicated. The only variables so far found to predict outcome are: first, the *type* of symptom—circumscribed phobias dating back to early childhood have done relatively well with behavior therapy, severe agoraphobia less well, compulsive rituals and writer's cramp least well of all; secondly, the *number* of symptoms—the more symptoms a phobic patient reports, the worse the outcome with behavior therapy. Thus in a restricted group of patients, a treatment can ignore underlying emotional factors, yet prove successful.

In other patients, however, emotional factors are obviously important and these are formulated better in psychodynamic than in learning theories. One woman developed her first symptoms when she rode on a bus to visit her rejected son dying in the hospital. During treatment a temporary remission of the phobias started after she had expressed her guilt about his death. However, she then relapsed and subsequently continued to ventilate her guilt without effect on the phobias, the guilt subsiding only when the anniversary of her son's death had passed. Clearly, the expression of emotion influenced the course of the patient's phobias, whether or not emotional conflict caused them in the first place.

Another case lends itself to both a learning theory and a psychodynamic explanation. A woman receiving behavior therapy for agoraphobia improved slightly at first, and was also less frigid. Her husband then resumed sexual relations, but when he fondled her breasts she felt sud-

den violent anxiety, with a fantasy of her father standing over her fondling her breasts when she was young. Concurrently, her agoraphobia
became much worse. Psychotherapists might argue that sexual conflicts
lay behind the phobias: learning theorists could argue that any factor
raising general anxiety would make the phobias worse, but does so regardless of the original cause of the phobia.

So far, only learning and psychodynamic points of view have been
considered, but there may be other factors influencing the course of
phobias. For example, Roth (1959) has suggested that disturbances in
temporal lobe function occur in some phobic anxiety states in which depersonalization is prominent.

The Varying Significance of Symptoms

Psychoanalytic theories assume that symptoms are rooted in the
development of the total personality, and therefore regard symptomatic
treatment which does not deal with presumed underlying "conflict" or
"neurosis" as superficial and likely to result in symptom substitution.
By contrast, learning theories assume that symptoms are maladjustive
habits which simply require unlearning or relearning. The consequences
of this view are that symptomatic treatment should suffice, and that
complex personality problems will be largely irrelevant to treatment of
the presenting symptoms.

The assumptions of both viewpoints require examination. The term
symptom covers many phenomena and different symptoms can have different origins. In a patient complaining of dyspnoea due to a pneumo-
thorax we do not ascribe this symptom to personality problems; in a
patient whose repeated depressions follow a trail of broken marriages
we are bound to see the symptom as part of a personality disturbance.
Somewhere between these two extremes lies an area where the significance of symptoms is unclear. It is in this area that disputes arise. If we
assume that *all* symptoms seen by a psychiatrist must have a bias in
disturbance of the total personality we can get into serious difficulties—an acute confusional state due to profound hypoglycemia is an obvious example where the psychiatrist needs to be aware that symptoms
can be largely irrelevant to personality difficulties. Serious difficulties
also arise if a child's aggressive behavior due to parental rejection is erroneously misread as pointing to temporal lobe epilepsy. Incorrect
treatment can result if either viewpoint is carried too far.

Equally the same symptom can have varying significance both in
general medicine and in psychiatry. Sunburn can be due to excessive
exposure—an isolated symptom, or due to drug sensitivity—a more
widespread condition, or due to one kind of porphyria—an underlying
disorder we can usefully call a disease. Anxiety may result simply from

an impending crucial examination, or be a sign of a phaeochromocy-toma, or result from underlying conflicts in a personality disorder. Any symptom the patient presents to the psychiatrist can variably result from simple or complex causes, and this spectrum of causation must be in the therapist's mind. Looking exclusively at one or other narrow band of this broad spectrum inevitably leads to misleading emphasis in certain cases.

Just as *all* medical symptoms are not the result of underlying disease, so also phobias, and other psychiatric symptoms have varying significance. This is exemplified by, for example, Fish's (1964) division of phobias into: (a) those which are conditioned or learned, e.g., fears of mice or frogs learned because a parent had a similar fear; (b) hysterical phobias which are unconsciously motivated, e.g., fears of going out alone; and (c) obsessional phobias.

Learning theory accounts fairly well for simple phobias, and for these behavior therapy is useful. However, learning theory accounts much less adequately for the phenomena of severe agoraphobia, and behavior therapy is of limited value. Learning theory, using ideas of stimulus generalization, sometimes explains how fears spread and recede, but does not clearly explain the onset of agoraphobia, nor the presence of other symptoms such as general anxiety, depression, depersonalization, obsessions, or frigidity. Similarly, psychodynamic theory cannot explain all the phenomena met in phobic patients, and leaves unanswered some of the same problems left by learning theory. Thus certain features can be explained by either theory, others better by one than by the other, and yet others remain unexplained by either.

In neither therapy does practice always follow closely from theory, and greater theoretical knowledge may not lead to better results. We analyzed results of behavior therapy in agoraphobia and simpler phobias (Marks and Gelder, 1965). The greater knowledge of learning theory possessed by staff psychologists apparently led to no better therapeutic results than those obtained by other therapists. This brings to mind Strupp's question (1960): "Is the expert psychotherapist more 'successful' than the novice? This . . . has not been answered to anyone's satisfaction." Thus knowledge of theory is not necessarily a major determinant of success in psychological treatments. This is not surprising when we know that theories are not yet adequate to describe events either in the disorders or in their treatment.

COMMON GROUND IN PRACTICE

Alexander (1963) commented of psychotherapy that "it is generally suspected that authors' accounts about their theoretical views do not

precisely reflect what they are actually doing when treating patients."
Our practical experience of behavior therapy has convinced us that in
this treatment also, practice does not always follow directly from theory.

Features Common to Both Behavior and Psychodynamic Methods

As we have seen, the main common feature of behavior therapies is
that all attempt direct modification of symptoms, unlike psychodynamic
therapies, which aim only indirectly at symptom relief, their emphasis
rather being on modification of feelings, motivation, and interpersonal
adjustment. Granted this, the two methods have several elements in
common (see Table 1). Both use advice and encouragement to some extent: in the more intensive psychotherapies this is restricted; in behavior
therapy the patient inevitably receives advice about everyday problems
as well as the specific advice about the most effective way of meeting his
fears. Symptoms are naturally discussed much more in behavior
therapy, and the therapist inevitably conveys an expectation of improvement to the patient.

Environmental manipulation also plays a definite part in behavior
therapy as it does in the briefer psychotherapies. In both, patients are
encouraged to recognize current sources of stress and repetitive patterns
of behavior. The behavior therapist will often point to stressful interpersonal relationships as well as responses conditioned to other sources of
anxiety. Wolpe (1958), for example, repeatedly mentions the importance
of interpersonal anxiety. Discussing the practice of behavior therapy,
Beech (1963) has noted that patients are often oblivious to important
motivations underlying their symptoms, citing a case whose writer's
cramp was aggravated in the presence of authoritarian figures—this was
only evident after interviews and tests.

Psychotherapists emphasize correct timing of graduated interpretations to prevent patients experiencing excessive anxiety; this is very
similar to behavior therapists gradually presenting anxiety-laden stimuli
during desensitization.

Features Peculiar to Each Approach

There are some psychotherapeutic methods which are seldom if
ever utilized in behavior therapies. Patients are not encouraged to recall
repressed memories; dreams are not analyzed, symbolic meanings or
unrecognized feelings never pointed out; the patient is not encouraged
to develop an intense emotional relationship with the therapist, and
what feelings he does develop are not analyzed.

Next there are techniques which are characteristic of behavior
therapy. The most important of these is the use of a graded series of
situations which provoke anxiety either in fact or in fantasy—the so-

TABLE 1. *Components in Psychological Treatments*

A. *Present in most treatments, including some psychodynamic methods*
  (i) "Nonspecific":   1. Placebo
                        2. Patient expectations
                        3. Suggestion
  (ii) More specific: 1. Encouragement, advice and reassurance
                        2. Environmental manipulation
                        3. Pointing out current sources of stress
                        4. Pointing out repetitive patterns of behavior

B. *Present in most psychodynamic methods, but not usually important in behavior therapy*
  1. Pointing out unrecognized feelings
  2. Understanding relationship with therapist
  3. Encouraging expression of feeling about therapist   } includes analysis of transference
  4. Relating present behavior to past patterns
  5. Interpreting fantasy and dream material
  6. Pointing out symbolic meanings
  7. Attempting modification of present personality

C. *Present in behavior therapies but not usually in psychodynamic methods*
  1. Emphasis on direct symptom modification
  2. Use of a hierarchy in practical retraining
  3. Use of a hierarchy in fantasy retraining
  4. Aversion techniques
  5. Positive conditioning
  6. Negative practice
  7. Other special techniques

D. *Present in several treatments, not necessarily psychodynamic*
  1. Relaxation and hypnosis
  2. Anxiety-reducing drugs
  3. Abreaction

called hierarchy. This hierarchy is used either for retraining in practice or for desensitization imagination during relaxation or hypnosis, as introduced by Wolpe. This method, systematic desensitization, is used mainly for phobias and is not exclusive to behavior therapy, because a somewhat similar method was used by Herzberg (1941) in his psychotherapy by graduated tasks. Wolpe's technique involves relaxation or hypnosis, and inevitably contains suggestion. It is important to recognize the role of this relaxation, hypnosis, and suggestion; how much desensitization contributes over and above this has yet to be determined, though in asthmatics Moore (1965) has shown that desensitization increases improvement in peak respiratory flow beyond that contributed by relaxation and hypnotic suggestion. Wolpe's emphasis on dealing with sources of interpersonal anxiety naturally overlaps considerably with other psychotherapeutic techniques.

Next most frequently used are aversion techniques, e.g., the use of electric shock or emetine in sexual and other disorders. These have very little in common with psychodynamic methods, but can still have their dynamic significance, as Pearce (1964) points out. Patients' relationships to therapists change during aversion, and they can enter a negative phase of resentment with depression. One shoe fetishist said, "I feel as though when this is taken from me there will be a big hole left inside me." Another patient of ours found it temporarily difficult to cooperate with her therapist as he stirred up feelings of antagonism she had earlier experienced toward her stepfather. These phenomena require recognition, even though they may be peripheral to the effective therapeutic events.

Lastly, positive conditioning in the treatment of enuresis by bell and pad, negative practice in the treatment of tics, and operant conditioning, as used in shaping small items of behavior in schizophrenics, all share little with psychodynamic methods.

The Role of Patient–Therapist Relationships

A multitude of clinical observations attest that important relationships develop between patient and therapist as behavior therapy progresses, just as they do in any prolonged treatment. The question is, how far do these contribute to the result of treatment?

Some evidence for this was obtained in our study of behavior therapy for severe agoraphobia (Marks and Gelder, 1965). With both behavior therapy and control treatments, those patients who were seen four or five times weekly showed more improvement than patients who were only seen once or twice weekly. In the behavior therapy group this finding might suggest that increased frequency of treatment provided more opportunities for deconditioning. However, as this was also found with controls, it seems that frequent contact with the therapist can also be helpful, and is one of many factors at work in behavior therapy. In a larger study of 77 patients who received behavior therapy (Cooper et al., 1965), we found that most patients were cooperative and had confidence in their therapists. This is a natural asset in any form of medical treatment, and it was not necessary to analyze such feelings to effect improvement. Intense feelings toward therapists did develop in seven patients, but these did not usually hinder therapy, nor were they obviously associated with the improvement obtained.

Conclusions

We have given examples to show that common ground exists first in that the patients' behavior in psychodynamic therapy can often be described equally well in the language of psychodynamics or of learning theory, which to some extent run parallel and have at times been united. Secondly, that the interview techniques of the psychodynamic therapist can be described in the same way. Thirdly, that certain aspects of the practice of behavior therapies contain elements also present in psychodynamic methods: placebo effects, suggestion, patients' expectations, encouragement, advice and reassurance, environmental manipulation, and the unraveling of current sources of stress, including repetitive patterns of behavior.

Different behavior therapies vary in the amount they have in common with psychodynamic methods—thus, desensitization in imagination overlaps considerably, especially when attention is paid to interpersonal anxieties, whereas positive conditioning for enuresis or aversion for homosexuality have little in common with other psychotherapies.

It is, however, important also to recognize the real differences of the two approaches in practice; a behavior therapist treating a patient for simple phobias does not ask him to associate or talk about most of his feelings, but instead concentrates on relaxing him and habituating him, actively but gradually, to the feared stimuli. Similarly, with enuresis the behavior therapist is concerned with the patient using the conditioning apparatus properly at home, and does not interview him at length after the history has been taken; feelings and motivations are peripheral to treatment in this instance. On the other hand, in a patient with prolonged depression following the death of the father no schedule of behavior therapy is easily applicable, and psychodynamic methods of encouraging the patient to talk about feelings for the parent are important for progress.

The two approaches can be complementary, not conflicting—some patients require the first approach, others the second, and yet others require a combined treatment. There are some pointers to the clinical indications for separate or combined treatment. We use both approaches in appropriate cases. Patients can be referred for behavior therapy when they have simple phobias, enuresis and reading disabilities where careful inquiry fails to show accompanying emotional disturbance, some cases of fetishism and transvestism, and clearly delineated problems suitable for a behavioral regime. Patients can be referred for psychodynamic psychotherapy when their difficulties appear to relate to unexpressed feelings and problems in interpersonal adjustment. A few patients can have both types of treatment when the problems require a combined approach. Psychotherapists can ask for their patients to have some behavior therapy as an adjunct, and vice versa.

Both approaches are here to stay, and it is to be hoped that each will develop. As Janet noted (1925), no one medical treatment can be expected to cure all medical complaints, rather we must seek to delineate the indications for and effect of each procedure. The same applies to psychological methods.

Summary

1. There are divergent opinions about the origins and status of psychodynamic and behavior therapies: some discern considerable common ground, others see them as mutually incompatible.

2. Behavior therapies aim at direct modification of symptoms, and claim a basis in learning theory, though their origins are in fact more complex. Psychodynamic methods aim at resolution of conflicts about feelings and interpersonal relationships, and only indirectly at symptom relief; they claim to spring from psychoanalytic theories but also have broader origins. Both approaches have influenced one another.

3. Learning theories start with simpler molecular items of behavior to explain complex behavior. Psychodynamic ideas start with complex molar behavior and analyze its components. Each is useful and necessary, and they have a common meeting point where the language of each can be translated into the other, especially in describing behavior during psychotherapy. Disagreements occur when theories are overgeneralized, and when the same data accord equally well with either approach.

4. Psychiatric symptoms, like medical ones, have varying significance. For example, simple phobias, can reasonably be described as faulty habits in the language of learning theories, and behavior therapy is useful for them. Others, however, e.g., most agoraphobias, are incompletely described by learning theories and for them behavior therapy has less value.

5. Practice does not always follow close on theory in either psychodynamic or behavior therapies. Some techniques are shared by the two therapies, others are peculiar to each. The amount of overlap and difference varies with particular methods under consideration.

6. Behavior and psychodynamic therapy are complementary, not conflicting. Certain disorders require the first, others the second, and yet others require a combined approach. Both can play a useful part in psychiatry.

Acknowledgments

We wish to thank Prof. Sir Aubrey Lewis for encouraging our work on behavior therapy; this was supported by a grant from the Medical

Research Council. Drs R. F. Hobson, M. Pines, H. H. Wolff, H. R. Beech, and S. Rachman kindly made helpful comments about the manuscript.

REFERENCES

Abell, R. G. and Cowan, J. (1964). The applications of modern learning theory to the psychoanalytic process. Paper given at *Learning Theory Symposium of 6th Int. Congr. Psychotherapy, London.*

Alexander, F. (1963). The dynamics of psychotherapy in the light of learning theory. *Amer. J. Psychiat.* 120, 440-8. [See also Chapter 1, this volume.]

Bandura, A. (1964). Behavioral modification through modelling procedures. In L. Krasner and L. P. Ullmann (eds.). *Research in Behaviour Modification.* London: Holt, Rinehart & Winston.

Beech, H. R. (1963). Some theoretical and technical difficulties in the application of behavior therapy. *Bull. Brit. Psychol. Soc.* 16, 25-33.

Berlyne, D. E. (1964). Emotional aspects of learning. In *Annual Review of Psychology,* vol. xv, pp. 115-42. (Ed. P. R. Farnsworth et al.)

Burnham, W. A. (1925). *The Normal Mind.* New York: Appleton.

Chomsky, N. (1959). Verbal behavior, by B. F. Skinner (a review). *Language,* 35, 26-58.

Cooper, J. E., Gelder, M. G. and Marks, I. M. (1965). Results of behavior therapy in 77 cases. *Brit. Med. J.* 1, 1222-5.

Dollard, J. and Miller, N. E. (1950). *Personality and Psychotherapy.* New York: McGraw-Hill.

Eysenck, H. J. (1960). *Behaviour Therapy and the Neuroses.* Oxford: Pergamon Press.

Eysenck, H. J. (1964). Psychotherapy or behavior therapy. *Ind. Psychol. Rev.* 1, 33-41.

Farrell, B. A. (1951). The scientific testing of psycho-analytic findings and theory. *Brit. J. Med. Psychol.* 24, 35-41.

Fish, F. J. (1964). *An Outline of Psychiatry.* Bristol: John Wright and Sons.

French, T. M. (1933). Interrelations between psychoanalysis and the experimental work of Pavlov. *Amer. J. Psychiat.* 89, 1165-203.

Freud, S. (1919). *Collected Papers, 2,* 392. London: Hogarth Press.

Gantt, W. H. (1944). *Experimental Basis for Neurotic Behaviour.* New York: Harper.

Gelder, M. G. and Marks, I. M. (1966). Severe agoraphobia. A controlled prospective trial of behavior therapy. *Brit J. Psychiat.* 112, 309-319.

Gelder, M. G., Marks, I. M., Sakinofsky, I. and Wolff, H. H. (1964). Behavior therapy and psychotherapy in phobic disorders: alternative or complementary procedures? Paper given at *Learning Theory Symposium of 6th Int. Congr. Psychotherapy, London.*

Grossberg, J. M. (1964). Behavior therapy: a review. *Psychol. Bull.* 62, 73-88.

Herzberg, A. (1941). Short treatment of neuroses by graduated tasks. *Brit. J. Med. Psychol.* 19, 19-36.

Hilgard, E. R. and Marquis, D. G. (1940). *Conditioning and Learning.* New York: Appleton-Century-Crofts.

Janet, P. (1925). *Psychological Healing,* vol. I. London: George Allen and Unwin.

Jersild, A. T. and Holmes, F. B. (1935). Children's fears. *J. Psychol.* 1, 75.

Jones, H. G. (1964). Basic principles of learning applied to behavior therapy. Paper given at *Learning Theory Symposium at 6th Int. Congr. Psychotherapy, London.*

Jones, M. C. (1924a). A laboratory study of fear: the case of Peter. *Ped. Sem.* 31, 308-15.

Jones, M. C. (1924b). The elimination of children's fears. *J. Exp. Psychol.* 7, 382-90.

Kanfer, F. H. (1961). Comments on learning in psychotherapy. *Psychol. Rep.* Monograph Supplement 6-V9, 681-699.

Kanfer, F. H. (1965): Vicarious Human Reinforcement: A glimpse into the Black Box. Chapter in L. Krasner and L. P. Ullmann (eds.). *Research in Behaviour Modification*. London: Holt, Rinehart & Winston.

Kimble, G. A. (1961). *Revised Version of Conditioning and Learning* (by Hilgard and Marquis), p. 473. London: Methuen.

Kardiner, A., Karush, A. and Ovesey, L. (1959). A methodological study of Freudian theory. *J. Nerv. Ment. Dis. 129*, 341-56.

Kubie, L. S. (1934). Relation of the conditioned reflex to psychoanalytic technique. *Arch. Neurol. Psychiat., 32*, 1137-42.

Leonhard, K. (1963). *Individualtherapie der Neurosen*. Jena: Gustav Fischer Verlag.

Liddell, H. (1958). History and prospects of the behavior farm laboratory at Cornell University. In W. H. Gantt (ed.): *Physiological Bases of Psychiatry*. Springfield: Charles C Thomas.

McDougall, W. (1923). *An Outline of Psychology*. London: Methuen.

Marks, I. M. (1965). Patterns of meaning in psychiatric patients. *Maudsley Monograph*, no. 13. Oxford University Press.

Marks, I. M. and Gelder, M. G. (1965). A controlled retrospective study of behavior therapy in phobic patients. *Brit. J. Psychiat. 111*, 561-73.

Massermann, J. H. (1943). *Behaviour and Neurosis*. Chicago: University Press.

Meige, H. and Feindel, E. (1907). *Tics and Their Treatment*. London: S. Appleton.

Metzner, R. (1961). Learning theory and the therapy of neurosis. *Brit. J. Psychol. Monogr.* Suppl. no. 33.

Moore, N. (1965). Behavior therapy in bronchial asthma: a controlled study of some factors. Unpublished dissertation for D.P.M., University of London and Institute of Psychiatry libraries.

Mowrer, O. H. (1950). *Learning Theory and Personality Dynamics*. New York: Ronald Press.

Pearce, J. (1964). Aspects of transvestism. Unpublished M.D. thesis, University of London.

Piers, G. and Piers, M. W. (1964). Modes of learning and the analytic process. Paper given at the *Learning Theory Symposium of 6th Int. Congr. Psychotherapy, London*.

Poore, G. V. (1878). An analysis of 75 cases of "writer's cramp" and impaired writing power. *Med. Chir. Trans. 61*, 111-45.

Roth, M. (1959). The phobic-anxiety depersonalization syndrome. *Proc. Roy. Soc. Med. 52*, 587.

Schilder, P. (1929). Conditioned reflexes. Cited by French (1933).

Shoben, E. J. (1949). Psychotherapy as a problem in learning theory. *Psychol. Bull. 46*, 366-92.

Strupp, H. H. (1960). *Psychotherapists in Action*. New York: Grune and Stratton.

Watson, J. B. (1916). Behavior and the concept of mental disease. *J. Phil. Psychol. and Scientific Method, 13*, 589-97.

Watson, J. B. and Rayner, R. (1920). Conditioned emotional reactions *J. Exp. Psychol. 3*, 1-14.

Wolf, E. (1964). The sociodynamics of functional psychiatric disorders. Paper given at *1st Int. Congr. Soc., Psychiatry, London*.

Wolpe, J. (1958). *Psychotherapy by Reciprocal Inhibition*. Stanford University Press.

Transference and Resistance Observed in Behavior Therapy

11

JOHN M. RHOADS, M.D., AND
BEN W. FEATHER, M.D., PH.D.

In this brief clinical paper, Rhoads and Feather present evidence countering the often-expressed statements (particularly by Wolpe and his followers) that neither transference nor resistance is encountered in behavior therapy. The authors demonstrate in three short but cogent clinical vignettes that these reactions can and do occur in the course of a strictly behavioral treatment model, as defined by Wolpe. Even more importantly, in two additional vignettes they indicate how combining psychodynamic understanding of these reactions with behavioral techniques makes it possible to overcome both transference and resistance obstacles.

Transference and Resistance Observed in Behavior Therapy

JOHN M. RHOADS, M.D., AND
BEN W. FEATHER, M.D., PH.D.

In the course of making observations on the results of behavior therapy by a therapist-observer method, we encountered two special types of difficulty. In the cases reported here the difficulties interfered significantly with treatment. We believe these problems must be anticipated and dealt with if therapy is to succeed.

The difficulties are best described by the terms *transference* and *resistance*. We define transference as the transfer to the therapist of attitudes appropriate to other persons past or present in the patient's life, and inappropriate to the therapist. By resistance we mean the failure of the patient to adhere to the therapeutic regime, and his active and/or passive interference with treatment. Wolpe and Lazarus believe that resistance does not exist in behavior therapy, and state that these (concepts) represent "popular alibis" utilized by certain therapists when treatment does not succeed (1968, p. 21). They deny the alleged omnipotence of the behavior therapist, stating: "the grade of acquiescence required is the same as in any other branch of medicine or education" (p. 23). Of the doctor-patient relationship they say:

> It is of first importance to display empathy and establish a trustful relationship. The patient must feel fully accepted as a fellow human being. . . . It may be desirable to defer the use of specific counterconditioning procedures when there is reason to think that the patient needs to unburden himself or requires enlightenment or reassurance. . . . We take leave to chide fellow behavioral scientists who . . . imagine that one can do without such personal influencing processes. (pp. 23-29)

This latter statement seems to us a case of calling the problem something else. This seems particularly true when they state:

> it is . . . sometimes helpful to apprehend the origins and development of patients' maladaptive reactions, and to examine and correct faulty attitudes

Reprinted from *British Journal of Medical Psychology*, 45:99-103, 1972, by permission of Cambridge University Press.

and misperceptions . . . the correction of misconceptions is often a necessary
forerunner to effective desensitization. . . . The same applies to patients with
mistaken attitudes to society, to particular people, or to themselves. (pp.
130-131)

We regard this as advocating a form of interpretative and educational
therapy, and in spite of their disclaimer we believe they correctly noted
the presence of countermotivations in their patients and were shrewd
enough to act on them.

Weinberg and Zaslove (1963) report on three patients whom they
desensitized to phobias. They noted that their subjects exhibited what
they felt was best expressed by the term *resistance*. In their project the
subjects did this by "involuntary" manipulations of the imaginal process, by variations of their hypnotic state, and by failing to practice relaxation at home. One dreamed of being cured and of not having to come
to the research appointments. Another attempted to waste time by talking about events quite peripheral to his problem.

The plan of this study was that whichever of us carried out the initial evaluation referred the patient to the other for behavior therapy. The
initial psychiatrist continued to see the patient, about one visit per three
behavior therapy sessions, in order to evaluate the response to treatment. An effort was made by the first psychiatrist to offer only supportive comments, in an effort to avoid contaminating the experiment with
interpretations.

The patient's responses varied from enthusiastic compliance with
the therapeutic regimen to those we felt were best described as resistance and negative transference. When the patient accepted his role as
such, was motivated unambivalently to be rid of his burdensome symptoms, and followed the instructions of the therapist, treatment proceeded rapidly and successfully. In the following cases where the patient
had negative feelings with respect to the method of treatment or about
the therapist, or where the symptom served a current need, the treatment ran into the same difficulty that Freud encountered, namely, that
patients obstinately refused to be cured and threw all sorts of obstacles
in the path of treatment.

Case 1. A single woman graduate student in her 20s was referred for behavior therapy
because of acute and chronic anxiety which interfered significantly with her ability to function. It was difficult to determine when her illness began, since she had been able to
conceal her shyness and inhibitions from her friends and teachers for years. As an undergraduate she had been able to avoid ever having to do public speaking, and was able to
escape being observed while carrying out technical procedures. As a graduate student, she
was no longer able to do so, as her work called for her to teach undergraduates, to act as a
demonstrator in laboratory experiments, and to confer with students about experiments.
She also had sexual problems. Asexual until entering graduate school, she tried heterosexual relations and found them unsatisfying. At best she regarded men as self-centered
beasts; more commonly, as passive ineffectual creatures. The latter concept coincided
closely with the actual personality of her father. Discouraged, she tried the alternative, but

homosexual relationships were no more satisfactory. Psychoanalytically orientated psychotherapy several times a week for a year met with no success. She criticized the method as too passive, urging that something else be done. It was suggested that she try behavior therapy. The behavior therapist instructed her in Wolpe's systematic desensitization. Hierarchies were constructed for her fear of being observed while carrying out the laboratory procedures. She practiced relaxation in a desultory fashion. During her therapy sessions she refused to carry out the desensitization procedure. She developed an intense dislike of the therapist, and communicated to the observer her detestation of the therapist and "his authoritarian ways." She consumed most of the time allotted with debates and disputations. She argued that the method was no good, and that the behaviorist should be treating her with a psychoanalytic approach, forgetting that she had argued with her former therapist to the contrary.

Her anxiety and refusal to cooperate increased, and after five sessions she broke off treatment and refused to return. Based on her history and on short follow-up by the observer, her attitudes toward the behavior therapist coincided with one aspect of her feelings about her father and to men to whom she might have some sexual attraction. As a teen-ager she had fantasied meeting a man unlike her father who would be aggressive and forceful and who would make her a woman, a state concerning which she had considerable fear and doubt. When confronted with a therapist who insisted that she lie down, relax, and deal with her fantasies, she inappropriately equated him with the beast-man of her fantasies and ran from him.

Case 2. A young married woman was referred for treatment of frigidity. Though married almost two years, she and her husband had never overcome her aversion to sex, and the marriage remained unconsummated. When she appeared with her husband she was dressed in a dowdy fashion, used no makeup, and acted contemptuously toward him. In contrast, when she appeared for her first appointment with the behavior therapist she wore a colorful miniskirt, makeup, and acted very kittenish. Initially she filled the behavior therapy sessions with clamorous complaints about her husband. The therapist repeatedly had to interrupt her declamations in order to give her instructions in the method. By the third hour it was apparent that she had not practiced relaxation, was making little progress in constructing hierarchies, but was quite openly jealous of the doctor's female assistant. She repeatedly interrupted his instructions with remarks to the effect that he was good-looking, and feared that he might take advantage of her while she was hypnotized. No mention of hypnosis had been made, nor was any such procedure intended. It was never possible to construct hierarchies for desensitization. The erotic attraction to the behavior therapist continued unabated, and treatment ended when she refused to return after six sessions. These attitudes corresponded to her behavior toward her father. To the observer, she gave a history of having acted quite seductively toward him, while being contemptuous and jealous of her mother (whom her husband resembled physically). She could not understand "what my father ever saw in my mother—or why he ever married *her*." She had frequent violent arguments with her father, but was never able to give any reason for the fights. The observer noted that they came at times when she was closest to him—for example, when she went on a trip to Europe with him while her mother remained at home. We believe treatment foundered on the resistance to facing an unresolved Oedipus complex, complicated by an erotic transference to the behavior therapist.

Case 3. The patient was a 42-year-old married woman admitted to the hospital because of dirt and germ phobias and a housecleaning compulsion. She had consulted a psychiatrist eight years previously for these and was treated unsuccessfully for two years with analytically orientated psychotherapy. For two years prior to admission she had no social activities because it took her so long to get ready; it was not worth the trouble. She described her marriage as happy. Systematic desensitization was instituted with hierarchies being constructed for her dirt and germ phobias. Within a week she was free of this group of symptoms, but she now disclosed her serious marital problems. By means of her compulsions she had been able to keep them out of awareness, and had been able to live with the situation. Her husband was difficult to deal with. Seemingly compliant, he always found a way to sabotage therapy. The patient, until then a minimal social drinker, began to drink excessively, to the extent that two additional hospitalizations were required during the next two years. During the last of these, her husband took the marriage counseling seriously, and the patient stopped drinking. At the time of writing she has been "dry" for three months. The phobias and compulsion never returned after the initial desensitization.

While the desensitization enabled the patient to abandon the phobias and compulsions, it did not provide her with a means of coping with the marital difficulties. Nor did a positive, and at times maudlin, transference help her to effect any changes in her destructive method of dealing with her husband's obstinacy. We interpreted both symptoms as efforts to call for help, to force her husband to see her point, while avoiding a possibly marriage-ending confrontation. Thus her illnesses served as partial solutions to an ongoing problem. We regarded this case as an instance of symptom displacement; one coping device having been removed, the patient shifted her reliance to another, since the underlying problem continued unchanged. This is the only instance of symptom substitution we have observed.

Case 4. The patient was a middle-aged physiologist who had been in psychoanalytically orientated psychotherapy for several years because of recurrent anxiety attacks. In the course of treatment he disclosed that he had a flying phobia, an odd symptom since he had formerly been a naval pilot. He was dissatisfied with his marriage. The phobia interfered with visits to his mistress, who lived so far away that he could visit her only by flying. Behavior therapy for the phobia utilized Wolpe's method of reciprocal inhibition with hierarchies constructed for his fears of assertiveness and exhibitionism. The patient also phobically avoided nearly all public gatherings. He feared he would do "stupid and noisy" things, such as standing up at a meeting of establishment types and shouting obscenities. After his first appointment and instruction in the method, he practiced assiduously. He missed the next two appointments, but called to make subsequent ones. When the behavior therapist brought up the matter of the missed appointments, he disclosed that he felt guilty about his reason for wanting to be desensitized to flying. He blurted out that he was disturbed in all areas of his life, and broke down and cried for the remainder of the hour. He refused to return to the behavior therapist. The observer discussed it with him and chose to respond to his description of the behavior therapist as "an authoritarian . . . [who was] threatening because I'm not used to anyone telling me what to do." In reality he frequently asked others to make decisions for him. The observer insisted that he go back and try at least once more. He kept the remainder of the appointments with the behavior therapist, but proceeded to miss the appointments with the observer, offering such excuses as "it slipped my mind completely until an hour past the appointment time." He worked through the hierarchies in the interviews and confronted some of his phobic situations successfully. These included flying, attending public meetings and public performances, and through generalization effect he was able to give lectures without taking tranquilizers. In this instance the resistance had a dynamic basis, namely, guilt feelings concerning an extramarital affair. There was also a transference problem involving his inability to cope with his ambivalence about "authority figures." Accepting an order from one authority figure to see another from whom he had run away (probably because of dependency temptation) enabled him to work through a desensitization to some symbolic representations of his deeper conflicts.

Case 5. A young male surgical technician was referred for treatment of acute anxiety attacks. These occurred when he was flying, and interfered with his moonlighting occupation of flying instructor. He was instructed in the method of relaxation and hierarchies were set up for his fears of being assertive with superiors, subordinates, and his family. He was seen ten times over a two-month period. His appointments were for 8:10 in the morning. He was always late, would apologize profusely, after which he would work conscientiously on the relaxation and desensitization procedures. Before beginning treatment he was having anxiety attacks nearly every time he flew; by the sixth treatment he was not having any at all. He was able to resume night flying, a disability he had not previously mentioned. He worked through hierarchies dealing with expression of anger, assertiveness, etc., until the eighth appointment when the therapist again chided him for arriving 35 minutes late. He disclosed that it was impossible for him to keep an 8:10 appointment for the following reasons: he had to drive one child to school, another child to kindergarten, his wife to work, and the baby to the sitter. The son who went to kindergarten could not arrive before 8:15 as the place did not open till then. His wife was due at work by 8:30, so he had to go to four locations, one not before 8:15, another no later than 8:30, before arriving for an 8:10 appointment with his psychiatrist! No interpretation was made, but we concluded that disclosure was made possible by a decrease of anxiety and confidence in the behavior therapist's tolerance as a result of exposure to him and to the desensitization procedure. In the tenth meeting the patient insisted that he was unable to afford further treatment. A review of his debts indicated that this was the case. This contrasted with his usual behavior, as he customarily ran up large bills because of his inability to say no. Between the ninth and tenth appointments the "worst possible thing that could happen while flying with a student" happened, a full power stall with the plane in a vertical climb. He was able to control his anxiety, keep his hands off the dual controls, and coach the student in what to do to bring the plane out of its earth-bound rendezvous.

In this case fear of assertiveness led to fear of flying (something his very stern and strict father had opposed his doing when he was a teen-ager). The desensitization procedure enabled him to be assertive with the behavior therapist as well as with his pupils, his partner (in the course of treatment he split with his overbearing partner), and his family. In this case the fear and the resistance coincided, and the desensitization to his fears of assertion made it possible for him to be assertive with the therapist!

DISCUSSION

The five cases described above are given in the chronological order in which they were treated by us. In the first three we insisted on not deviating from a strictly behavioral model, as defined by Wolpe. Partly as a result of these early cases, we concluded that the phenomena of resistance and transference resistance were interfering with our behavior therapy results, and that rigid adherence to a behavioral model was costing us success. Crisp (1966) observed transferences in the course of doing behavior therapy, and believed that they preceded alteration of symptoms. Freud first felt that resistance was an unwelcome complication of a task already difficult enough. He later realized that one could turn the liability into an asset because, like the transference, it reflected the patient's own style of defense. Better yet, material often not available in the form of memories was available in the form of behavioral repetitions in both transference and resistance. It was in those areas that the affect lay, and therefore in those areas that the neurosis could be worked out. Our failure to deal with either phenomenon led, in our opinion, to failures in the first three cases. By case 4 we had treated a number of intervening cases, and were less rigid in our approach. Accordingly, in case 4 the observer stepped out of his "neutral" role to insist that the patient return for further behavior therapy, exploiting a positive transference he knew existed. The fifth case displays how it was possible to continue the task of desensitization to fear of assertiveness in spite of an ongoing resistance. Perhaps the fact that the resistance was mutually recognized by the therapist and patient enabled it to be mutually tolerated until the patient was ready to deal with it.

REFERENCES

Crisp, A. H. (1966). 'Transference', 'symptom emergence' and 'social repercussion' in behavior therapy. *Br. J. Med. Psychol. 39*, 179-196.

Weinberg, N. H. and Zaslove, M. (1963). 'Resistance' to systematic desensitization of phobias. *J. Clin. Psychol. 19*, 179-181.

Wolpe, J. and Lazarus, A. A. (1968). *Behavior Therapy Techniques*. New York: Pergamon Press.

The Converging Paths of Behavior Therapy and Psychotherapy

12

R. Bruce Sloane, M.D.

In the following article Sloane examines three disparate psychotherapeutic approaches—psychoanalytical, behavioral, and Rogerian, and concludes that they have more likenesses than differences. (1) In all three, a relationship develops between patient and therapist that involves mutual expectancies, and in which the therapist overtly or covertly endeavors to get the patient to share or accept his beliefs. Moreover, in all three, the success of the therapy depends on both patient and therapist having certain personal attributes that tend to favor a good outcome. (2) In all three, past and present events are explored and "explanations" offered, although there are differences both quantitatively and in emphasis.

Moreover, although there are specific differences in technique—e.g., interpretation, counterconditioning (reciprocal inhibition), and the use or withholding of reward—they are not as totally different as one might assume, because they all represent aspects of learning with some degree of overlap in the actual process.

The Converging Paths of Behavior Therapy and Psychotherapy

12

R. BRUCE SLOANE, M.D.

Psychotherapy, like the elephant, tends to be difficult to define but easily recognized by all. However, despite this easy recognition its characteristics are to a greater or lesser extent shaped by the eye of the beholder. Moreover, as Gottschalk and Auerbach[17] have said: "Everyone knows what psychotherapy is. But it is easier to write a plausible convincing book explaining the subject and the method than to prove a single assertion about it with any degree of scientific rigor."

Psychotherapy clearly aims to bring about change in the way a person thinks and acts. Despite such a narrow goal the arena is large and filled with a diversity of approach and theory. Common to many of these approaches, however, are clinical skills encompassing case history taking, assessment and diagnosis, interviewing, and—depending on the particular technique—a greater or lesser amount of therapist skill.

Three disparate models, psychoanalytical, behavioral, and Rogerian, illustrate the range of methods.

Schlessinger and associates[36] stress two major factors in the psychoanalytic approach: (1) the existence of unconscious mental processes that need to be elucidated in order to understand the symptoms, and (2) the fact that the analyst and the patient influence each other in the course of this effort to understand. They add that:

> the essential contribution of the analyst is *interpretation*, a succinct statement pointing out the components and origins of the patient's conflicts and their hidden connections. . . . The function of this interaction is to produce *insight*, that is, to make conscious with affect the dynamic conflicts between the various structures of the mind . . . to deepen the understanding of the genetic roots of these conflicts. . . . Energy bound up in the defensive processes which maintain repression is freed and feelings that were repressed seek conscious expression as the adult ego struggles to make them acceptable and useful.

From *American Journal of Psychiatry,* 125:877-885, January 1969. Copyright 1969 by the American Psychiatric Association. Reprinted by permission.

In contrast, one group of behavior therapists[11,48] regards neurotic symptoms as learned (or conditioned) habits of reaction mediated by anxiety. The stimuli or cues to which anxiety is conditioned vary from patient to patient as a function of past experience. The maladaptive behavior of the patient that is termed the neurosis represents efforts to reduce anxiety by escape, avoidance, or other means. The therapy is then directed to the unlearning of the maladaptive behavior, in particular by counterconditioning techniques. Responses such as relaxing or aggressive or sexual ones that are antagonistic and therefore inhibitory to anxiety are systematically evoked in the presence of anxiety-producing thoughts (or "stimuli"). This "reciprocal inhibition" gradually weakens the bond between these stimuli and the anxiety. Thus expression of ego alien feelings is permitted, encouraged, or even instigated by the therapist and "extinguishes" the anxiety that is aroused by the usual realistic or imagined hostile reception.

A somewhat different approach of the operant conditioners[12,23,39] involves the use of reward. Their approach rests heavily on techniques of operant conditioning, on the use of "reinforcement" to control and shape behavior, and on the notion that symptoms, like all other behaviors, are maintained by their effects. By varying the contingency of the reward—e.g., the patient must respond in certain specified ways to the behavior of another individual in order to produce the reward—adaptive interpersonal behaviors can be developed as well.[3]

Yet a third approach is that of Carl Rogers and his school.[32] They suggest that it is not the special professional knowledge of the therapist, his intellectual conception of his therapy (his "school of thought"), or his techniques that are important. Rather, it is his personal attitudes in the relationship: in particular his empathy, his regard, and his liking for the patient. These in turn elicit traits from the patient of which his depth of "self-exploration" is the most crucial.

These various schools of psychotherapy would seem to have a number of items in common: (1) the relationship between the patient and the therapist; (2) a conversational content; and (3) techniques such as interpretation, counterconditioning, reward, and so on.

However, these processes and their underlying assumptions need to be examined in a variety of contexts. The first is that of the bias brought to psychotherapy by its participants, especially the therapist.

THE CONTROLLING SITUATION OF PSYCHOTHERAPY

Good psychotherapy, Masserman has said, is about as nondirective as good surgery.[26] The psychotherapist usually has clear ideas about how he would like his patient to behave. Such expectations may be couched in terms of self-actualization, greater maturity, less neurosis, insight, and so on. They may be more implicit than explicit but are certainly well formulated in his mind.

Rosenthal[34] has demonstrated the effect of examiner bias in obtaining desired results with animals as well as with human subjects. In humans his studies have shown that verbal conditioning may be an antecedent of biasing. He has also shown, however, that biasing is already in evidence at the beginning of a study before conditioning can, in fact, take place. He concluded that this bias was mediated in the brief predata gathering interaction during which the examiner greets, sets, and instructs the subject.

Goldstein[16] has illustrated the multifaceted influence of the mutual expectancies of therapist and patient. Frank[13] has pointed to the cultural factor contributing to favorable patient expectancy. There is an increasing acceptance in the United States that emotional illness is best treated by psychotherapy. It is also probable that, at this time, middle- and upper-class patients expect such psychotherapy to be psychoanalytically oriented.

Orne[29] has suggested:

> the subject's performance in an experiment might also be conceptualized as problem solving behavior; that is, at some level he sees it as his task to ascertain the true purpose of the experiment and response in a manner that will support the hypothesis being tested. Viewed in this light, the totality of cues that convey an experimental hypothesis to the subject become significant determinants of the subject's behavior.

Krasner[21] has illustrated the similarities of how the expectancies of either a patient or an experimental subject become intertwined with those of the therapist or experimenter. In this way the simple "desire to please" of the one becomes facilitated or inhibited by the goals of the other.

Frank[13] had added that in psychotherapy the patient's spontaneous behavior is his speech; the therapist reinforces certain verbalizations by cues of approval which may be as subtle as a fleeting change of expression or as obvious as an elaborate interpretation. In this way the therapist not only transmits desired verbal behavior but also some of his own expectations. If, for example, he expects the patient to get better soon the patient obediently responds.[37] Morever, Chance[7] found that the expectations regarding the role of the patient were very personal and characteristic to each clinician.

In the light of these considerations it seems likely that psychotherapy is dominated by the beliefs of the therapist and that its outcome is mediated by the success with which he can get his patient to share them.

THE RELATIONSHIP

The importance of the relationship between therapist and patient is stressed in all schools of psychotherapy, although it may be dignified by different titles and dealt with in different ways.

The Patient

In formal psychoanalysis it is expected that the patient will have feelings about the therapist that are derived in part from his previous formative emotional experiences. Such "transference" may be interpreted and forms an important technical part of the therapy.

In behavior therapy such feelings are made use of to facilitate instigation or reciprocal inhibition. Wolpe[49] illustrates how encouragement of assertion in a female patient was difficult even though "it had early become emotionally important to her to please the therapist." Crisp[8] has used measures of the transference to illustrate the progress of behavior therapy.

In Rogerian therapy it is probable that the patient's willingness to cooperate with the treatment and indulge in "self-exploration" in part determines its success. Thus although in Rogerian and behavior therapy "interpretation" of such feelings is not made, they remain important in the process. Strupp,[45] in fact, has suggested that the patient's willingness to behave in a dependent, childlike relationship to the parental authority of the therapist may be a fulcrum on which the success of treatment rests. Certainly such qualities make it easier for the therapist to like the patient and to exert his best efforts on his behalf.

The Therapist

Many studies of the process of psychotherapy have concentrated on the therapist's activity, emphasizing his personal characteristics.[9,22,44,45] The concept of the therapist as a "standard therapeutic instrument" has been replaced by an appreciation of his idiosyncrasies. There seems to be a general but as yet unconfirmed belief that the more experienced the therapist is and the more closely he resembles the "good" therapist, the better the results he will achieve.

The attributes of such a "good" therapist, who possesses understanding, empathy, flexibility, and a respect for the dignity and integrity of the patient, have seldom been subjected to systematic study.[18] Certainly the need for experience has been questioned by Poser.[30] Truax,[47] whose work is derived from Rogers, has been particularly concerned with qualities such as genuineness, unconditional positive regard, and accurate empathy in the therapist and their effect on "depth of self-exploration" in the patient and the outcome of treatment. His findings indicate that where there is a lack of these qualities therapeutic outcome is poor.

Similarly in behavior therapy "the patient enjoys the nonjudgmental acceptance of a person whom he perceives as possessing the necessary skills and desires to be of service."[50]

Common to all these approaches seems to be the warmth, tolerance, and acceptance of the therapist, which encourage relaxation in the patient.[5] In psychoanalysis the frequency of interviews, the recumbent position, and the use of dreams all foster regression; in this setting the patient can talk about the sources of his anxiety and learn to associate them with security.[38] This process bears a strong resemblance to the technique of counterconditioning described by Wolpe and Lazarus[50] as "reciprocal inhibition." If the response inhibitory to anxiety can be made to occur in the presence of an anxiety-evoking stimulus it will weaken the bond between the stimulus and the anxiety. In systematic desensitization the patient is invited to think of the least anxiety-provoking situation in the presence of deep relaxation. Although such relaxation is taught more directly than that occurring in psychotherapy, the end results may be the same. A reassuring comment in psychotherapy may inhibit a fear and diminish autonomic response in a very similar way.

Quite different kinds of reinforcement techniques were evolved by Skinner,[40] who viewed speech as a "verbal behavior" that follows the same degree of lawfulness as other behavior. This verbal behavior, which can be manipulated, is the crucial element in an interpersonal influencing situation such as psychotherapy. Skinner's view—that such verbal behavior is reinforced only through the mediation of another person—illustrates the importance of the social situation. Thus, a reinforcer as a rewarding act or stimulus cannot be separated from the person administering the reinforcement. As Krasner[20] says, this recognizes the obvious fact that some people are more effective behavior modifiers than others. Sapolsky[35] showed that there were differential effects in reinforcement that were dependent on the level of attractiveness of the examiner.

Psychotherapists of whatever persuasion use both positive and negative reinforcements in a variety of ways, slowly shaping the verbal behavior of their patients. However, this technique is used more directly by behavior therapists to remove and replace undesirable habits. Ayllon and Michael[2] have used social reinforcement to modify the behavior of mental hospital patients toward greater socialization such as knitting, playing the piano, sweeping, singing, and "normal" talk, going to the dining room, and self-feeding. Ferster and DeMyer[12] have used reinforcements such as food and candy to change the performance of autistic children.

In this context it is very probable that the special properties of the therapist, heightened by his patient's regard, will determine his effectiveness as a reinforcer.

Bandura[4] points out that although a certain amount of learning takes place through direct training and reward, a good deal of a person's behavioral repertoire may be acquired through imitation of what he observes in others. Affection and reward increase the secondary reinforcing properties of the model and thus predispose the imitator to pattern his behavior after the rewarding person. Also, models of high prestige are more effective than those of low prestige.

As Bandura says, during the course of psychotherapy the patient is exposed to many incidental cues involving the therapist's values, attitudes, and patterns of behavior. They are "incidental" only because they are usually considered secondary or irrelevant to the task of solving the patient's problems. Nevertheless, some of the changes observed in the patient's behavior may result not so much from the intentional interaction between the patient and the therapist but rather from the active learning by the patient of the therapist's attitudes and values, which the therapist never directly attempts to transmit.

Such modeling is probably similar to the mental sets imposed by the therapist. Rosenthal[33] found that in spite of the usual precautions taken by therapists to avoid imposing their values on their clients, the patients who were judged as showing the greatest improvement changed their moral values (in the areas of sex, aggression, and authority) in the direction of the values of their therapists, whereas patients who were unimproved became less like their therapists in values.

CONVERSATIONAL CONTENT

> The role of psychotherapy, regardless of the therapist's theoretical leanings, is to eliminate the anxiety and . . . to accomplish this goal, all therapists use the devices of conversing with a patient about his anxiety and the situations calling it forth. . . .[38]

Common to all therapies is this preoccupation with the patient's anxieties, whether they be his guilt, his inadequacies, or his omissions. The therapist is interested in both present and past events that lead to such feelings; emphasis is more on feelings than facts. As Shoben[38] points out:

> Even therapists like Rogers who . . . disclaims any interest in personal history . . . hardly prevent their patients discussing past experiences. . . . In a preliminary trial by the writer using material collected from twelve sessions with one case the greater part of a typical anamnestic form could be filled out from the transcriptions of the recordings.

It is probable, however, that earlier memories may be looked for more vigorously in psychoanalytic therapy and its derivatives. These may then be interpreted in the light of current behavior. However, this might be regarded as more a quantitative than a qualitative difference, and there remains a common denominator of content.

Conversely, although behavioral therapists depart from the springboard of eliciting anxiety to construct the hierarchies of a deconditioning technique, it is likely that they utilize many of the clinical skills of the more eclectic therapists. Breger[6] comments that a variety of activities occurs during behavioral treatment. These include discussions, explanation of techniques and of the unadaptiveness of anxiety and symptoms, hypnosis, relaxation, "nondirective cathartic discussions," and "obtaining an understanding of the patient's personality and background." In a similar way, Kanfer[19] points to a series of treatments by desensitization or conditioning techniques whose deceiving similarities are belied by the diversity of the individual protocol.

TECHNIQUES

Because of so many likenesses it may well be that the chief divergence in the therapies lies in the specific techniques engaged in.

Interpretation to Produce Insight

Psychotherapeutic insight occurs when the patient comes to recognize some of the previously unconscious roots of his attitudes, beliefs, feelings, conflicts, or behavior. This process is very similar to that described by early Gestalt psychologists, who considered that it was a large factor in human problem solving. In this process the numerous elements of a problem (or life situation) are suddenly (through some type of "closure") perceived to have a new meaning that has consequences previously unrecognized.

Brady[5] has suggested that insight can be as well conceptualized within the framework of learning as can psychoanalysis. Thus a neurotic difficulty can be viewed as an inappropriate emotional reaction due in part to stimulus generalization. The acquisition and extinction of conditioned emotional responses in humans are facilitated by being able to discriminate the conditions under which aversive stimulation occurs and has occurred in the past (awareness of stimulus contingencies). This insight allows the patient to discriminate between past and present experience and to decrease conditioned emotional responses. Such changed responses on the part of the patient may in turn elicit different responses from others in life. These may be more rewarding to the patient and therefore tend to maintain the process of improvement.

In a similar manner, Brady suggests that if intense anxiety is diminished, discriminatory behavior may be improved. Finally, he posits that a strong positive emotional response, which may follow some insights, is in itself inhibitory to the anxiety aroused by the material being considered. Thus extinction of an aversive conditioned emotional reaction that often follows the acquisition of insight. This, he suggests, may be part of the basis for the greater efficacy of "emotional" rather than "intellectual" insight.

However, it seems likely that insight is initially more idiosyncratic to the therapist than to the patient. Marmor[25] comments:

> But what *is* insight? To a Freudian it means one thing, to a Jungian another, and to a Rankian, a Horneyite, an Adlerian or a Sullivanian, still another. Each school gives its own particular brand of insight. Whose are the correct insights? The fact is that patients treated by analysts of all these schools may not only respond favorably, but also believe strongly in the insights which they have been given. . . . Thus each theory tends to be self-validating. . . . What the analyst shows interest in, the kinds of questions he asks, the kind of data he chooses to react to or to ignore, and the interpretations he makes, all exert a subtle but significant suggestive impact upon the patient to bring forth certain kinds of data in preference to others. . . . *What we call insight is essentially the conceptual framework by means of which a therapist establishes, or attempts to establish, a logical relationship between events, feelings, or experiences that seem unrelated in the mind of the patient.* In terms of the analyst's objectives, insights constitute the *rationale* by which the patient is persuaded to accept the model of more "mature" or "healthy" behavior which analysts of all schools, *implicitly* or *explicitly*, hold out to him.

Adams and associates[1] have shown that psychoanalytically derived interpretive statements can be used as verbal reinforcers to raise the frequency of a selected response class. In a later study Noblin and associates[28] demonstrated that even if the content of the interpretation were unrelated to the subject statement that it followed, it could act as reinforcer. Thus there is little to suggest that the relevance of interpretation is a central factor in modifying verbal behavior in a verbal conditioning situation.

In this light, insight tends to be merely the new "language" taught to the patient by the therapist. Nevertheless, it may still set the stage for a willingness by the patient to look at things differently and perhaps to behave differently. In this way it may break the circular and self-perpetuating habits of neurosis.

Counterconditioning

Although it is probable that counterconditioning is an important cause of the diminution of anxiety in the comforting presence of any therapist, it is possible that greater efficiency and technical virtuosity in accomplishing this may lie in the hands of the behavior therapist.

In addition to reciprocal inhibition techniques, aversive stimuli—particularly in sexual perversions and childhood autism[24,31]—have given encouraging results and extend the therapeutic armamentarium.

Extinction

Many conventional forms of psychotherapy probably rely heavily on extinction effects, although the therapist may not label them as such. Thus permissiveness or the "non-punishing audience" of Skinner[39] is considered by many to be a necessary condition for therapeutic change. It is expected that when a patient expresses thoughts or feelings that provoke anxiety or guilt, and the therapist does not disapprove, criticize, or withdraw interest, the fear or guilt will gradually be weakened or extinguished. These extinction effects are believed to generalize the inhibited thoughts to verbal and physical behavior as well.[10] In this way aversive stimuli generated by the patient's own behavior are gradually reduced and become less likely to arouse emotion.

However, extinction is likely to be less effective and more time-consuming than counterconditioning. Certainly the relatively long intervals between the interviews of orthodox psychotherapy would not facilitate such a procedure.

Reward and Punishment

As Bandura[4] points out, most theories of psychotherapy are based on the assumption that the patient has a repertoire of previously learned positive habits available to him, but these adaptive patterns are inhibited or blocked by the competing responses motivated by anxiety or guilt. The role of therapy is to reduce the severity of the internal inhibitory control, thus allowing the healthy patterns of behavior to emerge. Such a rationale may well apply to oversocialized neurotic patients but can scarcely be expected to apply to undersocialized extroverted ones, whose behavior reflects failure of the socialization process.

In fact it is probable that individuals learn differently; not all patients respond equally to reinforcements such as praise or censure. Sloane and associates[41] demonstrated that when some patients were given the positive verbal reinforcement "good," some responded and some did not. In general, the extroverted character-disordered persons responded; the anxious introverted did not. The distinction may lie in the perceived meaning of the situation, but individual differences in learning may be equally important.

In another study[42] Sloane and associates found that extroverted behavior-disordered persons showed less autonomic response to the "anxiety" of another person than introverted anxious ones and normal controls. Such an ability to intuit or "empathize" another person's feelings may be important in identification and the learning derived from this. It is likely that similar traits may distinguish one therapist from another and, as Truax suggests, determine his effectiveness as a healer.

CONCLUSION

It would seem that there are more similarities than dissimilarities among various psychotherapeutic approaches. The relationship and dialogue of the therapy are perhaps closer than their protagonists believe or describe. It is likely that the more the therapist believes in the correctness of his views, the better his results[14] will be. An enduring although false belief system might prove a powerful medicine.

In practice, some of the techniques of behavior therapy may ultimately be found more effective than those of orthodox psychotherapy. If, indeed, many of the changes in all forms of treatment are based on an unwitting application of learning principles, the necessary conditions for this to occur may be better designed by intent than by accident.

Much neurotic behavior seems to serve a variety of social purposes that dwarf the symptoms and are compatible with a theory of central mediators. However, such a theory is equally explained by one of central "cognitive maps"[27,46] as by a psychoanalytic one. Thus the "unconscious" may be viewed within the concept of neurotic conflict and defense "long chains of reinforcers," or strategies or programs acquired in learning the game of life. As Breger[6] has said, "unawareness" of the mediating strategies of behavior is more likely to be the rule than the exception. He uses the analogy of language in which the child can speak perfectly but is unable to give a description of the grammatical rules that govern the understanding and production of his language.

A valid criticism of the mathematical model, cognitive "image," or verbal learning approaches is their failure to demonstrate how behavior may be manipulated. However, this may merely be a result of the difficulty of designing suitable experiments to test these theories, rather than their incorrectness or implausibility. Nevertheless, the elegant parsimony and empirical justification of the stimulus response model commends it.

There are some common problems that remain to all forms of therapy. In particular, the link between the verbal behavior of the therapeutic session and the social behavior of real life remains obscure. Behaviorists such as Goldiamond and associates[15] have been active in trying to ensure that this process does in fact take place by carrying the therapy into the environment itself.

Similarly, the removal of overlearned patterns of behavior and the acquisition of new ones, although they may occur in the therapeutic situation, need to be applied to reality.[25] These social aspects of the working through process may proceed inefficiently or aberrantly and may require structuring. Stevenson[43] has advocated "direct instigational" planning of the daily life during psychotherapy. Certainly the technical aspects of converting ameliorative intrapsychic change into ameliorative social change deserve greater study than they have been afforded in the past. Moreover, the range of effective reinforcing stimuli such as praise and censure, and the effect of these on the variables of personality, remain both unstudied and of crucial importance, regardless of the therapeutic endeavor engaged in.

Summary

Despite apparent diversities there are common threads to all psychotherapies, including the behavioral ones.

The judgmental clinical skills of interviewing and assessment are necessary to all therapists. Therapists also share a belief in the efficacy of their own procedure that proselytizes, arouses hope, and improves the prognosis.

All treatments involve a relationship between the therapist and the patient—a dialogue and a number of techniques which differ from "interpretation" to "counterconditioning." It is chiefly in these technical aspects that the therapies differ, but they may, at a practical level, approach the same goal by a somewhat different pathway. "Insight" may be as well conceptualized within the framework of learning theory as of psychoanalysis. An ability to discriminate the conditions under which anxiety has occurred in the past is likely to lead to a decrease of conditioned emotional responses in the present and future. Moreover, some construe "insight" as an idiosyncratic rationale by which the patient is persuaded to accept the treatment goals of the therapist. Despite growing experimental evidence, the importance of the expectancies induced in the patient by the therapist have been underestimated.

All therapists tend to eschew scientific rigor when they are faced with clinical demands. Few practice *exactly* what they preach. Explanation, exhortation, and instigation are undoubtedly used in varying degrees in all psychotherapies, although they may be dignified by different titles.

Clearly the greatest barrier to the integration of present-day therapies lies in their differing theoretical assumptions. The "dictionary constructs" of the past have done little to alleviate these idiological distinctions. Perhaps the empirical research of today may provide the forum out of which may come the psychotherapy of tomorrow.

References

1. Adams, H. E., Noblin, C. D., Butler, J. R., and Timmons, E. O.: The differential effect of psychoanalytically derived interpretations and verbal conditioning in schizophrenics (Abstract), *Amer. Psychol.* 16:404, 1961.

2. Ayllon, T., and Michael, J.: The psychiatric nurse as a behavioral engineer, *J. Exp. Anal. Behav.* 2:323-334, 1959.
3. Azrin, A. H., and Lindsley, O. R.: The reinforcement of cooperation between children, *J. Abnorm. Soc. Psychol.* 52:100-102, 1956.
4. Bandura, A.: Psychotherapy as a learning process, *Psychol. Bull.* 58:143-159, 1961.
5. Brady, J. P.: Psychotherapy, learning theory, and insight, *Arch. Gen. Psychiat.* 16:304-311, 1967.
6. Breger, L., and McGaugh, J. L.: Critique and reformulation of "learning theory" approaches to psychotherapy and neurosis, *Psychol. Bull.* 63:338-358, 1965. [See also Chapter 4, this volume.]
7. Chance, E.: *Families in Treatment.* New York: Basic Books, 1959.
8. Crisp, A. H.: Transference symptom emergence and social repercussions in behavior therapy: a study of 54 treated patients, *Brit. J. Med. Psychol.* 39:179-196, 1966.
9. Dollard, J., and Auld, F., Jr.: *Scoring Human Motives: A Manual.* New Haven, Conn.: Yale University Press, 1959.
10. Dollard, J., and Miller, N. E.: *Personality and Psychotherapy.* New York: McGraw-Hill, 1950.
11. Eysenck, H. J., ed.: *Behavior Therapy and the Neuroses.* New York: Pergamon Press, 1960.
12. Ferster, C. B., and DeMyer, M. K.: The development of performance in autistic children in an automatically controlled environment, *J. Chron. Dis.* 13:312-345, 1961.
13. Frank, J. D.: The dynamics of the psychotherapeutic relationship, *Psychiatry* 22:17-39, 1959.
14. Frank, J. D.: *Persuasion and Healing.* Baltimore, Md.: Johns Hopkins Press, 1961.
15. Goldiamond, I., Isaacs, W., and Thomas, T.: Applications of operant conditions to reinstate verbal behavior in psychotics, *J. Speech Hearing Dis.* 25:8-12, 1960.
16. Goldstein, A. P.: *Therapist-Patient Expectancies in Psychotherapy.* New York: Pergamon Press, 1962.
17. Gottschalk, L. A., and Auerbach, A. H.: *Methods of Research in Psychotherapy.* New York: Appleton-Century-Crofts, 1966.
18. Holt, R. R., and Luborsky, L.: *Personality Patterns of Psychiatrists.* New York: Basic Books, 1958.
19. Kanfer, F. H., and Phillips, J. S.: Behavior therapy: a panacea for all ills or a passing fancy? *Arch. Gen. Psychiat.* 15:114-128, 1966.
20. Krasner, L.: Behavior modification research and the role of the therapist, in Gottschalk, L. A., and Auerbach, A. H., eds.: *Methods of Research in Psychotherapy.* New York: Appleton-Century-Crofts, 1966.
21. Krasner, L., and Ullmann, L. P.: *Research in Behavior Modification.* New York: Holt, Rinehart & Winston, 1965.
22. Lennard, H. L., and Bernstein, A.: *The Anatomy of Psychotherapy.* New York: Columbia University Press, 1960.
23. Lindsley, O. R.: Characteristics of the behavior of chronic psychotics as revealed by free-operant conditioning methods, *Dis. Nerv. Syst.* 21:66-78, 1960.
24. Lovaas, O. I., Schaeffer, B., and Simmons, J. Q.: Building social behavior in autistic children by use of electric shock, *Journal of Experimental Research in Personality* 1:99-109, 1965.
25. Marmor, J.: Psychoanalytic therapy as an educational process, in Masserman, J. H., ed.: *Science and Psychoanalysis,* vol. 5. New York: Grune and Stratton, 1962.
26. Masserman, J. H.: Experimental and humanitarian approaches to the therapy of behavior disorders, *Canad. Med. Ass. J.* 95:616-621, 1966.
27. Miller, G. A., Galanter, E., and Pribram, K. H.: *Plans and Structure of Behavior.* New York: Henry Holt & Co., 1960.

28. Noblin, C. D., Timmons, E. O., and Reynard, M. C.: Psychoanalytic interpretations as verbal reinforcers: importance of interpretation content, *J. Clin. Psychol. 19*:479-481, 1963.

29. Orne, M. T.: On the social psychology of the psychological experiment, *Amer. Psychol. 17*:776-783, 1962.

30. Poser, E. V.: The effect of therapists' training on group therapeutic outcome, *J. Consult. Psychol. 30*:283-289, 1966.

31. Raymond, M. S.: Case of fetishism treated by aversion therapy, *Brit. Med.J. 2*:854-857, 1956.

32. Rogers, C. R.: Some learnings from a study of psychotherapy with schizophrenics, *Pennsylvania Psychiatric Quarterly* 3-15, 1962.

33. Rosenthal, R.: Changes in some moral values following psychotherapy, *J. Consult. Psychol. 19*:431-436, 1955.

34. Rosenthal, R.: On the social psychology of the psychological experiment, *Amer. Sci. 51*:268-283, 1963.

35. Sapolsky, A.: Effect of interpersonal relationships upon verbal conditioning, *J. Abnorm. Soc. Psychol. 60*:241-246, 1960.

36. Schlessinger, N., Pollock, G. H., Sabshin, M., Sadow, L., and Gedo, J. E.: Psychoanalytic contributions to psychotherapy research, in Gottschalk, L. A., and Auerbach, A. H., eds.:*Methods of Research in Psychotherapy*. New York: Appleton-Century-Crofts, 1966.

37. Shlien, J. M., Mosak, H. H., and Dreikurs, R.: Effect of time limits: a comparison of two psychotherapies, *J. Counsel. Psychol. 9*:31-34, 1962.

38. Shoben, E. J., Jr.: Psychotherapy as a problem in learning theory, *Psychol. Bull. 46*:366-392, 1949.

39. Skinner, B. F.: *Science and Human Behavior*. New York: Macmillan Co., 1953.

40. Skinner, B. F.: *Verbal Behavior*. New York: Appleton-Century-Crofts, 1957.

41. Sloane, R. B., Davidson, P. W., Staples, F., and Payne, R. W.: Experimental reward and punishment in neurosis, *Compr. Psychiat. 6*:388-395, 1965.

42. Sloane, R. B., Staples, F., and Payne, R. W.: Individual differences in social behavior in neurosis, read at the 122nd annual meeting of the American Psychiatric Association, Atlantic City, N. J., May 9-13, 1966.

43. Stevenson, I.: Direct instigation of behavioral change in psychotherapy, *Arch. Gen. Psychiat. 1*:99-107, 1959.

44. Strupp, H. H.:*Psychotherapists in Action*. New York: Grune and Stratton, 1960.

45. Strupp, H. H., and Williams, J. V.: Some determinants of clinical evaluations of different psychiatrists, *Arch. Gen. Psychiat.2*:434-440, 1960.

46. Tolman, E. C.: *Collected Papers in Psychology*. Berkeley: University of California Press, 1951.

47. Truax, C. B., and Carkhuff, R. R.: Significant developments in psychotherapy research, in Abt, L. E., and Riess, B. F., eds.: *Progress in Clinical Psychology*, vol. 6. New York: Grune and Stratton, 1964.

48. Wolpe, J.: *Psychotherapy by Reciprocal Inhibition*. Stanford, Calif.: Stanford University Press, 1958.

49. Wolpe, J.: Reciprocal inhibition as the main basis of psychotherapeutic effects, in Eysenck, H. J., ed.: *Behavior Therapy and the Neuroses*. New York: Pergamon Press, 1960.

50. Wolpe, J., and Lazarus, A.: *Behavior Therapy Techniques*. New York: Pergamon Press, 1966.

Neurosis and the Psychotherapeutic Process

Similarities and Differences in the Behavioral and Psychodynamic Conceptions

JUDD MARMOR, M.D.

This is a discussion by Marmor of the previous paper by R. Bruce Sloane. Dr. Marmor agrees that behavior psychotherapy and the dynamic psychotherapy indeed converge in clinical practice. However, significant differences do exist in terms of theoretical orientation concerning the nature of neurosis and the nature of the psychotherapeutic process.

13

Neurosis and the Psychotherapeutic Process

Similarities and Differences in the Behavioral and Psychodynamic Conceptions

Judd Marmor, M.D.

Dr. Sloane's article is a thoughtful and valuable effort at identifying the common denominators in behavior psychotherapy and dynamic psychotherapy. (Incidentally, his title tends to suggest that behavior therapy is not a form of psychotherapy; such an implication is not warranted.) In the main, I agree with his conclusions, particularly in his thesis that "many of the changes in all forms of [psychotherapy] are based on an unwitting application of learning principles."

It seems to me, however, that he has been somewhat less critical than he should be of the theoretical assumptions on which the behavior therapies rest, especially when he commends the "elegant parsimony and empirical justification of the stimulus-response model." Parsimony in a theory is "elegant" only if the theory encompasses all of the data it must explain. If it ignores essential data it becomes inadequate, rather than parsimonious.

SHORTCOMINGS OF THE S-R MODEL

It is open to serious question whether or not the stimulus-response model has empirical justification, even in simple conditioning experiments with lower animals. When applied to the interpersonal and intrapsychic reactions of human beings, however, a stimulus-response model becomes a simplistic kind of reductionism that cannot begin to do justice to the complex variables that are involved. Breger and McGaugh, in their excellent "Critique and Reformulation of 'Learning-Theory' Approaches to Psychotherapy and Neurosis" [Chapter 4, this volume], have beautifully delineated the shortcomings of the S-R model, particularly in its failure to take into account the central mechanisms that make "stimulus equivalence" and "response-transfer" possible.[1]

Reprinted by permission from *International Journal of Psychiatry*, 7:514-519, July 1969.

Designating the therapeutic transaction between patient and therapist in terms of "conditioning" does not per se make the explanation more "scientific." To define neurosis, as Eysenck does, as "simple learning habits" and to state that "there is no neurosis underlining the symptom but merely the symptom itself—get rid of the symptom and you have eliminated the neurosis"[2] is like defining an elephant in terms of what comes easiest to hand, and represents a retrogression from the sophisticated open-systems thinking that has been influencing psychiatry in recent years. Dynamic psychiatrists are beginning to recognize that psychopathology does not reside simply in the individual, but also in the nature of his relationships with other persons and with his milieu. Hence the growing emphasis of family therapy, conjoint marital therapy, group therapy, and on the amelioration of the unfavorable socioeconomic factors that are the breeding ground for so many of our human personality disorders. To see the locus of psychopathology only in the individual leads to the dangerous grounds of thought-and-behavior control in which the emphasis becomes one of using therapeutic techniques to adjust the individual to his environment regardless of how distorted, intolerable, or irrational that environment might be.

But even if we restrict our focus only to what goes on within the individual himself, the theoretical point of view represented in its extreme form by Eysenck and Wolpe seems to me to be quite inadequate. It overlooks all of the complexities of thought, symbolism, and action that must be accounted for in any comprehensive theory of psychology and psychopathology. To assume that what goes on subjectively within the patient is irrelevant and that all that matters is how he *behaves* is to discard half a century of important psychodynamic insights. In saying this, I am not defending all of psychoanalytic theory. I have been as critical as anyone of certain aspects of classical Freudian theory and I am in full accord with those who argue that psychodynamic theory needs to be reformulated in terms that conform more closely to modern theories of learning and neurophysiology. Current knowledge suggests that the brain functions as an infinitely complex information receiver, retriever, processor, and dispatcher. A stimulus-response theory of human behavior cannot do justice to this process. It is what goes on in the central "black box" *between* stimulus and response that constitutes the core challenge to psychiatric theory, and no theory that ignores the complexities of the processes within that "black box" can be considered an adequate one. It is to Freud's eternal credit, regardless of the limitations of his theoretical assumptions, that he was the first to develop a rational investigative technique for, and a meaningful key to, a beginning understanding of this vast uncharted realm that exerts so profound an influence on *both* our perceptions *and* our responses.

Role of Insight

Sloane has also—quite unintentionally, I am sure—misrepresented my views concerning insight by quoting a paragraph from one of my papers and concluding from this that "insight tends to be *merely* [italics mine] the new 'language' taught to the patient by the therapist."[3] In a subsequent paper in which I explored the subject of insight more thoroughly, I commented that my earlier paragraph was "subject to the misinterpretation that insights given by analysts of different schools may be capriciously different, and that they do not necessarily have any relationship to the actual realities of the patient's life and behavior. Such an interpretation would be misleading. . . . The insights given . . . all bear a definite relationship to clinical reality."[4] They all refer to observed or inferred patterns of clinical behavior in the patient, and under these circumstances insight, in part at least, represents a form of cognitive understanding about the patient's or other people's behavior that is capable of adding to his capacity to function more adaptively. Indeed, in some instances insight may lead to what Karl Buhler has called an "a-ha" experience, and result in an immediate reorientation toward more adaptive behavior. My basic earlier point was that the *particular theoretical frame of reference* in which the insight was given (Freudian, Jungian, Adlerian, Sullivanian, etc.) was not *specific* to the success of psychotherapy, since patients were capable of responding equally well within different theoretical orientations.

The Patient–Therapist Relationship

In any psychotherapeutic relationship—including the behavior therapies—we start with an individual who presents a problem. This problem may be in the form of behavior that is regarded as deviant, or it may be in the form of subjective discomfort, or in certain distortions of perception, cognition, or affect, or in any combination of these. Usually, but not always, these problems motivate the individual or someone in his milieu to consider psychiatric treatment for these problems. This decision in itself establishes an *expectancy* in the individual that is quite different than if, say, "punishment" rather than "treatment" were prescribed for his problems. The expectancy is an essential part of *every* psychotherapeutic transaction at its outset, regardless of whether the patient presents himself for behavioral or dynamic psychotherapy. The patient, in other words, is not a neutral object in which certain neurotic symptoms or habits have been established. Expectancy is a complex process. It encompasses factors that Frank has demonstrated as being of major significance in psychotherapy—the *faith*, *trust*, and *hope* that the patient brings into the transaction.[5] It is based in large part on previously learned perceptions about authority or help-giving figures, perceptions that play a significant role in the degree of receptivity or nonreceptivity that the patient may show to the message he receives from the psycho-therapist. Psychoanalysts have traditionally referred to these represent-ing expectations as aspects of transference, but, regardless of what they are called, they are always present and constitute an integral part of every psychotherapeutic relationship. (Even in "simple" conditioning studies, experimenters like Liddell, Masserman, and Pavlov have called attention to the significance of the relationship between the experimen-tal animal and the experimenter.) Transference is not, as some behavior therapists seem to think, something that is "created" by the thera-pist—although it is true that transference distortions may be either in-creased or diminished by the technique the therapist employs. The way in which the therapist relates to the patient may reinforce certain maladaptive perceptions or expectations, or it may teach the patient that his previously learned expectations in relation to help-giving or author-ity figures are incorrect.

Thus, a therapist who behaves in a kindly but authoritarian manner may confirm the patient's expectancies that authority figures are om-nipotent and omniscient. This increases the patient's faith and facilitates his willingness to give up his symptoms, to please the powerful and good parent-therapist, but it may not alter his childlike self-image in relation to authority figures. *Depending on the therapist's objectives, this may or may not be of importance.*

What I am indicating, in other words, is that a so-called positive transference facilitates symptom removal, but if the patient's emotional maturation is the goal, what is necessary eventually is a "disolution" of this transference—which means teaching the patient to feel less childlike not only in relation to other authority figures but also to the therapist himself.

Closely related and interacting with the patient's expectancies is the therapist's *social role*. As a professional person he is endowed by the help-seeking patient with presumptive knowledge, prestige, authority, and help-giving potential. These factors play an enormous role in strengthening the capacity of the therapist to influence the patient, and is another element in the complex network that makes up the phenome-non of transference.

Also, the real attributes of both patient and therapist, their actual physical, intellectual, and emotional assets and liabilities, and their re-spective value systems enter into the therapeutic transaction. Neither the patient nor the therapist can be regarded as a stereotype upon whom any particular technique will automatically work. Their idiosyncratic variables are always an important part of their transaction.

Nature of the Psychotherapeutic Process

In all dynamic psychotherapies, then, the following processes take place in varying degrees and admixtures:

1. A release of tension via the initial catharsis in a setting of faith, hope, and expectancy. *This also takes place in behavioral therapies in the process of taking the initial history.*

2. Suggestion and transmission of values via the therapist's interpretations, confrontations, questions, and by his nonverbal reaction as well. *Suggestion and implicit transmission of values also take place in the behavioral therapies, regardless of claims to the contrary.* They need not be overt, and indeed, are probably most potent when they are covert. Wolpe's technique, which he has documented both in print and in film, abounds in covert as well as overt suggestion.[6] First, the technique of relaxation itself is closely related to hypnotic technique. Second, the patient is assured that he will feel better as a result of following the process outlined to him. There is repeated implicit and explicit suggestion that his anxiety will diminish as he reconstructs particular kinds of fantasies. Third, there is also direct transmission of values, as when Wolpe says to a young patient, "You must learn to stand up for yourself." The rationale for this, according to Ullmann and Krasner,[7] is the hypothesis that self-assertion diminishes anxiety. They indicate that therapists in behavioral therapy point out the irrationality of the patient's fears and encourage the individual to insist on his "legitimate human rights." This is obviously not very different from what goes on in dynamic psychotherapies and does not become more "scientific" by virtue of the fact that it "is given a physiological basis by Wolpe who refers to it as excitatory."

3. Trial and error learning and relearning via insight. "Look what you were doing." "There, you've gone and done it again."

4. Gestalt learning via insight.

5. Reconditioning and desensitization via the suggestion and transmission of values as indicated above, and also through the corrective emotional experience in the patient–therapist transaction. It is in this area that behavior therapists have made their greatest contribution. They have focused heavily on desensitization and have demonstrated the therapeutic value of such an emphasis in achieving symptom remission. This is particularly true of Wolpe's techniques and of the Masters and Johnson technique of treating sexual inadequacies. My thesis, however, is that the other factors I have mentioned—faith, hope, expectancy, transference, suggestion, and the transmission of certain values—are taking place also. They should not be minimized and cannot be ignored in any comprehensive theory concerning the nature of the psychotherapeutic process.

6. Learning by imitation. This takes place subtly and often without

the awareness of either patient or therapist. It has been variously described under such concepts as "identification with the therapist" or
"introjection of bits of the therapist's superego." *Some of this undoubtedly
takes place in the behavior therapies also.*

7. Repeated reality testing. This, in effect, consists in practicing
new adaptive techniques and in reinforcing them through positive feedback from both the therapist and the environment. *This latter factor is also
heavily emphasized in the behavior therapies with considerable value.* This aspect of the process plays a particularly important role in Skinnerian reward-punishment forms of therapy.

CONCLUSION

We see, therefore, that in both behavior therapies and dynamic psychotherapies a complex kind of learning process occurs that does not
lend itself to simple categorization within stimulus-response or reward-punishment models only. The challenging problem in psychotherapy today is not to polarize our therapeutic attitudes either for or
against either behavior therapy or dynamic psychotherapy. The technique employed should depend on the patient's needs as determined by
careful psychodynamic diagnostic evaluation. If symptom relief is what
is primarily needed, an emphasis on behavior therapy may well be indicated. On the other hand, if the core of the patient's problem rests in
symbolic distortions of perception, cognition, affect, or subtle disturbances in interpersonal relationships, the sources and nature of which
are out of his awareness, then the more elaborate reeducational processes of dynamic psychotherapy may be necessary. Indications for one
approach do not necessarily rule out the other. Marks and Gelder[8] and
Brady,[9] among others, have demonstrated that the use of both behavior
and dynamic therapy in the same patient, either concurrently or in sequence, often seems to bring about better therapeutic results than the
use of either approach alone. Indeed, dynamic psychotherapists have
for years been using such a combination of approaches when they prescribe drugs for the direct control of certain symptoms while pursuing a
psychotherapeutic approach concurrently.

In my opinion, then, behavior therapies and dynamic psychotherapies, far from being irreconcilable, are complementary psychotherapeutic approaches. The line of demarcation between them is by no
means a sharp one, and as Breger and others have shown, behavior
therapists do many things in the course of their conditioning procedures
that duplicate the activities of dynamic psychotherapists.[1]

These include, as Sloane says, "discussions, explanation of techniques and of the unadaptiveness of anxiety and symptoms, hypnosis, relaxation, 'nondirective cathartic discussions,' and 'obtaining an understanding of the patient's personality and background.' '' The process in both approaches is best explicable in terms of current theories of learning, theories that go beyond simple conditioning explanations and encompass central cognitive processes also. The fact that in some types of disorders one approach may be more effective than the other should not surprise us, and presents no contradiction. Just as there is no single best way of teaching all pupils all subjects, there is no single psychotherapeutic technique that is optimum for all patients and all psychiatric disorders.

REFERENCES

1. L. Breger and J. L. McGaugh, Critique and reformulation of 'learning-theory' approaches to psychotherapy and neurosis, *Psychological Bulletin*, 63:338-358, 1965. [See also Chapter 4, this volume.]
2. H. J. Eysenck (ed.), *Behavior Therapy and the Neuroses* (New York: Pergamon Press, 1960).
3. J. Marmor, Psychoanalytic therapy as an educational process, in J. H. Masserman (ed.), *Science and Psychoanalysis*, Vol. 5 (New York: Grune and Stratton, 1962).
4. J. Marmor, Psychoanalytic therapy and theories of learning, in J. H. Masserman (ed.), *Science and Psychoanalysis*, Vol. 7 (New York: Grune and Stratton, 1964). [See also Chapter 3, this volume.]
5. J. D. Frank, *Persuasion and Healing* (Baltimore, Maryland: Johns Hopkins Press, 1961).
6. J. Wolpe, *Psychotherapy by Reciprocal Inhibition* (Stanford, California: Stanford University Press, 1958).
7. L. P. Ullmann and L. Krasner (eds.), *Case Studies in Behavior Modification* (New York: Holt, Rinehart & Winston, 1965).
8. I. M. Marks and M. G. Gelder, A controlled retrospective study of behavior therapy in phobic patients, *British Journal of Psychiatry*, 111:561-573, 1965; Common ground between behavior therapy and psychodynamic methods, *British Journal of Medical Psychology*, 39:11-23, 1966. [See also Chapter 10, this volume.]
9. J. P. Brady, Psychotherapy by a combined behavioral and dynamic approach, *Comprehensive Psychiatry*, 9:536-543, 1968. [See also Chapter 15, this volume.]

Behavior Therapy

Observations and Reflections

14

MARJORIE H. KLEIN, PH.D.,
ALLEN T. DITTMANN, PH.D.,
MORRIS B. PARLOFF, PH.D.,
AND MERTON M. GILL, M.D.

In this article a group of psychoanalytically oriented clinicians and theoreticians report on their findings after a week of intensive observations of the work of two of the leading practitioners of behavior therapy, Joseph Wolpe and Arnold Lazarus. Their observations lead them to a number of significant conclusions:

1. *Behavior therapies are quite varied and diverse, even when subsumed under a single rubric like "systematic desensitization"—i.e., they include assertiveness or expressiveness training, manipulation of behavior outside the treatment setting, education in learning principles, indoctrination and exhortation.*
2. *Suggestion plays a major role in these therapies, with manipulation of the patients' expectations and attitudes.*
3. *As the clientele for behavior therapy has broadened to include "less good" cases, its process is becoming longer and more complicated, with concomitant lowering of success rates.*

Behavior Therapy

Observations and Reflections

Marjorie H. Klein, Ph.D.,
Allen T. Dittmann, Ph.D.,
Morris B. Parloff, Ph.D.,
and Merton M. Gill, M.D.

Like many clinicians and researchers today, we have been impressed by claims made for behavior therapy: its superior effectiveness, straightforwardness, efficiency, flexibility, and objectivity. In order to learn more about how behavior therapists function we undertook to spend a period of time observing ongoing behavioral treatment under the guidance of two of its most prominent proponents, Joseph Wolpe and Arnold Lazarus. In this paper we wish to present some questions, comments, and inferences based on observations of their clinical activities which we were privileged to make during a typical week at the Eastern Pennsylvania Psychiatric Institute. Over 5 working days we saw both private and demonstration sessions for cases in various stages of treatment, and occasionally were able to interview patients. We had access to tape recordings of other treatment sessions, attended staff meetings and case conferences, and discussed many issues with both Wolpe and Lazarus. We are aware that 1 working week is in many ways an unusual length of time for outsiders to visit a clinical operation, but realize that a different week may have brought different patients and yielded other impressions.

At the outset we wish to express our appreciation for the extraordinary cooperation of our hosts and our deep respect for their unusual openness. Wolpe and his associates were both patient and helpful in their efforts to answer our questions, many of which we must admit were less than gentle and friendly and reflected our own psychoanalytically oriented training, experience, and biases. In the interests of accuracy in writing this paper, we sent drafts to both Wolpe and Lazarus, and they made a number of comments about it. Many of these concerned misstatements of fact on our part, and we have incorporated these by

Reprinted by permission from *Journal of Consulting and Clinical Psychology*, 33:259-266, 1969. Copyright 1969 by the American Psychological Association.

making the necessary corrections. Others were comments about interpretation, and we have, with their kind permission, included them in the article, separated from the body of our text by the use of smaller type size identifications of the commenters. We are greatly indebted to Wolpe and Lazarus for making this method of presentation possible.

Therapy as practiced by Wolpe and his colleagues is among the most widely used form of behaviorally oriented treatment. It was first described fully by Wolpe in 1958, with a more technique-oriented exposition including new developments recently available (Wolpe and Lazarus, 1966). Complete unanimity of approach to theory and technique is not to be found in any so-called school of psychotherapy, and behavior therapists are no exception. Even the two we visited are quite different on some issues, Lazarus being a good deal more eclectic in his choice of techniques. Still, there are some basic general principles. The chief of these has to do with reciprocal inhibition, in which the fear response (or some other maladaptive response) to those situations which form the basis for the patient's complaint is inhibited by an incompatible response, usually a positive one. The positive responses most frequently used are relaxation and self-assertion. Relaxation is brought about by a modification of Jacobson's technique, and for each symptom the patient is instructed to imagine situations like those he fears, arranged in hierarchical order from least to most fear-producing. When the patient is able to imagine each situation and remain relaxed the therapist goes on to the next hierarchy scene. Where self-assertion is used as the new response, the patient is instructed in the relevant procedures for performance between sessions. Treatment is considered successful when all major symptomatic complaints are reorganized in this fashion.

Although most of what we encountered has been spelled out explicitly in the writings of Wolpe and others, some of what we saw surprised us and led us to understand the literature more fully when we returned to it later. In addition, there were a few impressions which have not, as far as we know, been spelled out completely in any publication. We shall note these as we come to them and state them rather tentatively. We shall begin with a description of the range of patients who came in during our week of observation and of the techniques we saw employed and shall go on to discuss the implications of what we have seen for research in psychotherapy and for programs of clinical training.

PATIENTS

Consistent with Wolpe's emphasis that his method has wide applicability, cases we observed under treatment went well beyond simple phobias or social anxieties (cases for whom behavior therapy has been thought to be a specific) to include a broad range of complex psychoneurotic problems, character neuroses, or borderline psychotic problems (acute psychoses are excluded). Many had been resistant to prior therapeutic efforts. To the clinician of ordinary persuasion a number of these patients would seem to have extremely poor prognosis and present a formidable challenge. They were not particularly gratifying patients for the behavior therapist either. These patients were often unwilling or unable to meet what are considered the basic requirements for behavior therapy or to perform correctly the therapeutic tasks that were assigned. In some of the more complex cases we observed (and in others we were told about) the patients were not optimally relaxed or would at times exaggerate or misreport their levels of relaxation. On occasions inquiry would reveal that the hierarchy scene actually "imagined" was considerably different from that which the therapist had presented. As a consequence new cues or response dimensions were often introduced, reducing or heightening anxiety levels spuriously. In addition, compliance with the very specific instructions for response performance outside the therapy setting seemed equally difficult at times to obtain or to verify.

In general, it was our impression that broadening the clientele for behavior therapy to include "less good" cases has introduced inevitable strain on the method and potential depression of its outcome rate. It should be noted that behavior therapists have not by plan increased the range of problems they treat. Rather, as they have become better known, they have been referred a broader spectrum of patients, a number of whom, as we have said, had experienced unsatisfactory results in the care of others.

TECHNIQUES

From our acquaintance with the literature we knew intellectually at least that behavior therapists do not work in a unitary fashion and indeed take pains to vary their approach from case to case. We were surprised to find, however, that within most cases, too, a number of manipulations were routinely employed. Even where desensitization was the primary technique, others such as assertiveness or expressiveness training, manipulation of behavior outside the treatment setting, and education in learning principles were also included. With the more complex cases the spectrum of techniques became even broader. In addition to desensitization involving a variety of hierarchies, many variants of assertion and expression, often elaborate role-playing and behavioral programs of homework were devised to correct response deficiencies. Along with these specific procedures we found also that patients were given a good deal of indoctrination, teaching, and exhortation, apparently intended to provide a rationale for the treatment and to enhance motivation.

These remarks may well sound like complaints by outsiders that behavior therapists use a "shotgun" approach. But such an accusation would be unfounded, since the many techniques do have a unity in the behavior therapist's view in that they are thought either to produce reciprocal inhibition of anxiety or to alter stimulus-response contingencies. It would make no more sense to insist that the behavior therapist be limited to one behavioral manipulation than it would to insist that another kind of therapist restrict himself to one content area or interview technique. It is appropriate, however, to note the apparent contradiction between the proliferation of methods in behavior therapy and the popular conception, based partly on hope, partly on the behavior therapists' writings, that this is a simple and straightforward treatment of the neuroses. It is also appropriate for us to look into the research implications of a many-method approach, as we shall do later on in this paper.

The popular notion of simplicity in behavior therapy covers not only treatment techniques but diagnostic procedures as well. Many people suppose that the therapist begins by clearly and systematically defining the patient's problems in terms of manageable hierarchies and then selects appropriate responses to be strengthened or weakened. We found little support for this conception of behavior therapy diagnosis in our observations. Indeed the selection of problems to be worked on often seemed quite arbitrary and inferential. We were frankly surprised to find the presenting symptomatic complaint was often sidestepped for what the therapist intuitively considered to be more basic issues. Most surprising to us, the basis for this selection seemed often to be what others would call dynamic considerations. The distinction between "secondary" (that is, the superficial) and "primary" (the more basic, underlying) was even made openly on occasion by behavior therapists: The words we have put in quotes or their terms. The literature, of course, gives no hint of this development.

> JW: This conveys the impression that the writers assume that "more basic" in a behavioral sense is the same thing as the psychoanalysts mean. This is really quite incorrect. For example, it may be found that a person's fear of enclosed spaces is based on a fear of developing certain physical symptoms that may lead, as he believes, to his death, and he avoids enclosed spaces because once within them he cannot easily run out and seek help. It is the fear of his symptoms that would then be the primary focus of this person's treatment. What is involved here is the pinpointing of the time stimuli to anxiety, but these are still extrinsic, and no reference is made to "intrapsychic mechanisms."
>
> AAL: One must be careful when using a term like "dynamic trends." A behavior therapist may trace a patient's anxiety to faulty identification with an inadequate father coupled with excessive sibling rivalry, compounded by ambivalence engendered at the hands of an inconsistent mother. However, these basic and formative interpersonal encounters are then taken at face value and do not presuppose additional "dynamics" such as "castration anx-

iety," "incestuous wishes" or "death wishes," etc. As to the statement, "The behavior therapy literature, of course, gives no hint of this development," may I refer you to Lazarus (1966).

We also learned that behavior therapists prefer to structure hierarchies on dimensions of time and space (for example, "a month before an examination," and leading up to the time of an examination; "standing in a hall a mile away from the hospital" and gradually approaching it; treading water in a pool 5 feet deep and 5 feet from the edge," working up to greater depths and distances). The examples of hierarchies reported in the behavior therapy literature are generally much more flexible and lifelike than the ones we encountered during our visit.

One point which the behavior therapist's writing makes quite clear but which did not strike us until our visit has to do with the ongoing evaluation of the patient progress. Because behavioral treatment is posited as highly specific, it follows that success depends on the patient's exact and close cooperation with the therapist's instructions. It is therefore very important for the therapist to test this cooperation repeatedly during treatment. The therapist must also constantly assess the patient's progress on hierarchy dimensions. With the possible exception of role-playing, the therapist is dependent in this evaluation upon the patient's report both of progress outside treatment and of events within the sessions themselves. Since there are no independent procedures for evaluating or verifying his report, the patient has considerable leeway to bias his report in order to please, frustrate, or otherwise manipulate the therapist, or to meet some personal expectation. And the form of much of the feedback from the patient (i.e., lifting his finger if he feels an increase in anxiety during desensitization or doing nothing if he does not) gives the therapist very few cues for distinguishing valid from invalid reports. Thus the therapist must use considerable intuition to assess progress and correct the treatment plan. This all serves to highlight a very basic discrepancy between the theoretical orientation of behavior therapy and its actual practice. While the theory clearly calls for the manipulation of overt behavior, the therapist typically deals primarily with the patient's report of his image of that behavior.

> JW: We all have "images" of everything we talk about. If a patient says that he has a feeling of anxiety, this is presumed to be his image of some responses within him. Except insofar as this kind of image cannot be shared by another observer, there is no difference between such a report and the report of something perceived in the world outside the subject. Either *could* be false: but what would motivate patients to mislead their helpers? And what instinct would make them all lie according to the same rules with regard to their emotional responses to repetitions of an image—that is, they report either that anxiety is weak and progressively diminishes, or that it is strong and does not?
>
> AAL: It is incorrect to state that, "the theory calls for manipulation of

overt behavior." All forms of behavior are covered by the theory, including "thinking behavior."

Perhaps the most striking impression we came away with was of how much use behavior therapists make of suggestion and of how much the patient's expectations and attitudes are manipulated. Behavior therapists are not at all silent on this point in their descriptions of technique, but the literature did not prepare us for the unabashed suggestions that therapists directed toward their patients. The major arena for suggestion is in the orientation period of treatment. Here the therapist tells the patient at length about the power of the treatment method, pointing out that it has been successful with comparable patients and all but promising similar results for him, too. The patient is provided with a detailed learning-theory formulation of the etiology of his problems and is given a straightforward rationale for the way in which the specific treatment procedures will "remove" his symptoms. The patient's motives and values may also be considered so as to "correct misconceptions" which block desirable courses of action or restrict the effect of treatment. Indeed, it seemed to us that treatment plans and goals were laid out in such a detail that the patient was taught precisely how things would proceed and what responses and changes were expected of him all along the way. A quite complete account of these procedures may be found in Wolpe and Lazarus (1966, pp. 16-20).

> AAL: Both Wolpe and I have explicitly stated that relationship variables are often extremely important in behavior therapy. Factors such as warmth, empathy, and authenticity are considered necessary but often insufficient.

Although Wolpe and other behavior therapists are reluctant to ascribe therapeutic effectiveness to these features of the relationship it is difficult for us to believe that they do not constitute an important part of the treatment. Certainly the explicit, positive, and authoritative manner with which the therapist approaches the patients seems destined if not designed to establish the therapist as a powerful figure and turn the patient's hopes for success into concrete expectations. The introductory education in learning theory, in addition, must function to make the treatment more plausible and provide a simple and coherent frame of reference for the patient's understanding of his difficulty. Further, the focus of the treatment philosophy on the role of external psychonoxious environmental factors in the formation of the patient's problems must be quite reassuring for many patients. At the very least the therapist's evident willingness to assume major responsibility for correcting the patient's problems may be especially important in helping him overcome inertia and start on the path to change.

> JW: Paul's (1966) study in which psychoanalytically oriented therapists obtained significantly better results with desensitization than with either

their own insight methods or with another clearly structured method indicates a relatively small role for the factors suggested here.

The Course of Treatment

As behavior therapists have gained more experience with their methods and behavior therapy has been more widely used, a number of complementary trends seem to have emerged; techniques have become more polished, tending to shorten the treatment of specific cases, but at the same time patients with more complicated problems have been seeking behavior therapy, tending to lengthen treatment. In the first years of Wolpe's experience with behavior therapy the average number of interviews per case rose from 25 (Wolpe, 1952, p. 827) and 26 (Wolpe, 1954, p. 217) to 45 (Wolpe, 1958, p. 218), but declined sharply thereafter: Lazarus reports an average of 14 interviews per case in 1963 (Lazarus, 1963, p. 75). At the present time it is our impression that the length of treatment is on the increase again. Some of the patients we observed had been in treatment for over a year. In others the number of interviews per week had increased dramatically. One patient was being seen four times a week, and this had been going on for approximately 9 months. We felt that these trends reflected the shift in the case load to include more complex or seriously disturbed cases. Also related are changes over the years in reported outcome rate. From the over 90% improvement originally reported (see Wolpe, 1952, 1954, 1958) the claims have been modified to approximately 80% (Lazarus, 1963), with some of Wolpe's associates now reporting 70% rate. These figures cannot be taken literally as they were not derived from data specifically designed to yield comparative outcome rates—indeed, the last figure is purely anecdotal. What we wish to convey by referring to them is that behavior therapy seems to be taking longer and showing less spectacular successes. Why this should be so could be the topic of extensive study. It should be noted, however, that these trends are familiar ones among psychotherapies as they are introduced and find their way.

One final impression about the course of treatment: It is interesting to note that the ongoing argument between behaviorist and other methods concerning symptom substitution seems to be taking a new turn. When confronted with a patient who is successfully treated for his initial array of problems but continues to report disabling complaints, the therapist talks not of symptom substitution but of faulty or inadequate treatment. It may be argued, for example, that (a) the original formulation of the case did not consider the correct stimulus contingencies; (b) "secondary" anxieties may have masked the more "primary" or situational pervasive anxieties; or (c) the patient did not comply with the instructions or work hard enough to extend his learning outside the treatment setting. While it may be commendable for behavior therapists to assume primary responsibility for slow or uneven progress in their patients, the distinction between backsliding due to inadequate treatment and symptom substitution is certainly not as obvious to outsiders (especially to dynamically oriented ones) as it is to behavior therapists. In any case it is a distinction which is difficult to verify.

> JW: Symptom substitution means replacement of one symptom by another. It is not symptom substitution if a patient complains of symptoms that he had before treatment began, though other symptoms have been removed by therapy. "Backsliding" is in no sense commonly observed.
>
> AAL: "Symptom substitution" is an unfortunate term. It presupposes that unresolved unconscious complexes result in the terminal manifestation of new problems. Patients can always acquire new aberrant responses (e.g., when faced with inimical life situations). Is this "symptom substitution?"

Research Implications

In this section we shall consider a number of implications our observations have for behavior therapy research. It should be clear, and let us stress it if it is not, that these problems are by no means unique to research in behavior therapy. Indeed, what struck us most forcefully was the fact that the issues and research problems which confront behavior therapy are the same familiar ones which have long troubled all psychotherapy research.

The first and most obvious research problem behavior therapists must face is a consequence of the diversity of their techniques. While it is true, as we said earlier, that behavior therapists believe all of their techniques are united in their derivation from theories of learning, the question of the exact function and effectiveness of each technique is still an empirical one. Research questioning which of the many techniques is best suited to which patient, and which produces which result, would teach behavior therapists how to make their treatment more effective and efficient.

In making these points let us stress again that we are not criticizing behavior therapy for its technical variety; the range of patients seen certainly calls for flexibility in treatment, and the underlying experimental and empirical philosophy demands constant technical adjustments. Nonetheless, it remains that the question of the theoretical utility of a many-faceted method, whatever its theoretical persuasion and whatever its clinical value, has never been adequately dealt with in psychotherapy research. Thus the fact of variety in behavior therapy makes it as difficult to talk of behavior therapy as a single method of treatment to be evaluated and compared with others as it is to talk of a single method of insight therapy. The subtleties and variations within methods may be as important as the unifying theories. It may be possible to compare therapeutic approaches on some dimensions—behavioral symptoms versus unconscious conflicts as the "core" of neurosis, for example, in comparing behavior and insight therapies—but it must be remembered that the dimensions are theoretical ones. They may relate only indirectly to the specific therapist activities during the treatment session, and there may be equally important variables that may be overlooked because they do not happen to be in the theoretical spotlight.

In our earlier section on technique we emphasized the role of suggestion in behavior therapy practice. We did this because we were surprised at the extent and consistency of its use. The research implications are obvious: Even though these factors are not called techniques, in that they do not follow from the theoretical framework, they nevertheless have an effect on the patient, and these effects must somehow be understood and differentiated from the effects of the theoretically important "techniques."

> JW: Suggestion is nothing but the use of words to obtain the responses that are associated with these words. If deliberate evocation of responses in this way brings about habit change, it is just as much behavior therapy as habit change through responses otherwise contrived. Words are probably used with this intent more consciously by behavior therapists than most other therapists.

> AAL: The statement that suggestion as a technique does not follow from the theoretical framework is not correct. "Suggestion" can only have an effect by virtue of responses already in the person's repertoire (i.e., previously conditioned cues) which the suggestions come to elicit. Furthermore, if suggestion enables the person to attempt new responses, these may have positive effects. One thus endeavors quite deliberately to maximize the "placebo effect."

Again, this problem is not unique to behavior therapy, but again, it is the popular notion that behavior therapy is simple and straightforward, behaviorally oriented, and thus untrammeled by these side effects. In practice, all therapists make suggestions, by telling their patients about the methods they employ, and by explaining why they believe these methods will be helpful. The particular behavior therapists we observed were experienced clinicians (whose training included dynamic methods), and they went about their business very confidently and skillfully. Much of what they did was what any clinician does in dealing with patients, and they did it by second nature, so to speak. The point is that all of these activities, the second-nature ones, the overt suggestions, the specific "technique"—all must be examined for their effects on the patient.

> AAL: Recent experimental results lead me to endorse the authors' contentions here. Indeed, even the results of a specific technique like systematic

desensitization cannot be accounted for solely in terms of graded hierarchies
and muscle relaxation.

The more complex cases highlight some other difficult questions for assessing the outcome of behavior therapy. It is generally assumed that the behavior therapist, basing his judgment on change in manifest symptoms, enjoys a simpler criterion of outcome than does the "dynamic" therapist, whose criteria are cast in such inferential terms as conflict resolution or structural personality change. But the apparent objectivity of symptomatic change is lost when the behavior therapist treats patients who present complex symptom pictures. Unless all symptoms are successfully removed, one must decide in assessing outcome whether all symptoms are to be equally weighted, whether only those symptoms mentioned at intake should be counted, or whether complaints emerging later should be given secondary status. Questions like these are certainly not news to behavior therapists, any more than they are to therapists of other persuasions. In fact, it looks as if they may have already begun to work toward some answers although perhaps unwittingly: The differentiation between "primary" and "secondary" problems which we mentioned earlier may be a first try at ordering symptoms for therapeutic attack. That this differentiation was made on the dynamic basis was our inference from our observations. Whatever the basis, it must be defined more clearly before it can be used in designing research studies.

One more research implication of the complex cases: Behavior therapists have relied almost exclusively on patient reports, both for evaluating the success of manipulations within a given session and for assessing the outcome of the entire case. In general it was our impression that the more disturbed patients were especially unlikely to give reliable reports. The problem seemed to make it difficult for therapists to handle these patients clinically. It brings about insuperable difficulties in comparing patients with each other in a research study, or for that matter in comparing two reports collected at different times from the same patient. The obvious way out of this problem is to rely more heavily on external measures, preferably behavioral ones, as criteria for the success of treatment.

Implications for Clinical Practice and Training

At present there is a clearly discernible trend in a number of training institutions to emphasize behavior therapy considerably, in both theory and technique. We are concerned that such training practices not provoke an overreaction against "dynamic" theory and practice. It may be well to recall that the innovators of behavior therapy have each had con-

siderable training and experience with classical psychodynamic orientations.

> JW: It seems to be suggested here that previously acquired psychoana-
> lytic knowledge plays an integral part in the practical repertoire of behavior
> therapists. Earlier passages have implied that because the behavior therapist
> is not always content with "a simple mechanical acceptance of the patient's
> statements regarding his fears and anxieties," and may go into probing activ-
> ities for the sake of clarification to establish the antecedents, this is ipso facto
> psychoanalytic. It *is* in a sense *analytic*, but in every important respect repug-
> nant to whatever is specific to the psychoanalytic theory of neurosis, and
> different from the practices of psychoanalytic therapy.

Despite their present enthusiasm for behavior therapy the fact remains that previously acquired skills still form an integral part of their
repertoire. The effect is perhaps most clearly evident in the selection of
patient-relevant hierarchies, which we have stressed before. Recall also
our observations that Wolpe and his associates make very effective use
of the patient-therapist relationship to establish a context in which the
specific behavioral techniques can be utilized most effectively. Although
the behavior therapist would not wish to ascribe his results to any
"dynamic" theories he may have learned in the past, it is clear that many
clinical decisions in the treatment are based on an understanding of
some functional organization of behavior, and an appreciation of the
power of the relationship.

The danger for training programs as we see it is that the trainee will
be exposed principally to learning theory and behavioral techniques
without being adequately trained in other areas of psychology. It is
especially those clinical skills of interviewing and diagnosis, and those
theoretical skills that grow with knowledge of a wide range of therapeutic theories that prevent training from becoming sterile and one-sided.
Without these skills the training will severely limit the competence of the
therapist and restrict the quality of research and theoretical development
possible within the field. Training programs which do not specifically
attempt to develop a broad range of clinical skills are in danger of reducing the effectiveness of the entire profession.

> JW: With regard to the statement that behavioral training should avoid
> being one-sided, the answer is that a very good knowledge of all kinds of
> reactions and interactions is highly desirable. Our position is that it is not
> important to know a great deal about theories, but enough to obtain a histori-
> cal perspective for present-day practices. From the point of view of the prob-
> lems presented by patients, only propositions that have some scientifically
> meaningful, factual support are worth anything at all. If behavior therapists
> have tended to ignore propositions from the psychoanalytic field, it has been
> because of a dearth of them that qualify for respect on this criterion.
>
> AAL: Do we need only a knowledge of general psychology and
> therapeutic theories to be effective clinicians or do we need in addition a
> course in sensitivity training and rational thinking combined with a mélange
> of specific techniques?

Little benefit to the field of psychotherapy is to be gained from developing yet another closed system of treatment. We believe that the stimulus provided by the behavior therapist's apparent willingness to examine the consequences of his procedure may be a positive one for the field. Perhaps ultimately the greatest contribution the behavior therapist can make to psychotherapy theory and practice is his dedication to making both the process and the outcome of treatment as objective and as efficient as possible. If the discrepancies between behavior therapy and other therapies can be subjected to empirical tests, then our ultimate aim of achieving a more effective theory of personality change may also be served.

References

Lazarus, A. A. The results of behavior therapy in 126 cases of severe neurosis. *Behaviour Research and Therapy*, 1963, *1*, 69-79.

Lazarus, A. A. Broad-spectrum behavior therapy and the treatment of agoraphobia. *Behaviour Research and Therapy*, 1966, *4*, 95-97.

Paul, G. L. *Insight vs. Desensitization in Psychotherapy*. Stanford, California: Stanford University Press, 1966.

Wolpe, J. Objective psychotherapy of the neuroses. *South African Medical Journal*, 1952, *26*, 825-829.

Wolpe, J. Reciprocal inhibition as the main basis of psychotherapeutic effects. *A.M.A. Archives of Neurology and Psychiatry*, 1954, *72*, 205-226.

Wolpe, J. *Psychotherapy by Reciprocal Inhibition*. Stanford, California: Stanford University Press, 1958.

Wolpe, J., and Lazarus, A. A. *Behavior Therapy Techniques: A Guide to the Treatment of Neuroses*. Oxford: Pergamon Press, 1966.

15

Psychotherapy by a Combined Behavioral and Dynamic Approach

JOHN PAUL BRADY, M.D.

Dr. Brady was one of the early clinicians to demonstrate the fact that behavioral and dynamic therapies need not be viewed as polar opposites: Psychodynamic factors may operate in behavioral therapies, and behavioral factors in dynamic therapies. He conceptualizes a continuum between the two, with the patient's problem being the key factor that should determine where, on the continuum, the therapy should be selected.

Behavioral therapists and dynamic therapists tend to view neurosis in a different fashion. The former stress symptoms and overt behavioral patterns while the latter stress the underlying conflicts. This apparent lack of agreement on what constitutes illness and, therefore, adequate assessment of change, often precludes comparative studies of outcome. The two forms of treatment may bring about changes in different aspects of the patient's life, suggesting a therapeutic rationale for simultaneous or sequential treatment. For example, a purely behavioral approach might be best for an anorgasmic woman with primary sexual inhibition, a purely dynamic treatment where the problem is secondary to unresolved nonsexual problems, and a combined approach where both the factors are operative.

Too often therapists are inclined to fit the patient to the treatment rather than to develop a flexible stance centered about a comprehensive understanding of the problem and treatment needs. The openness and flexibility of Dr. Brady's approach is well worth serious consideration and study.

Psychotherapy by a Combined Behavioral and Dynamic Approach

John Paul Brady, M.D.

Behavior therapy refers to an approach to psychological disorders which stresses a behavioral analysis of the patient's adjustment difficulties and employs a number of psychotherapeutic techniques which focus fairly directly on the removal or amelioration of maladaptive behaviors or psychological states. Many of these techniques, such as the systematic desensitization treatment of neurosis[1] and the anticipatory avoidance treatment of homosexuality,[2] involve the direct application of principles derived from experiments in learning (learning theory). Others, such as the treatment of tics and stuttering by "negative practice," seem more empirical in nature although they too are often rationalized in learning-theory terms.

In contrast, the psychotherapeutic approach currently in most common use in the United States focuses less on the patient's presenting symptoms than on the intrapsychic conflicts and interpersonal relationships which are presumed to give rise to his specific neurotic difficulties. This group of techniques also has some empirical basis but is derived to a large extent from psychoanalytic theory and practice. Treatment in which these techniques are emphasized is usually termed *dynamic* or *psychoanalytically oriented psychotherapy*.

DIFFERENCES IN THEORY

Some therapists of exclusively psychodynamic or behavioral orientation hold that the assumptions which underlie the two treatment approaches are antithetical and mutually exclusive. These therapists often

From *Comprehensive Psychiatry*, 9:536-543, 1968. Reprinted by permission of Grune and Stratton, Inc., and the author. This research was supported in part by Research Scientist Award K3-MH-22, 682 from the National Institute of Mental Health, U.S. Public Health Service.

suggest that the considerable overlap in the way patients are actually treated by exponents of behavioral and dynamic methods is the basis for the fact that each form of treatment produces favorable results in some patients. Thus it has been argued that favorable results in behavior therapy are due to suggestion, transference, or other processes rather than specific conditioning procedures.[3] Others attribute the improvement associated with dynamic psychotherapy to the unplanned reciprocal inhibition of neurotic responses.[1] However, many authors hold that the psychological theories which underlie the two approaches are not mutually exclusive but rather different levels of conceptualization and analysis of the same phenomena. Apropos of this view are efforts to reexamine concepts and principles of psychoanalytic theory and practice from the viewpoint of learning theory. Concepts such as displacement, repression, and insight which are central to dynamic theory have been meaningfully analyzed in conditioning terms.[4-6] The purpose of such reformulations has not been to replace one terminology or frame of reference with another. Rather, the object has been to gain new perspectives on psychotherapeutic phenomena which may help clarify important theoretical issues and suggest innovations in treatment which are amenable to clinical investigation.

Many psychoanalytic writers also have argued for reformulations of analytic theory by means of learning models. However, these writers generally prefer the more cognitive theories of learning than the conditioning or "stimulus-response" models which form the basis of most behavior therapists' concepts of neurosis and treatment procedures.[7-10] However, these knotty problems of theory will not be discussed further; rather, attention will be turned to differences in practice between the two approaches.

DIFFERENCES IN PRACTICE

Dynamic psychotherapists have often recommended techniques and procedures which, in somewhat different form, constitute one or another procedure of behavior therapy. In fact, Freud stated that the patient with severe agoraphobia hardly ever overcomes his problem "if one waits till the patient lets the analysis influence him to give it up."[11] Rather, concurrent with analytic treatment, the patient must go out alone and struggle with his anxiety. This suggestion of Freud touches upon a group of behavior therapy techniques in which the anxiety elicited by certain situations is gradually reduced by having the patient expose himself to the situation, in real life or in imagination, in a gradual manner and under conditions in which the anxiety may be inhibited by other responses.[12] In recent years many therapists have described techniques conducted within the framework of traditional dynamic psychotherapy which are closely akin to behavior therapy procedures. For example, Stevenson described such techniques as assigning a patient the task between sessions of asserting himself more in a relationship in which he is usually overly passive.[13] This kind of direct instigation of behavioral change is closely related to a behavioral technique usually termed *assertive training*.[1] Such innovations in traditional dynamic therapy are becoming more frequent.[12] Of course, the difference between these innovations and behavior therapy proper is that in the latter learning principles are applied in an explicit and systematic manner to fashion more effective methods of behavior modification.

It has been pointed out by a number of writers that the influence of the behavior therapist on the course of his patient's illness is not restricted to the specific conditioning procedures involved.[14,15] In obtaining a detailed account of the patient's difficulties and adjustment before specific treatment is instigated, the patient may obtain a clearer picture of his illness and factors that are important in its maintenance. In addition much emotional support and suggestion may be conveyed. Such factors continue to operate during the course of treatment as there is usually considerable therapist-patient interaction in addition to the administration of conditioning procedures. Much of this interaction is potentially therapeutic and may include interpretative as well as supportive elements. Thus techniques which are used in a more focused and systematic manner in dynamic therapy are present here as well and doubtlessly contribute to the efficacy of behavior therapists' treatment.

From the foregoing it appears that the degree to which the treatment of a particular patient involves indirect techniques which relate to the patient's feelings, thoughts, and relationships versus efforts toward the direct modification of symptom-behavior varies on a continuum. Idealized psychoanalytic therapy would be at one end of this continuum and therapy conducted solely by an inanimate conditioning machine at the other. It would seem reasonable that different patients have different needs and might best be treated by approaches corresponding to different points on this continuum.

Some therapists believe that behavior therapy is best suited for certain patients but that dynamic therapy is the method of choice for others. In the course of careful clinical investigations Marks, Gelder, and their colleagues have attempted to delineate some of the relative indications for each approach in the treatment of phobic patients.[15-18] A number of writers have described the use of both behavior therapy and dynamic therapy for the same patient, either concurrently or in sequence.[14,15,17,19] The flexibility inherent in these approaches to the treatment of neurotic patients is appealing. However, the problem of establishing criteria for choice of treatment approach is a difficult one, involving complex theoretical issues which probably can only be solved by careful clinical investigations. This is also difficult because behavior therapists and dynamic therapists are often unfamiliar with the terminology and procedures each other use. Further, they often differ in their methods of evaluating patients, assessing improvement, and, in fact, what they consider the illness to be. In this paper, no comprehensive discussion of these problems will be attempted but one issue of special importance will be briefly discussed. This concerns the notion of neurosis.

The Concept of Neurosis

The controversy in the literature over the relative efficacy of behavior therapy and dynamic therapy has been confused by different uses of the term *neurosis*.[20] Behavior therapists usually mean by neurosis the collection of specific behavioral and psychological symptoms the patient displays. For example, a housewife with a typical agoraphobia may report and display anxiety in a variety of situations, such as leaving her house alone and riding on public conveyances, which restricts her movements and activities a great deal. Of course, not everyone is equally disposed to develop a neurosis of this kind, even under the same degree of "environmental stress." This predisposition to neurosis, whether it be primarily genetic or experiential in origin, some behavior therapists term *neuroticism*. Thus the patient with agoraphobia may be a generally anxious and dependent person. Indeed, the agoraphobia may be maintained in part by its effects on her husband, tending to keep him at her side and thus fulfilling some of her excessive dependency needs. The behavior therapist would focus his treatment on the agoraphobic symptoms, perhaps in a treatment program to decondition the anxiety associated with going out alone, being on a public conveyance, etc. Some behavior therapists would in addition deal directly with the patient's dependency on her husband. In any case the therapist would anticipate that relieving the specific agoraphobic symptoms would facilitate general improvement in the patient's adjustment. Self-confidence and self-esteem would be increased by mastery of the problem and more adaptive means of dealing with current stresses would be expected to emerge.

In contrast, the dynamic therapist would not consider the agoraphobic symptoms the neurosis but merely a manifestation of the neurosis. Rather, the neurosis would be regarded as certain underlying conflicts. Depending on the clinical details of the case (and to some extent on the therapist's theoretical orientation), these conflicts might be viewed as chiefly sexual in nature or primarily as conflicts arising from unresolved dependency needs and aggressive strivings. An understanding of these conflicts would in turn involve an understanding of the patient's character structure. Thus it seems what the behavior therapist terms *neuroticism* is close to what the dynamic therapist terms *the neurosis*; in both instances the propensity to develop certain maladaptive feelings and behaviors which compromise the patient's adjustment. The dynamic therapist would focus his treatment on these propensities and work toward their diminution. Again depending on his orientation, style of dynamic therapy, and the intensity of therapy planned, he might think more in terms of altering the patient's character structure or resolving current intrapsychic and interpersonal conflicts. His expectation would be that the specific agoraphobic symptoms will improve when progress is made with the underlying conflicts and/or character structure.

It is essential to keep these differences in mind in assessing the relative efficacy of behavioral and dynamic treatments. Otherwise, lack of agreement on what constitutes the illness and adequate assessment of change precludes any meaningful comparison of results. This indicates the necessity of evaluating multiple aspects of patients' adjustment in comparative studies since it may be that behavior therapy techniques bring about improvement in some areas whereas the impact of dynamic psychotherapy is greater on other areas of the patient's life. Indeed, some comparisons of the results of behavior therapy and dynamic therapy in the treatment of phobic patients suggest that this is the case.[18] This suggests further that some patients might be best treated by a combined approach. Perhaps in certain instances this would mean behavioral techniques for specific neurotic symptoms which are currently restricting the patient's activity and are an immediate source of discomfort and concern. Dynamic psychotherapy might be directed at less focused maladaptive tendencies the patient demonstrates in his relationships with others.

A Combined Behavioral and Dynamic Approach

The present writer has developed an innovation in the systematic desensitization treatment of severe sexual frigidity which involves the use of subanesthetic doses of I.V. Brevital (methohexital sodium) to facilitate the deconditioning process.[21,22] It has been the only treatment in those cases in which primary sexual inhibition seemed central to the patient's adjustment difficulties. Marital and other adjustment problems are usually present in these women as a consequence of their frigidity. Successful treatment of the frigidity is usually followed by general improvement in these other areas of the patient's life.

In other patients with a complaint of frigidity it is apparent that current sexual difficulties are not primary or central, but rather the result of other neurotic problems, especially ones involving the marital relationship. In these instances, progress in resolution of marital or other difficulties by psychotherapy is often accompanied by improvement in sexual adjustment.

However, there remain women in whom both primary sexual inhibition and unresolved nonsexual conflicts play a major role in the frigidity. A case will be briefly described to illustrate this situation and its treatment by a combined behavioral and dynamic approach.

The patient was a 25-year-old nurse who was frigid during the two years of her marriage. Petting before marriage produced some embarrassment and distress, but she did not anticipate the severe negative reactions which occurred during intercourse after marriage. At times these reactions were mild, permitting her to complete coitus but rarely bringing pleasure and never ending in orgasm. At other times intense anxiety would develop, making it necessary to terminate relations. Sometimes during these latter encounters, phantasies of a sadomasochistic nature would intrude themselves in which she would see herself being "abused" by her husband with other men looking on. Although accompanied by sexual arousal, the phantasies would lead to more anxiety and termination of coitus. After a year with little change in symptoms, the patient entered psychotherapy which focused on early experiences and her relationship with her husband. It seems that her father had been an impatient and physically abusive man who ran the family in an autocratic manner and demonstrated affection toward no one. The patient's mother reacted to these abuses with the attitude of a martyr and was close and affectionate with all her children. The patient recognized that her sexual problems were probably related to the poor model her father presented of a husband and lover and, at the same time, unresolved aspects of her relationship with him. She recognized also her tendency to overreact to her husband's somewhat critical manner. An accountant with many obsessive-compulsive personality traits, the husband was inclined to be a little demanding and controlling with his wife but was a generally warm and affectionate person.

The frigidity did not yield to psychotherapy, however, and other aspects of their adjustment worsened. The patient felt progressively more discouraged and inadequate, and her husband became less tolerant of the problem as he, too, experienced a growing feeling of frustration and inadequacy. Therapy was terminated after nine months because the couple moved to Philadelphia.

The problem remained the same during the four months before the couple was seen by the present writer. After assessing the present status of the problem, it was decided to make a direct approach to the frigidity since progress in other areas seemed unlikely so long as this very disruptive symptom persisted. To this end the frigidity was treated by systematic desensitization as described by Wolpe[1] and Lazarus[23] but modified by the use of I.V. Brevital. This procedure has been reported elsewhere and will not be described in detail here.[21,22,24] In brief, the patient was gotten into a deeply relaxed and tranquil state with the aid of Brevital. Then she was instructed to vividly imagine a series of sexual scenes with her husband beginning with the initial sexual approach and ending with coitus. However, she was permitted to progress from one scene of the series or hierarchy to the next only if no appreciable anxiety was experienced. With this patient it required 17 sessions of 30 minutes each over a period of three months for her to be able to vividly imagine continuing coitus with her husband without negative affects of any kind. During the course of the desensitization therapy, there was steady improvement in her sexual adjustment. By the time the desensitization treatment was completed, the couple regarded their sexual adjustment as satisfactory for the first time. Negative emotional reactions were no longer occurring but the patient was yet to experience an orgasm. This improvement in the sexual relationship was accompanied by a general improvement in both wife and husband and in the marriage. However, some residual problems were still in evidence, centering around the husband's overly controlling tendencies. The author then saw the patient in weekly sessions over a period of four months in which her relationship with her father was reexplored with an effort to work through those feelings which seemed to be contributing to her sensitivity to the husband's behavior. The husband was also seen several times to help him understand his wife's needs for independence and autonomy. Following this period of short-term psychotherapy, the total situation improved further, including the sexual adjustment. The patient experienced an orgasm for the first time during the last month of therapy and has continued to do so with coitus about 90% of the time. At present, two years after both courses of treatment were completed, the sexual and general marital adjustment has remained good, as has the individual adjustment for both man and wife.

Needless to say, this one case does not prove the efficacy of combined treatment of this sort. It is cited merely to demonstrate its feasibility. It is possible that all aspects of the problem presented by this patient and her husband could have been treated by behavior therapy procedures. It is possible also that a good result would have been attained by a longer trial of dynamic psychotherapy alone. However, the data of the case strongly suggest that the combined approach was an efficient way to deal effectively with the problem presented by this patient.

Summary

Much of the psychological theory underlying behavior therapy and dynamic therapy are not contradictory or mutually exclusive but are different levels of conceptualization of the same phenomena. There seems to be much overlap in the way patients are actually treated within the frameworks of these two approaches. It is argued that for some patients an effective therapeutic regimen may be one that includes both a behavioral and dynamic course of treatment. The feasibility of such a combined approach is illustrated by a case report of a woman whose severe frigidity was first treated by Brevital-aided systematic desensitization. This brought about an increase in her sexual responsiveness and improvement in her general adjustment. Following this, problems in relationships with her husband and others were the focus of short-term dynamic psychotherapy. This was followed by further improvement in her sexual functioning as well as improvement in other aspects of her adjustment.

References

1. Wolpe, J.: *Psychotherapy by Reciprocal Inhibition*. Stanford, Calif., Stanford University Press, 1958.
2. Feldman, M. P., and MacCulloch, M. J.: The application of anticipatory avoidance learning to the treatment of homosexuality. *Behav. Res. Ther.* 2:165-184, 1965.
3. Glover, E.: Critical notice. *Brit. J. Med. Psychol.* 32:68-74, 1959.
4. Brady, J. P.: Psychotherapy, learning theory, and insight. *Arch. Gen. Psychiat.* 16:304-311, 1967.
5. Dollard, J., and Miller, N. E.: *Personality and Psychotherapy*. New York, McGraw-Hill, 1950.
6. Miller, N. E.: Theory and experiment relating psychoanalytic displacement to stimulus-response generalization. *J. Abnorm. Soc. Psychol.* 43:155-178, 1948.
7. Alexander, F.: The dynamics of psychotherapy in the light of learning theory. *Amer. J. Psychiat.* 120:440-448, 1963. [See also Chapter 1, this volume.]
8. Marmor, J.: Psychoanalytic therapy and theories of learning. *In* Masserman, J. H. (Ed.): *Science and Psychoanalysis* VII. New York, Grune and Stratton, 1964. [See also Chapter 3, this volume.]
9. Miller, G. A., Galanter, E., and Pribram, K. H.: *Plans and the Structure of Behavior*. New York, Henry Holt, 1960.
10. Piers, G., and Piers, M. W.: Models of learning and the analytic process. *6th Int. Congr. of Psychotherapy, London, 1964*. Basel, S. Karger, 1965.
11. Freud, S.: Turnings in the ways of psycho-analytic therapy. *Collected Papers*, Vol. II. London, Hogarth Press, 1953, pp. 399-400.
12. Freeman, H.: The current status of behavior therapy. *Compr. Psychiat.* 6:355-368, 1965.
13. Stevenson, I.: Direct instigation of behavioral changes in psychotherapy. *Arch. Gen. Psychiat.* 1:99-107, 1959.
14. Crisp, A. H.: "Transference," "symptom emergence," and "social repercussions" in behavior therapy. *Brit. J. Med. Psychol.* 39:179-196, 1966.
15. Marks, I. M., and Gelder, M. G.: Common ground between behavior therapy and

psychodynamic methods. *Brit. J. Med. Psychol.* 39:11-23, 1966. [See also Chapter 10, this volume.]

16. Gelder, M. G., and Marks, I.: Severe agoraphobia: A controlled prospective trial of behavior therapy. *Brit. J. Psychiat.* 112:309-319, 1966.

17. Gelder, M. G., Marks, I. M., and Wolff, H. H.: Desensitization and psychotherapy in the treatment of phobic states: A controlled inquiry. *Brit. J. Psychiat.* 113:53-73, 1967.

18. Marks, I. M., and Gelder, M. G.: A controlled retrospective study of behavior therapy in phobic patients. *Brit. J. Psychiat.* 111:561-573, 1965.

19. Lazarus, A. A.: The results of behavior therapy in 126 cases of severe neurosis. *Behav. Res. Ther.* 1:69-79, 1963.

20. Bookbinder, J. J.: Simple conditioning versus the dynamic approach to symptoms and symptom substitution: A reply to Yates. *Psychol. Rep.* 10:71-77, 1962.

21. Brady, J. P.: Brevital-relaxation treatment of frigidity. *Behav. Res. Ther.* 4:71-77, 1966.

22. Brady, J. P.: Comments on methohexitone-aided systematic desensitization. *Behav. Res. Ther.* 5:259-260, 1967.

23. Lazarus, A. A.: The treatment of chronic frigidity by systematic desensitization. *J. Nerv. Ment. Dis.* 136:272-278, 1963.

24. Brady, J. P.: Brevital-relaxation treatment of neurosis. *Proceedings of the Symposium on Higher Nervous Activity (Madrid)*. Madrid, Spain, Sept. 9, 1966.

16

The Use of Psychotherapy and Behavior Therapy in the Treatment of an Obsessional Disorder

An Experimental Case Study

EUGENIA L. GULLICK, PH. D., AND
EDWARD B. BLANCHARD, PH.D.

Behavior therapists are much more oriented toward an ongoing and systematic measurement of change in target behaviors or symptoms than are dynamic therapists. The latter, focusing upon underlying conflicts, are more apt to view change as a more slowly evolving and global phenomenon. This case study is of a patient hospitalized for depression and obsessional thoughts, and treated by sequential and concurrent behavioral therapy and psychotherapy. The former included "thought stopping" and "assertion training," while the latter included group therapy, insight-oriented psychotherapy, and "attribution therapy." This aspect of the therapy was primarily organized around helping the patient to understand his symptoms as a response to anxiety arising from stress in daily life. No mention was made of systematic attempts to relate the stress to the presence of unconscious dynamic conflicts.

The methodology employed to relate behavioral change with specific intervention is subject to debate. However, the goal of attempting to assess the therapeutic efficacy and efficiency of specific techniques in a given patient is worthy of consideration and further study. In the patient presented, the combination of therapeutic approaches was successful in a relatively short period of time in relieving extremely debilitating symptoms.

The Use of Psychotherapy and Behavior Therapy in the Treatment of an Obsessional Disorder

An Experimental Case Study

EUGENIA L. GULLICK, PH. D., AND
EDWARD B. BLANCHARD, PH.D.

Recently, several workers in the field of behavior therapy[3,10] have suggested combining empirically validated principles of psychotherapy with those of behavior therapy into what has been termed *broad spectrum behavior therapy*.[4] Basic to this new "technical eclecticism"[5] is the systematic application of whatever techniques are effective in dealing with a patient's problems.

The present paper presents a case study of the successful treatment of an obsessional disorder through the combination of insight-oriented psychotherapy and behavior therapy. Also included are some of the principles of clinical research in behavior modification, illustrated through the use of the single subject reversal design. Through the systematic monitoring and recording of target behaviors, it was possible to examine the relative efficacy of various aspects of the treatment program during the course of the study.

Case History. The patient was a 33-year-old, married, Caucasian male, with a Ph.D. in plant physiology. He was admitted to the psychiatric unit of the University of Mississippi Medical Center with a chief complaint of recurring thoughts that he had blasphemed God. This symptom first occurred 3 weeks prior to admission when he had been baptized in the Pentecostal church, but had not experienced a feeling of "being saved." He had joined this fundamentalistic church after a 2-year-long "religious crisis" during which time he was seeking "to acquire religion." This crisis period coincided with the completion of the work for his Ph.D. and his being employed as a research administrator for a state agency.

The chief symptom, the obsessive thoughts about having "blasphemed God," had so incapacitated him for the 10 days prior to admission that he could not work or even participate minimally in family activities. He also had moderately severe initial and terminal sleep disturbances and his appetite was diminished. He had taken to shaking and striking his head with his palms in an effort to banish the obsessional thoughts.

From *Journal of Nervous and Mental Disease*, 156:427-431, 1973, The Williams & Wilkins Co. Reproduced by permission.

Method

Data Collection

Data collection was started the day after the patient was admitted to the hospital and consisted of having him record the length of time between obsessional thoughts (which were self-defined). This method of recording the number of obsessional thoughts has the advantage of yielding an accurate tally while preventing the patient from focusing on the number of obsessions; this procedure was followed throughout the course of his hospitalization.

Treatment Techniques

Several different techniques were applied sequentially in the treatment of the patient, each of which is described briefly below. At times a second technique, usually a specific behavior therapy technique, was applied concurrently with the ongoing psychotherapy.

Baseline. During this 3-day phase no therapeutic interventions were applied other than having the patient become adjusted to the open ward milieu. The ward was an acute treatment unit for children and adults which at any one time contained a mixture of patients with psychotic, neurotic, alcoholic, and behavior disorder diagnoses. Group therapy sessions for the entire patient population, as well as weekly ward government meetings, were held.

Psychotherapy. The first treatment phase consisted of nine daily psychotherapy sessions. The focus of each of the psychotherapy phases of this case was to help the patient achieve insight into the nature of his problem while offering him support and encouragement, particularly for verbalizations of intentions to change some distressing aspects of his environment.

Thought Stopping. In addition to psychotherapy sessions the technique of "thought stopping," described by Wolpe[9] for the treatment of obsessional disorders, was introduced. Briefly, it consists first of having the therapist shout "stop" in the midst of one of the patient's ruminations. This usually disrupts the rumination. Next the patient is instructed to shout "stop" himself, first aloud, then covertly, as a way of disrupting the ruminative chain. This technique was applied for 5 days.

First Reversal. Since the patient was being treated in experimental fashion, a control phase, or reversal, was instituted. During these 3 days, the patient was not seen in psychotherapy. Thus this phase served as a control for the nonspecific effects[1] of "being in therapy" by removing them temporarily. It was, of course, not possible to remove any "insight" which the patient might have achieved. Moreover, the patient continued to be in the ward milieu, making this a good control for "being in therapy."

Psychotherapy and Second Reversal. Psychotherapy was reinstituted along the lines described above for 3 more days. Next, a second control phase was instituted during which time psychotherapy was again discontinued. Then psychotherapy, including attribution therapy, was again instituted on a daily basis and continued until the patient's discharge 11 days later.

Attribution Therapy. Since there was little improvement when psychotherapy was reinstated, the focus was changed for the next 9 days to one utilizing attribution therapy, as described by Valins and Nisbett.[8] The latter consists of the systematic applications of the theory and research on the social psychology of the attribution of causation to the clinical area. It deals in particular with the locus of causality.

In the specific application to this case it was pointed out to the patient that his chief symptom, the obsessional thoughts, was the result of his being anxious and could be considered an avoidance response. Moreover, it was pointed out that he became anxious primarily as a result of outside stresses, in particular the demands of his job. Thus, he was led to *reattribute* the meaning of obsessional thoughts from a sign that something was wrong with him (e.g., such as his initial interpretation that he had failed in his attempt to become a Christian) to a sign that there was some stress in his environment to which he should attend because it was causing him to become anxious. Hence, there was a shift in the locus of causality of the symptom from himself to his environment. The patient was reminded of this reattribution on a daily basis and was instructed to reinterpret his immediate history in that light.

Finally, because of clinical indications, the patient was given a course of assertive training, as described by Lazarus[2] and McFall and Marston,[6] during the final 4 days of hospitalization. In these sessions the patient was asked to describe anxiety-arousing situations, particularly as related to his job; next, assertive responses were first modeled by the therapist and then attempted by the patient with feedback given him by the therapist on the adequacy of his performance.

Posthospitalization Treatment. The patient was discharged after 33 days of hospitalization. He was then seen weekly in a therapy group which emphasized the learning of assertive responses. He was also seen briefly by his primary therapist before group sessions both to monitor his progress and to reemphasize attribution therapy.

RESULTS

The number of obsessive thoughts is plotted in Figure 1 for each of the phases of the study. In this figure we have a day-to-day description

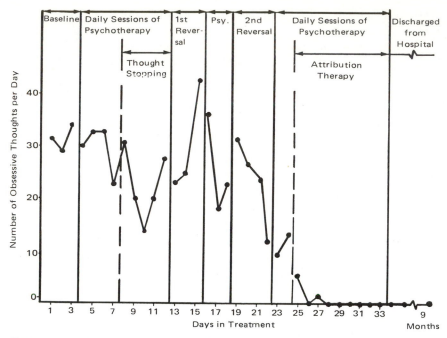

FIGURE 1. Number of daily obsessional thoughts as a function of experimental conditions.

of target symptoms which enabled the therapist to make decisions as to efficacy of a particular treatment procedure.

During the baseline phase, the patient had an average of 31 incidents of obsessive thoughts per day. During the first four psychotherapy sessions there was a slight decrease in number of obsessive thoughts as the patient achieved some insight into the nature of his problem. He even verbalized, "I know why I'm doing these things, now I want to learn how to stop them." The addition of thought stopping to psychotherapy led to an initial decrease in number of obsessive thoughts, but overall it was ineffective.

The first reversal, or control phase, for the nonspecific effects of being in therapy, provided some confirmation that the latter was effective. For the 3 days in which the patient was not seen there was a steady rise in the number of daily occurrences of obsessive thoughts to 41. Reinstitution of psychotherapy without thought stopping led to a decrease in obsessions to a level of about 20 per day.

In the second reversal a somewhat puzzling set of events occurred. The number of obsessions initially rose and then dropped dramatically to a new low of 13 per day. The patient was on leave from the hospital for the last 2 days of the reversal phase, and activities at home may have countered his tendency to obsess.

Two more psychotherapy sessions led to no further reduction. With introduction of attribution therapy in the context of psychotherapy for the next 5 days, the rate of obsessive thoughts dropped to zero. A mild depression which had been present intermittently throughout his hospitalization also lifted.

The final treatment phase, assertive training, was introduced because there were definite clinical indications that this form of treatment was needed to enable the patient to return to work and function fully.

Follow-up Data

During the first 2 months after discharge there were two recurrences of the obsessive symptoms, three obsessive thoughts on 1 day and four on another occasion. Brief conferences between the patient and the therapist which focused on the reattribution theme revealed stresses in the patient's job. He was able to cope with these adequately by his report. Since that time he has discontinued group psychotherapy; a follow-up at 9 months after discharge revealed the patient to be functioning well with no further return of obsessive symptoms.

DISCUSSION

As is well known, obsessive-compulsive neuroses do not usually respond well to psychotherapy, but when they do, the course of therapy is typically quite protracted.[7] It is therefore heartening to find such a thorough remission of symptoms as a result of 5 weeks of hospitalization and short-term follow-up on an outpatient basis. This remission is probably due to a combination of two sets of factors: (1) good prognosis due to very brief duration of symptoms prior to treatment and a large degree of environmental stresses present; and (2) the second set of factors, the main topic of this paper, is the judicious combination of insight-oriented psychotherapy with several behavior therapy techniques. This case illustrates that both approaches can be used with benefits simultaneously and serves to validate Lazarus's[3,4] call for "broad spectrum behavior therapy."

An important aspect of this study is that it highlights the advantages of monitoring the target symptoms on a systematic basis. Through having the patient record the latency of each episode of obsessive thoughts, it was possible to obtain daily frequency counts on the number of obsessive thoughts. Using this information enabled us to make decisions on treatment. For example, it was possible to observe the effects of using a well-known behavior therapy technique, thought stopping, within the context of psychotherapy. Following a basic principle of the behavior therapy approach, i.e., systematic specification and measurement of target behavior and reliance on empirical verification of the efficacy of a procedure, it was possible to terminate use of an ineffective technique. Likewise, we were able to determine by this monitoring that another technique, attribution therapy, was very successful and to continue to focus on its use.

REFERENCES

1. Frank, J. D. *Persuasion and Healing*. Johns Hopkins Press, Baltimore, 1961.
2. Lazarus, A. A. Behavior rehearsal *vs.* non-directive therapy *vs.* advice in effecting behavior change. *Behav. Res. Ther.*, 4: 209-212, 1966.
3. Lazarus, A. A. *Behavior Therapy and Beyond*. McGraw-Hill, New York, 1971.
4. Lazarus, A. A. Broad spectrum behavior therapy and the treatment of agoraphobia. *Behav. Res. Ther.*, 4: 95-97, 1966.
5. Lazarus, A. A. In support of technical eclecticism. *Psychol. Rep.*, 21: 415-416, 1967.
6. McFall, R. M., and Marston, A. R. An experimental investigation of behavior rehearsal in assertive training. *J. Abnorm. Psychol.*, 76:295-303, 1970.
7. Nemiah, J. C. Obsessive-compulsive reaction. In Freedman, A. M., and Kaplan, H. I., Eds. *Comprehensive Textbook of Psychiatry*, pp. 912-927. Williams & Wilkins Co., Baltimore, 1967.
8. Valins, S., and Nisbett, R. E. *Attribution Processes in the Development and Treatment of Emotional Disorders*. General Learning Press, New York, 1971.
9. Wolpe, J. *The Practice of Behavior Therapy*. Pergamon, New York, 1969.
10. Woody, R. H. *Psychobehavioral Counseling and Therapy: Integrating Behavioral and Insight Techniques*. Appleton-Century-Crofts, New York, 1971.

Concurrent Psychotherapy and Behavior Therapy

Treatment of Psychoneurotic Outpatients

R. TAYLOR SEGRAVES, M.D., PH.D., AND
ROBERT C. SMITH, M.D., PH.D.

Since few therapists are proficient in both psychoanalytically oriented psychotherapy and behavior therapy, the feasibility of concomitant but separate treatment programs for the same patient, by different therapists, is an extraordinarily important clinical issue. Both analytic and behavioral purists have hypothesized a host of disruptive consequences and yet there are certain patients whose symptoms are so highly disruptive as to make this an important therapeutic consideration. The authors report on three such cases referred for behavior therapy for a disruptive target symptom (anxiety attacks, phobia, fetish) during the course of psychoanalytic psychotherapy. Not only were complications minimal, but the two therapies were synergistic, with the behavior therapy initiating change and the psychotherapy functioning to make it more permanent. We commonly think of symptom relief following rather than preceding the elaboration and resolution of etiological conflict, yet for these patients the behavioral resolution of their symptoms facilitated the development of transference reactions and insights related to the unconscious material previously "bound" by the symptom. There were few problems associated with the simultaneous treatment by separate therapists, and these were easily resolvable.

Concurrent Psychotherapy and Behavior Therapy

17

Treatment of Psychoneurotic Outpatients

R. Taylor Segraves, M.D., Ph.D., and
Robert C. Smith, M.D., Ph. D.

The empirically oriented psychotherapist frequently faces a dilemma in deciding a responsible course of treatment for a given neurotic outpatient. The typical neurotic outpatient who enters treatment with a combination of both specific behavioral symptoms and more diffuse interpersonal problems has traditionally been treated by one of the verbal-insight or verbal-relationship types of psychotherapy. The evidence regarding the efficacy of these therapies is unclear, although most clinicians "subjectively know" that certain patients respond rather dramatically to this type of therapy with a major shift in their subjective experience of the world, as well as in their behavior. There is some empirical evidence to substantiate this, as Bergin,[1] in his review of psychotherapy outcome research, concluded that on the average, one can expect a slightly positive outcome from one of the traditional psychotherapies, but that this average outcome for a group of patients probably reflects both highly positive and negative results in different patients. On the other hand, a burgeoning literature in behavior therapy suggests that a set of effective procedures exists for the treatment of certain specifiable psychological symptoms such as phobias,[2] stuttering,[3] fetishes,[4] obesity,[5] sexual dysfunction,[6] and obsessive-compulsive rituals.[7] Unfortunately, in these clinical conditions the presenting target symptom may represent only a fragment of the patient's emotional and interpersonal difficulties.

Thus, a focus of concern and debate among contemporary clinicians has been on which type or combination of types of therapeutic interventions should be used. In the recent past, much of this discussion centered around attacks by representatives of one school of thought on the

Reprinted by permission from *Archives of General Psychiatry*, 33:756-763, June 1976. Copyright 1976 by the American Medical Association.

results and flaws of the opposing theoretical system,[8,9] and appeared to serve political as well as scientific motivations.[10] More recently, eclectic therapists have struggled for some sort of synthesis between learning theory and psychoanalysis.[11-13] Another approach has been for one therapist to attempt to combine effective treatment strategies from different theoretical sources in an optimal package for the individual patient. Arnold Lazarus[14] and his development of multimodal therapy, and Lee Birk et al.,[15] with their combining of group psychotherapy and aversive conditioning, would be examples of this approach. There are fewer reports discussing the problems of incorporating therapies from different theoretical systems when more than one therapist is involved. Woody[16] has reported successful outcomes in patients referred to him for behavior therapy by psychoanalytically oriented colleagues. Unfortunately, he did not discuss the problems and advantages of the "shared patient" approach in any detail. Smith and Carlin[17] discussed the problems of incorporating contingency management into a traditional psychiatric hospital setting.

The lack of precise information about the effectiveness of the shared patient approach is unfortunate. Because of the polemical nature of the debate between behavior therapists and analytically oriented therapists, many practicing therapists are probably proficient in only one of the two schools of therapy. A typical psychiatric outpatient who has a combination of both specific and diffuse interpersonal difficulties probably receives a variant of one of the traditional verbal psychotherapies in most psychiatric outpatient settings, although certain of his difficulties might well respond to one of the behavioral approaches. Thus, a practical clinical question, potentially having considerable importance, is whether patients in traditional psychotherapy can profitably be referred to a colleague for symptom removal therapy. This article will focus on this practical clinical question—what are the difficulties and advantages of referral of a patient in psychoanalytically oriented psychotherapy to a behavior therapist?

A second and related purpose of this project is to observe the consequences of symptom removal from the perspective of a dynamically oriented psychotherapist. A substantial body of evidence indicates that symptom removal seldom, if ever, leads to symptom substitution or clinical deterioration.[18] These studies would almost lead one to infer that a symptom exists in isolation from the remainder of a patient's mental life and interaction with his environment. Thus, a secondary purpose of this project is to examine the evidence for attitude and behavior change concomitant with symptom removal in areas of the patient's life not directly linked with the symptom. This information would be of importance to the referring psychotherapist, as the impact of symptom removal could effect subsequent events in psychotherapy.

METHOD

Within the psychiatry department at the University of Chicago, both authors have been involved in numerous cases involving simultaneous treatment of the same patient by two different therapists. However, this report will be limited to three patients formally admitted to this clinical series. One of the authors (R.C.S.) agreed to refer patients in psychoanalytically oriented psychotherapy to the other author (R.T.S.) for behavior therapy. The conditions of referral were that all patients he had in psychotherapy who also had specifiable symptoms amenable to behavior therapy would be referred at times he deemed appropriate from the standpoint of psychotherapeutic considerations. The other author accepted for referral all patients who had conditions he judged amenable to respondent conditioning techniques. After referral, both therapists remained incommunicado regarding the patients unless a specific problem arose. This was done to approximate the conditions of clinical practice, and to make the therapists independent observers as much as possible.

After experience with the initial case, the authors decided to administer several questionnaires to provide an additional independent source of information to either corroborate or refute clinical impressions and observations. These scales included the Hopkins Symptom Check List (HSCL),[19] the Profile of Mood Scales (POMS),[20] the Wolpe Fear Survey Schedule (WFSS),[21] and an Osgood Semantic Differential (OSGOOD).[22] The POMS and HSCL were employed to independently monitor subjectively experienced distress in the patients. The WFSS was used to assess changes in ratings of phobic stimuli. The OSGOOD was used to measure changes in concepts thought to be clinically important for each patient. Patients were asked to rate relevant concepts on the OSGOOD with a series of bipolar scales. Results were computed on three factors computed from these scales: evaluative (good vs. bad), activity (passive vs. active), and potency (strong vs. weak). Each OSGOOD contained eight or nine concepts: two concepts directly related to the symptom being treated (e.g., chicken, egg), four or five concepts not overtly related to the target symptom (e.g., housewife, father), and two control or neutral concepts (Europe, earnest). These scales were administered by the behavior therapist on three occasions: before the behavior therapy began (initial), at the termination of behavior therapy (termination), and at four- to six-month follow-up (follow-up). Because of the small sample size, these scales were not used to assay statistical significance of change.

REPORT OF CASES

Case 1. Mr. P. was a 45-year-old Protestant minister who sought psychiatric help because of profuse perspiring and anxiety attacks. The typical attack occurred while he was actively conducting religious services, and consisted of his inexplicably becoming extremely anxious and perspiring so profusely that his hair, face, beard, and clerical gown became drenched in perspiration. The patient had certain self-doubts about the value and validity of the religious services he conducted, and feared that members of the congregation would notice his perspiration as a sign of his hypocrisy. The perspiration appeared to be more intense when his senior colleague, who was going to retire next year, was also present during services, and the sweating also occurred occasionally in ministerial social situations when he was identified as a clergyman and treated with some favor. Mr. P. dated the onset of his sweating to an incident when, as a college undergraduate, he had gone to visit one of his professors and had tried to impress this professor with his interest and knowledge in the professor's field of interest. Although he was successful in his stated purpose, Mr. P. suddenly became extremely anxious and started perspiring profusely. He left the professor's office and avoided all future contact with this man. Mr. P. reported that he had undergone 18 months of psychodynamically oriented psychotherapy in another city without alleviation of his sweating. In light of the ineffectiveness of the previous psychotherapy for this specific symptom, the psychotherapist referred Mr. P. to the behavior therapist after about two months of once-a-week psychotherapy. He also continued to be seen in weekly psychodynamic psychotherapy.

Because of the failure of a behavioral analysis to clearly identify eliciting stimuli for the perspiration, the behavior therapist arranged a systematic desensitization to a temporal hierarchy of imagined scenes during the religious services. This series of imagined scenes began with the minister imagining being in his office 10 minutes prior to the service, and then progressed through the service in minute detail. Otherwise the desensitization was fairly standard, with muscle relaxation being induced by training in progressive relaxation, and aided by 4 mg of diazepam (Valium) taken orally. The rationale of this treatment is to countercondition the stimuli that elicit anxiety, and this is accomplished by a gradual exposure to these stimuli while in a state of deep relaxation.

The early systematic desensitization sessions proceeded unremarkably, with concomitant reduction in sweating during the early part of the actual religious services. However, treatment with Mr. P. then entered a phase where he reported marked fluctuation in his perspiration during services, and some unusual interactions occurred between the behavior therapist and Mr. P. Mr. P. had canceled the previous behavior therapy session to attend a funeral, and prior to beginning the desensitization, the behavior therapist casually inquired if the funeral had been for anyone close to the patient. Mr. P. seemed surprised and pleased by the question, replied that it was a distant relative, and then began a brief discussion about a television talk show concerning psychiatry. A brief superficial discussion of the philosophy of psychiatry discussed on the television show followed, and suddenly Mr. P. blushed and began to perspire profusely. On questioning, Mr. P. stated that he knew practically nothing about psychiatry and was afraid that the behavior therapist would realize what a "phony" he was. The behavior therapist was genuinely surprised by this occurrence, dealt with it at face value, stated that the patient seemed quite knowledgeable, and shifted their attention back to the desensitization, which proceeded extremely slowly that session. In the following session, a similar incident occurred after Mr.

P. initiated a conversation about cartoons in the *New Yorker* magazine. Mr. P. remained tense during this session as well, and progress was problematic during this and the sessions of the subsequent week. A meeting between the behavior therapist and the psychotherapist was arranged to discuss these problems. Shortly thereafter, Mr. P. again began progressing through the desensitization hierarchy and reporting relief from perspiration in real life.

Progress through the remainder of the hierarchy was unremarkable, except that Mr. P. required numerous repetitions of two particular scenes before achieving anxiety-free visualization. The first of these involved his noticing two church elders standing in the congregation during a responsive reading, with stern, disapproving facial expressions. The second scene involved his performing an altar service with his older colleague and a female church custodian. After struggling repetitively to elicit and maintain this visual image, he suddenly remarked that he was puzzled to find himself angry at the custodian and his older colleague. The therapist encouraged him to maintain the visual image. Suddenly, Mr. P. remarked, "You know, I have trouble imagining that scene because I keep remembering that slut custodian wandering about the church in a loose housecoat, and also her face kept resembling my mother's. You know, I just remembered that my mother used to always do that at home."

Mr. P. was then able to visualize the scene without difficulty, and finished his course of systematic desensitization without further incident. At the termination of behavior therapy, which had lasted for 18 sessions, Mr. P. began to speak of the religious service as being filled with deep historical meaning and significance, was puzzled over his previous feelings of hypocrisy, reported that his perspiration was no longer a problem, and said, "You're winning, but that's OK." Inquiries by the behavior therapist and the psychotherapist at several points up to eight months after the termination of treatment indicated that the marked decrease in sweating had been maintained.

About the same time that the two therapists had arranged a meeting to discuss the slow and problematic progress in behavior therapy, the issue of competition came up in the psychotherapy sessions. When the patient's competitive fantasies were explored, it became clear that therapy itself was seen as competition on multiple levels. Although Mr. P. wanted to be cured of his sweating attacks, he also felt that "getting better" was also "losing a game"—i.e., if the patient got better, the therapist was the victor and the patient had been defeated. Mr. P. also felt that there must be competition between the behavior therapist and the psychotherapist. The patient also discussed competitive feelings and fears about displacing his senior colleague in the church. In one session, he seemed uncomfortable as the psychotherapist began to make a tentative interpretation; he interrupted and effectively stopped the therapist by his own effusive talking. With the therapists' help, Mr. P. was able to become aware of his "uncomfortable feeling" of competition with the psychotherapist, the interaction that had elicited it, and the characteristic way in which he dealt with the feeling.

After two further sessions in which these competitive feelings were explored and clarified, the patient began to report renewed progress in behavior therapy. As he made progress in the behavior therapy, he once again expressed some concern about how the psychotherapist was feeling about the success of behavior therapy. Shortly after the termination of the behavior therapy, although the patient reported a sustained marked reduction of sweating during the religious service, Mr. P. was concerned that the behavior therapist may have felt bad because he had been unable to completely cure the patient of all of his symptoms. These instances provided additional stimuli to reexplore the feelings of competition and rivalry as they related to both the therapist and other interpersonal relationships.

Mr. P. continued to undergo weekly psychotherapy for eight months after the termination of behavior therapy. During this time, Mr. P. became more aware of his need to control situations, and of the mechanisms he used to deal with his anxiety when he felt he could not control the situation. The patient also spent more time recalling the character of his silent but still affectionate father, and the long competitive struggle with his younger brother for primacy in their parents' love and approval. He also came back to feelings about replacing his older colleague, and challenged one of the policies of the association of clergy in his local area. Toward the termination of psychotherapy, his feelings of dependency on the psychotherapist were discussed, and the ways Mr. P. tried to take more active control of the termination were explored.

This case is an excellent example of behavior therapy and psychotherapy complementing one another. Clearly, the direct uncompromising attack on the target symptom by the pragmatic behavior therapist elicited many of Mr. P.'s learned responses (transference reactions) to authority figures. The structured, controlled setting of behavior therapy elicited in detail almost the identical emotional reaction in which the symptom had first occurred, and also evoked associations suggesting an oedipal origin to his anxieties regarding competition. This full-blown "transference reaction" occurred in only six weeks of contact with the behavior therapist, and never occurred in the more permissive atmosphere of psychotherapy. More importantly, Mr. P.'s experience in behavior supplied much meaningful material for psychotherapy. As discussed in the case summary, experiences in behavior therapy elicited a discussion of Mr. P.'s fantasies regarding competition, memories of sibling rivalry, and his tendency to control interpersonal situations to avoid these anxieties. Behavior therapy reached an impasse approximately halfway through systematic desensitization, and progress in behavior therapy occurred only after a discussion of the issue of competition occurred in psychotherapy. Clinically, both therapists felt that this discussion facilitated Mr. P.'s renewed progress in behavior therapy.

Three potential difficulties were encountered in this case. After behavior therapy started producing therapeutic results, Mr. P. began evaluating the efficacy of psychotherapy. The fact that a therapeutic alliance had already been established prior to referral precluded this from becoming a serious problem. A related difficulty could have been more serious. When Mr. P.'s progress in behavior therapy reached an impasse, the therapists met to discuss a unified approach. Although this meeting was arranged to discuss therapeutic tactics, in retrospect it also seemed to serve a covert purpose of helping the therapists resolve their own feelings of competition. Although both therapists work in the same clinical setting and are social acquaintances of three years' duration, an element of distrust arose. Specifically, the psychotherapist wondered if the behavior therapist was trying to take over the case, and the behavior therapist wondered what "misguided" analytic interpretations had led to Mr. P.'s difficulty in behavior therapy. These difficulties were fortunately easily resolved by the meeting. The fact that the "transference reaction" occurred outside of the psychotherapy setting may be of concern to clinicians of a more traditional psychoanalytic orientation. Although the development of the transference reaction was atypical in that sense, a careful reading of the case reveals that the transference reaction once elicited by behavior therapy then transferred to the psychotherapy setting, where a clearer explication of the internal eliciting stimuli was accomplished.

Case 2. Ms. S. was a 23-year-old schoolteacher who entered therapy with two complaints: depression over her unsatisfactory relationships with men, who she felt used and abused her, and a secondary complaint of a bird phobia. She was involved with a married man who she felt was treating her unfairly, and she was becoming more depressed as this relationship continued. The bird phobia did not greatly interfere with her daily work and social life. She avoided camping trips and picnics, became nauseated at the sight of poultry, had recurring frightening dreams of being in cages with chickens, and washed her hands three or four times after touching eggs. However, she experienced the phobia subjectively as proving that she was a neurotic, silly woman.

The first seven months of twice-weekly psychodynamically oriented psychotherapy focused primarily on the patient's feelings of depression and her relationships with men. The psychotherapist attempted with only moderate success to help the patient become aware of some of the ways she became involved in frustrating relationships with men. However, her "underlying" problems did not appear to have been substantially affected, and the patient mentioned the bird phobia several times and expressed some interest in treatment for this condition. When the behavior therapist had an opening, she was referred to him for treatment, while continuing to undergo twice-weekly psychotherapy.

Behavior therapy consisted primarily of a traditional course of systematic desensitization to a hierarchy of imagined scenes involving increasing physical proximity to birds. Systematic desensitization was supplemented with homework *in vivo* desensitization assignments (e.g., read a book on birds, visit a pet shop) and followed by three sessions of *in vivo* desensitization and modeling (the therapist touched a duck in his office and had the patient do likewise). In all, the patient was seen for 11 behavior therapy sessions on a once-a-week basis.

Progress in systematic desensitization was unremarkable, except that progress was slow initially because of extreme anxiety accompanied by leg cramps. Later sessions were followed by waves of nausea and migraine headaches. These problems were easily circumvented by slowing the rate of hierarchy progression.

After the patient achieved anxiety-free visualization of touching a bird, the behavior therapist brought a live caged duck to his office. In the first session the therapist modeled touching the duck. In the second session, although extremely anxious, Ms. S. said that she felt she could now touch the duck. Prior to touching the duck, the patient made an unusual comment. "You know it's funny. I want to touch the duck, but somehow feel that it's wrong. It reminds me of dating in high school when I desired intercourse, but always said no." Subsequently, she touched the duck and cried with relief. In the next and last behavior therapy session, Ms. S. spontaneously reported a dream that had occurred the night after touching the duck. In the dream her uncle, wearing only a loose bathrobe in the patient's presence, had ripped open the neck of a cooked goose by jamming his fingers down the throat of the bird, and the ripped flesh was red rather than white. On awakening after the dream, the patient had said to herself, "Of course, that was a vagina." She subsequently stated that her attitude toward sex and her father had somehow changed; she no longer idealized her father as much, and now felt that sex without "love" was acceptable. The behavior therapist did not make any comments about this dream or the associated attitude change, but constantly shifted the focus back to the behavior therapy tasks. During the follow-up, at several points up to 1½ years after behavior therapy, there was no evidence of return of the bird phobia, and the patient would now eat fowl dishes in restaurants and had allowed birds to build a nest on her window. The patient also experienced a tremendous rise in self-esteem, stating, "I'm no longer a silly, neurotic woman with a phobia."

During the initial stages of behavior therapy, Ms. S. continued to discuss her relationships with men, emphasizing her role as victim and only reluctantly questioning the role of her own behavior in initiating and maintaining these relationships. About midway through the course of behavior therapy, Ms. S. began to bring up memories of attempted childhood seduction in the psychotherapy sessions, material that had not surfaced previously. For example, when she was 6 or 7 years old, a boyfriend of the family maid tried to seduce her by enticing her with food and then manually stimulating her mons pubis area. She remembered being sexually stimulated, but her main feeling was that of being overwhelmed and helpless to take action. In another childhood incident, she accepted the invitation of a school bus driver to sit on his lap and he began to undress her. She again reported that she had felt helpless, although she eventually did get off the bus. She denied that any of her own wishes or impulses were involved in these incidents.

After touching the duck in behavior therapy, Ms. S. reported fairly dramatic changes. In the subsequent psychotherapy session, she stated that a heavy depression had lifted. A number of significant dreams occurred in the week after touching the duck. In one, she dreamed of a letter about her father's death and the subsequent funeral. In association to this dream, Ms. S. commented on her change in attitude toward her father, stating that she felt more neutral toward him and viewed him less sentimentally. She recalled that her father was still touching and kissing her when she was 17 or 18 years old, and that he would charge her with being hysterical when she cried or complained about this. During this time, Ms. S. began to experience and express anger more readily toward men and toward her father, and began to see herself in a less passive role. During the two weeks after completion of behavior therapy, Ms. S. began to break off relationships with her married boyfriend, reported an active effort to attract a man on an airplane flight, went to work without a brassiere one day, and reported that she felt less overwhelmed and helpless in the face of sexual stimulation.

In subsequent psychotherapy, which lasted for 1½ years after the termination of behavior therapy, some of the dramatic changes that followed symptom removal, such as the changed attitude toward her father and the more frank acknowledgment of her own sexual feelings, were maintained. Some of the other changes, such as Ms. S.'s more active pursuit of men and her "giving up" the image of being a helpless victim in sexual encounters, appeared to be more transient, and reemerged as issues in psychotherapy. The memories of attempted childhood seduction came up again on numerous occasions, and were discussed in greater depth. Ms. S. accused the therapist of charging her with luring or provoking these men, and her anger and sullenness became even more intense when the therapist acknowledged his own feelings of being sexually stimulated by her at times. In discussing this interaction, the patient became more observant of her own provocative behavior, and reported being able to see the therapist as a man rather than a God-like doctor. As a man, he could have sexual feelings that she could arouse, but she didn't have to sexually submit to him. This change in attitude to a more active responsibility and acknowledgment of her own sexual feelings, which had emerged immediately after the behavior therapy, appears to have now become a permanent change.

Ms. S. showed rather remarkable decreases in self-reported distress immediately after successful symptom removal on both the POMS and HSCL scales. These changes were largely maintained, with little additional change at six months' follow-up. Changes on the WFSS were remarkable. Selected data from the POMS is reproduced in Table 1 for illustrative purposes.

Data from the OSGOOD Semantic Differential were less clear, but appeared to demonstrate a shift toward a more positive evaluation of the concept "chicken," a more negative evaluation of "father," and a more potent conception of "housewife." The other concepts did not demonstrate notable shifts relative to the control concepts. Selected data from the OSGOOD scales are reproduced in Table 2.

The changes on the questionnaire data appeared to parallel the attitudinal changes noted in psychotherapy.

Although the relatively brief course of behavior therapy was successful in removing the bird phobia, it also appeared to have many other effects on the patient's life and on the psychotherapy sessions. The marked effect of the behavior therapy on other aspects of Ms. S.'s feelings and behavior (which were not directly connected with the bird phobia on a manifest level) is clearly evident from the dramatic changes that followed almost immediately on removal of the phobia. These effects were documented as follows: (1) symbolically in the patient's dreams; (2) in her reports to the psychotherapist of changes in her feelings toward significant people in her life and her behavior of actively attracting men; and (3) in the questionnaire responses, which showed considerable reductions in anxiety and depression, and changes in her evaluation of others. Removal of the phobia seemed to coincide temporarily with a change in her subjective view of the world. Specifically, she seemed to assume responsibility for her own sexual feelings, and to adopt a more active role in her relationships with men. This later change occurred immediately after removal of the bird phobia, then receded in subsequent months, and was reactivated and consolidated by additional work in the psychotherapy sessions.

Again, it appears that successful behavior therapy mobilized feelings and memories significant to the origin of phobia, as well as providing symptomatic relief. This mobilization of feelings and associations appeared to facilitate and accelerate progress in psychotherapy. Also, both therapists were surprised to report that neither was aware of any therapeutic difficulty due to the presence of concurrent therapy. Ms. S. apparently viewed each therapy as having a separate purpose and treated each accordingly. Whether the absence of difficulty in concurrent therapy was due to a patient characteristic or due to the therapists being more comfortable working together is uncertain.

Case 3. Mr. B. was a 31-year-old engineer who entered psychotherapy with a chief complaint of a wet-boot fetish. However, at the time he entered psychotherapy, his most pressing problem was his anxiety and depression over his marital difficulties and impending divorce. Mr. B.'s memory of pleasure associated with wet feet or boots dated from age 5. At the time his brother was born, he was sent to a neighbor's house to stay. On the way to the neighbor's house, he accidentally got his feet wet and enjoyed the sensation. He remembered more instances between the ages of 5 and 12 where he got his feet wet on purpose and found this exhilarating. The first clear sexual feeling associated with the fetish occurred in early adolescence, when a female cousin asked him to go wading with her. He later had his first masturbatory experience after getting his feet wet. His heterosexual experience prior to marriage was limited, and he was impotent on the wedding night. However, he was able to have an erection on the next day after his wife got her feet wet by accident. Thereafter, their sexual life was satisfactory for several years, although occasionally Mr. B. would have to fantasize wet shoes or have his wife get her feet wet before being able to have intercourse. Later in the marriage, the severity of his wet-shoe fetish appeared to covary directly with the severity of marital discord.

Although his fetish was one of Mr. B.'s initial complaints on entering therapy, it was not a prominent issue during the first seven months of psychotherapy. In this phase of psychotherapy, Mr. B.'s depressive reaction accompanying the separation from his wife and his ways of coping with the impending divorce were explored. Therapeutic intervention was directed at the martyr role Mr. B. assumed, and at his attachment to the image of an innocent victim. His inability to express anger to his wife or toward most other people in his life became clear. During this initial phase of psychotherapy, Mr. B. became somewhat more aware of these chronic ways he mediated his transactions with others, his depression had receded, and he became slightly more assertive toward his wife in dealing with divorce proceedings. Since the patient himself saw the fetish as a persistent problem and noted it as a major reason why he was afraid to establish any new relationships with women, the psychotherapist felt that a behavior therapy approach to attacking the symptom directly might be a useful adjunct to the psychotherapy.

The behavioral treatment of Mr. B.'s fetish consisted of a masturbatory reconditioning regimen. After a diagnostic interview, Mr. B. was told that wet shoes had fortuitously become associated with sexual arousal, and that the point of masturbatory reconditioning would be to shift sexual arousal to more socially acceptable sexual objects. He was instructed to masturbate at home, starting with any sexually arousing fantasy that he liked, but always, at the point of ejaculatory inevitability, to switch to a fantasy not involving wet shoes or wet feet. The treatment plan consisted of having the patient begin masturbation to fetish scenes, but to progressively and gradually switch to the nonfetish images at times further and further prior to ejaculation, until he could eventually masturbate to orgasm without using the fetish scene at all.

During the early weeks of behavior therapy, the patient became concerned about violent dreams and fantasies. For example, he reported that he sometimes had to introduce fantasies of forcible seduction or rape in order to ejaculate, and that he had repetitive dreams of tornadoes killing people. The behavior therapist treated this in a matter-of-fact way, saying that aggression and sexuality are frequently linked, and that this is nothing to be worried about. Later, Mr. B. mentioned trancelike sleep-waking states of being afraid of a prowler in his bedroom, brought up concerns about homosexuality, and wondered if he had been using his fetish as a way of coping with overpowering females. The behavior therapist noted that these were interesting observations but not really relevant to removing the fetish.

By the termination of behavior therapy (14 sessions over a six-month period), Mr. B. reported that he was much less stimulated by scenes or fantasies involving his fetish, and was more stimulated by fantasies of nude women and sexual intercourse. He did complain that his pleasure during masturbatory orgasm never quite reached the peak pleasure he experienced during the period when his fantasies were almost totally fetishistic. At this time, he was masturbating solely to nonfetish images.

Inquiries by the behavior therapist or the psychotherapist at several points up to one year after the end of behavior therapy showed no increase in fetishistic fantasies. After the termination of behavior therapy, Mr. B. began dating again for the first time. Although these relationships had not progressed to the state of sexual intercourse, Mr. B. felt less threatened by the fetish in relation to women, and stated that the fetish was no longer a problem in his dating eligible females.

During the period of behavior therapy, Mr. B. was seen two to three times per week in intensive individual psychotherapy. Soon after the start of behavior therapy, memories surrounding the fetish became more prominent in the psychotherapy sessions. Mr. B. dwelled on the period he spent in France, when his wife started an affair with a local doctor. He remembered that his preoccupation with his fetish increased substantially during this period, and that he felt helpless to do anything about the affair. He also brought up an unexplained feeling of sympathy or friendliness he felt for the French doctor during this time. This memory progressed into a discussion of various topics covertly concerned with homosexuality. With a few leads from the psychotherapist, Mr. B. himself came to the interpretation that these events and memories indicated a concern over homosexuality, and he commented that he always felt that being a homosexual was worse than having a fetish. He remembered how he had been surprised by the "oversolicitousness" of the behavior therapist, who had given Mr. B. his home phone number to call if he became too restless, and accepted the interpretation that "solicitation" may have had a homosexual meaning to him. Shortly after these sessions, Mr. B. reported that he was able to sleep better and was no longer restless at night, although he did continue to be bothered, for a few weeks, by some anxiety after each masturbatory assignment. The theme of homosexuality reappeared in dreams and associations many times in the psychotherapy sessions, but did not again become so bothersome.

As the behavior therapy progressed, Mr. B. began to express his thoughts about an important change in his self-image, which he himself associated with the effects of behavior therapy. Since he was now more able to control his fetish on his own volition, he now felt responsible for his use of the symptom. He could no longer see himself as an innocent victim. He began then to reflect on how he and his wife had been engaged in a sadomasochistic relationship on many levels. He described how he used the fetish as a way of degrading his wife, and how she also used it as a club over his head. Mr. B. slowly began to see how his wife was currently trying to manipulate him, and he began to resist some of her ploys.

In later sessions, Mr. B. complained about feeling generally more anxious and depressed at times, and realized that now he could not completely cover up both pleasant and unpleasant affects that he previously had not consciously experienced in most situations. He felt a bit uneasy about these changes, but stated that he would not want to go back to the way he had been.

The issue of competition between the therapists came up briefly in the psychotherapy sessions. After Mr. B. reported some difficulty going along with the behavior therapy program, it became clear that he saw the therapists as if in competition for him. This preoccupation did not remain central to the patient's therapy, and a number of weeks later he challenged the behavior therapist to a game of handball and asked the psychotherapist to join him for a cocktail.

Mr. B. continued in individual psychotherapy for one year after the termination of behavior therapy, and is still in therapy at the time of this writing. He has continued to become more aware of his feelings of annoyance and anxiety in interpersonal situations, and to become less passive. He has had several dating relationships, although none have progressed to intercourse. His fantasies of aggressive women have again become more prominent. The boot fetish itself, and Mr. B.'s concern about homosexuality, did not again become prominent issues.

The psychological scales of both the POMS and HSCL showed substantial, although transient, elevations in subjectively reported distress. At follow-up, these values had returned toward baseline values. Changes on the WFSS scale were unremarkable. Selected data from the POMS questionnaire are reproduced in Table 1.

Scores on the OSGOOD showed a slightly more negative evaluation of mother and wife at the termination of behavior therapy, although these values returned to baseline at follow-up. The concept "mother" decreased markedly on the potency factor at follow-up. Concepts related to the target symptoms—shoe and boot—showed only marginal changes. Clinically, it appeared that these questionnaire changes paralleled Mr. B.'s recognition of his anger at women. Selected data are reproduced in Table 2.

Again we see an example of psychotherapy and behavior therapy appearing to facilitate one another rather than being competitive treat-

TABLE 1.   Changes in Mood Scores (POMS) Before and After Behavior Therapy*

Patient	Factor	Time of testing		
		Initial	Termination	Follow-up
Ms. S.	Anxiety	20	3	3
	Depression	28	1	1
	Anger	33	0	11
Mr. B.	Anxiety	7	19	11
	Depression	9	20	11
	Anger	6	22	9

*Each score represents the sum of scores from several items making up each factor. Each item is scored on a 4-point scale, from 1 (not at all) to 4 (extremely).

TABLE 2. Changes in Evaluation of Concepts on the OSGOOD Semantic Differential

Patient	Factor	Concept	Time of testing		
			Initial	Termination	Follow-up
Ms. S.	Evaluative*	Control†	5.9	5.3	4.9
		Chicken	1.6	3.6	3.6
		Father	5.3	5.0	3.6
	Potency	Control	5.5	5.8	5.5
		Housewife	2.5	5.0	5.5
Mr. B.	Evaluative	Control	3.5	4.1	4.3
		Mother	3.9	1.4	3.1
		Wife	4.3	1.4	3.1
	Potency	Control	2.0	4.0	3.0
		Mother	6.0	5.5	2.0

*Each number represents the average factor score from 3 to 4 scales that define the OSGOOD factors: evaluative, activity, potency. Each scale was scored on a 0-to-6 range, with high scores indicating good, active, and strong, respectively.
†Mean of two combined control concepts.

ment strategies. The rather direct, uncomplicated behavioral approach appeared to facilitate Mr. B.'s awareness of anger at women (as evidenced by changes in psychotherapy and on the quantitative indices), to precipitate his fears about homosexuality, and, more importantly, to directly attack his image of himself as a passive victim by giving him volitional control over his fetish. Psychotherapy was useful in alleviating Mr. B.'s increasing fears about homosexuality as behavior therapy progressed, and in desensitizing Mr. B.'s fantasies about the competition between the two therapists. More importantly, psychotherapy appeared to work to consolidate and extend the cognitive changes elicited by behavioral change.

Rather surprisingly, again neither therapist was aware of any detrimental effect to his therapeutic regime by the presence of concurrent therapy by a therapist of a different theoretical school. The increase in feelings of anxiety, depression, and anger that may have been stimulated by the behavioral therapy did not interfere with the patient's progress in psychotherapy, but rather seemed to provide an opportunity to make the patient aware of some of the important feelings he had previously "repressed." The transient rise in anxiety and depression receded toward baseline during subsequent psychotherapy, but the patient still seemed more sensitive to feelings of anxiety when they arose in some interpersonal or professional situations.

It would appear unnecessary at this point to emphasize that behavioral change appeared to have had important impacts on feelings and attitudes unrelated to the target symptom on a manifest level.

COMMENT

The primary purpose of this article was to evaluate the practical difficulties and advantages in referring a patient in psychoanalytically oriented therapy for concurrent therapy of a specific symptom by a behavior therapist. Both authors were surprised to find that the actual difficulties appear to be minimal. Anticipated difficulties, such as the patient having difficulty with a split therapeutic alliance, the patient trying to pit one therapist against the other, and the patient precipitously withdrawing from psychotherapy after symptom removal, all failed to occur. Instead, the difficulty that did appear to arise was a problem of competition between the therapists. The problem of competition between cotherapists has been adequately discussed in the group therapy literature,[23] and will not be repeated here, as the same issues appear to be involved. Suffice it to say that the authors found a brief meeting to reestablish contact and communication essential to the successful continuation of this project. This was necessary although both therapists are social friends belonging to the same university hospital faculty. This would suggest that therapists from different agencies, of different professional affiliations, and who were not personally acquainted, might find concurrent therapy of this sort more difficult, and perhaps should anticipate arranging some form of regular contact between the therapists. This difficulty could, of course, be avoided if the same therapist conducted both types of treatment.

The question of the advantages of concurrent therapy of this sort is clearly related to the second question asked in this project, about the possible indirect consequences of symptom removal. From the available literature it would appear that behavior therapy and psychotherapy would be essentially independent tasks, with behavior therapy perhaps aiding psychotherapy by removing crippling symptoms and engendering a sense of competence and renewed self-esteem. Clearly, in these cases, symptom removal appeared to evoke memories which psychoanalytic theory would posit as causally related to the origin of the symptoms. More importantly, in these three cases, the symptoms appeared to be key factors in the way the patients organized their subjective views of the world, and removal of these symptoms rather dramatically opened the way for a new subjective reorganization. Successful behavior therapy elicited this change, but psychotherapy then aided in making the change permanent. For example, the woman with a bird phobia had entered psychotherapy because of her unsatisfactory heterosexual relationships. Material elicited during psychotherapy suggested that this passivity was related to her denial of her own sexual feelings. Subsequent events in behavior therapy suggested that her phobia of birds was integrally involved. While preparing to touch a bird during *in vivo* desensitization, this patient spoke of the supposed fear-eliciting phobic object in a most peculiar way, as if it were a sexual object toward which she had ambivalent feelings—"I feel as I did in high school when I desired sexual intercourse with my boyfriend, but felt that I shouldn't." After touching the bird, she subsequently spoke of changing her attitude toward her father and having resented his sexual overtures. At the same time, she reported feeling less passive toward men, and began reporting more active moves in her relationship with men. Psychotherapy was necessary to help her maintain these changes. From this and the other two cases, it would appear that behavior has its internal cognitive referents, and that change of behavior may lead to internal symbolic change. These conclusions are, of course, speculative, because of the small sample size and because we cannot rule out the possibility of psychotherapy rather than behavior change as the principle variable. Also, the documented changes on the semantic differential were small, and could have occurred by chance.

This pilot investigation suggests the importance of further work in this area. It is hoped that other clinicians will begin concurrent therapy of this sort, and report their findings. The suggestion that psychotherapeutic change in some patients can be accelerated by a two-pronged simultaneous attack on the actual behavior and its internal cognitive mediating events is of considerable practical importance, and needs to be investigated in a more rigorous fashion. Similarly, clinical investigation as to the relative efficacy of the differing therapeutic approaches in certain subpopulations, such as the chronic "externalizers" who appear to be poor candidates for traditional psychotherapy, would appear warranted. Our unanticipated finding that successful behavior therapy of target symptoms appears to be temporally related to changes in feelings and cognitions, which were initially not overtly associated with the target symptom, suggests that symptomatic behavior occurs in clusters. One approach to systematic description of these clusters would be to begin clinical series of patients undergoing behavior therapy alone, while independently assessing nontarget behavior, thoughts, and feelings. Isolated symptom removal therapy might be an excellent experimental paradigm to employ in order to start objectively specifying links between external behavior and internal cognitive-emotional events, and perhaps to start experimentally testing certain psychoanalytic hypotheses about these interrelationships. The recent work by Wahler[24] on behavior clusters in deviant child behavior is an example of a possible research design.

References

1. Bergin A: The evaluation of therapeutic outcomes, in Bergin A, Garfield S (eds): *Handbook of Psychotherapy and Behavior Change*. New York, John Wiley & Sons Inc, 1971.
2. Marks IM: *Fears and Phobias*. London, William Heineman Ltd, 1969.
3. Brady JP: A behavioral approach to the treatment of stuttering. *Am J Psychiatry* 125:843-848, 1969.
4. Marks IM, Gelder MG: Transvestism and fetishism: Clinical and psychological changes during faradic aversion. *Br J Psychiatry* 113:711-729, 1967.
5. Stunkard A: New therapies for the eating disorders: Behavior modification of obesity and anorexia nervosa. *Arch Gen Psychiatry* 26:391-398, 1972.
6. Jones WJ, Park PM: Treatment of single-partner sexual dysfunction by systematic desensitization. *Obstet Gynecol* 39:411-417, 1972.
7. Meyer V: Modification of expectations in cases with obsessional rituals. *Behav Res Ther* 4:273-280, 1966.
8. Eysenck HJ, Rachman S: *The Causes and Cures of Neuroses*. London, Routledge & Kegan Paul Ltd, 1965.
9. Breger L, McGaugh JL: Critique and reformulation of learning theory approaches to psychotherapy and neurosis. *Psychol Bull* 63:338-358, 1965. [See also Chapter 4, this volume.]
10. London P: The end of ideology in behavior modification. *Am Psychol* 27:913-920, 1972.

11. Feather BW, Rhoads JM: Psychodynamic behavior therapy: Theory and rationale. *Arch Gen Psychiatry* 26:496-502, 1972. [See also Chapter 20, this volume.]
12. Birk L, Brinkley-Birk AW: Psychoanalysis and behavior therapy. *Am J Psychiatry* 131:499-510, 1974. [See also Chapter 9, this volume.]
13. Hunt HF, Dyrud JE: Commentary: Perspective in behavior therapy. *Res Psychother* 3:140-152, 1968.
14. Lazarus A: *Behavior Therapy and Beyond.* New York, McGraw-Hill Book Co Inc, 1971.
15. Birk L, Huddleston W, Miller E, et al: Avoidance conditioning for homosexuality. *Arch Gen Psychiatry* 25:314-323, 1971.
16. Woody RH: Conceptualizing the shared patient: Treatment orientation of multiple therapists. *Int J Group Psychother* 2:228-233, 1972.
17. Smith RC, Carlin J: Behavior modification using interlocking reinforcement on a short-term psychiatric ward. *Arch Gen Psychiatry* 27:386-389, 1972.
18. Nurnberger JI, Hingtgen JN: Is symptom substitution an important issue in behavior therapy? *Biol Psychiatry* 7:221-236, 1973.
19. Derogatis LR, Lipman RS, Rickels K, et al: The Hopkins Symptom Checklist: A self-report symptom. *Behav Sci* 19:1-15, 1974.
20. McNair DM, Loor M, Droppleman LF: *EITS Manual for Profile of Mood Scales.* San Diego, Calif, Educational and Industrial Testing Service, 1971.
21. Wolpe L, Lang PJ: A fear survey schedule for use in behavior therapy. *Behav Res Ther* 2:27-30, 1964.
22. Osgood CE, Suci GJ, Tannenbaum PH: *The Measurement of Meaning.* Urbana, Ill, University of Illinois Press, 1957.
23. Heilfron M: Co-therapy: The relationship between therapists. *Int J Group Psychother* 19:366-381, 1969.
24. Wahler RG: Some structural aspects of deviant child behavior. *J Appl Behav Anal* 8:27-42, 1975.

Concurrent Sex Therapy and Psychoanalytic Psychotherapy by Separate Therapists

18

Effectiveness and Implications

ALEXANDER N. LEVAY, M.D.,
JOSEF H. WEISSBERG, M.D., AND
ALVIN B. BLAUSTEIN, M.D.

Innovators of new treatment methods usually wish to maintain the "purity" of their approach. It is equally certain that this will be only a temporary state of affairs, with the new method eventually becoming amalgamated with other clinically effective techniques. So it was with Masters and Johnson's position that all other treatment should be discontinued during the period of sex therapy. In this paper Levay and his associates report on the introduction of a program of sex therapy, utilizing a second therapist, during ongoing psychoanalytic psychotherapy.

Their experience with a two-therapist approach is consistent with the findings of others, namely, that there are both resolvable complications and often rewarding therapeutic opportunities. With adequate communication and respect, and with minimal competition, each therapist was able to maintain the integrity of his or her own treatment program while at the same time complementing and enhancing the other treatment. If their experiences can be replicated by other teams, this is an important finding since therapists are often not schooled in both treatment methodologies. Even if one were equally experienced with both treatment methods, the clinical experience reported here suggests that at times there may be distinct advantages to having separate therapists who are both working toward the relief of targeted sexual symptoms.

Concurrent Sex Therapy and Psychoanalytic Psychotherapy by Separate Therapists

Effectiveness and Implications

ALEXANDER N. LEVAY, M.D.,
JOSEF H. WEISSBERG, M.D., AND
ALVIN B. BLAUSTEIN, M.D.

LITERATURE REVIEW

There are specific references in the literature to similar therapeutic approaches, although many related issues have been dealt with by various authors:

Flescher's (1968, 1958) "Dual Therapy" technique involves the treatment of one patient by a male and female therapist on alternate days. He states that many transference and countertransference problems are elucidated and resolved more easily by this technique.

Woody reports two cases of integrated aversion therapy and supportive psychotherapy by separate therapists in an inpatient setting. The patients suffered from specific perversions (transvestitism and fetishism) and were reported as benefiting from the dual approach. Kaplan reports on the sequential and alternating use of sex therapy and psychoanalytic psychotherapy by the same therapist. There are, in addition, several clinical and theoretical reports (Birk and Brinkley-Birk; Gullick and Blanchard) on the combined use of behavioral and psychoanalytic psychotherapeutic techniques by the same therapist. The literature reveals a paucity of discussions, even on an experimental basis, of concomitant treatment of one patient by two therapists.

METHODOLOGY

In the context of a psychoanalytic research study group, a couple with sexual problems was selected, one of whom—the wife—was already

Reprinted by permission from *Psychiatry*, 39:355-363, November 1976. Copyright 1976 by the William Alanson White Psychiatric Foundation, Inc.

involved in psychoanalytic psychotherapy. The couple was referred to a
sex therapist, a psychoanalyst who had received formal training at the
Reproductive Biology Research Foundation in St. Louis. The couple was
informed of the existence of the study and apprised of its purposes.
Their permission was secured to tape-record all sex therapy and psychotherapy sessions for the duration of the study, and to allow both
therapists and all study group members to listen to the tapes. Sex
therapy sessions were scheduled weekly for four months. The psychotherapy with the wife was continued on a twice-weekly basis. The study
group met monthly and heard representative segments of both therapies
from the previous month. Six months after the termination of sex
therapy, the couple was interviewed by a third research group member
for an in-depth evaluation of their treatment experience and the results,
including the effect of the study.

THE SEX THERAPY

Sex therapy is a structured, step-by-step educational experience in
functional sexual behavior for a couple. The couple, rather than the dysfunctional individual, is the patient. Both members of the couple are
treated as equal partners in the problem, even if one of them does not
suffer from an explicit dysfunction. The treatment goal is the establishment of functional sexual behavior based on mutual pleasure, rather
than a specific resolution of the individual dysfunction itself. Treatment
goals are individually tailored at the onset of therapy to be consistent
with the couple's expectations, backgrounds, and realistic limiting factors. Once these goals have been set and mutually agreed upon, the
couple is expected to abide by the treatment rules and expectations for
the duration of the treatment, even if some of these may not meet with
their preferences or be consistent with their previous therapeutic experience. Patients' treatment behavior is evaluated throughout the treatment
and corrected whenever necessary. The focal point of the treatment is
the assignment of specific tasks for the bedroom in graded sequence.
These represent essential component parts of functional sexual behavior. By reviewing with the couple how each of these exercises was
performed and experienced, the therapist is enabled to correct "mistakes," such as undue emphasis on performance and goal orientation.
Among frequently encountered "mistakes" are exaggerated emphasis
on the partner's satisfaction at the expense of one's own pleasure, and
preoccupation with achieving erection, ejaculatory control, and orgasms. Stress is laid on the here and now, and on the conscious individual experience as well as on the interpersonal interaction. No attempt
is made to avoid expressing value judgments regarding functional be-

havior. New assignments are not made until previous ones are performed comfortably and with pleasure. Special techniques are employed at appropriate times, such as the squeeze method for ejaculatory control and the use of vaginal dilators in the treatment of vaginismus. Throughout the therapy much information is provided on sexual anatomy, physiology, and psychology. The therapist actively encourages open, honest, nonjudgmental communication. The therapist plays an active and supportive role throughout. During the course of treatment all sexual activity is limited to that prescribed by the therapist.

The original Masters and Johnson method called for a two-week daily treatment regimen. For a number of practical as well as therapeutic reasons, this has been modified in many clinics to a once-a-week therapy in which the two-week program is spread out over a three- to four-month period. Masters and Johnson feel that all couples must be treated by male-female cotherapy teams. This, too, is handled by many as an option, essential only in a minority of cases.

Couples have a screening interview, as much to establish their suitability for this type of treatment as to help them gain a realistic view of their problem, the therapy, and the therapist. Some of the more frequently encountered contraindications are lack of motivation, especially to work out the sexual problem for oneself; marital problems precluding cooperation between partners; ongoing extramarital relationships; inability of one or both partners to cooperate with the therapist; major life crises; and psychotic or prepsychotic states. Next, in separate sessions, a complete history is elicited as indirectly as possible. The sexual history emphasizes not only dysfunction, but also positive and pleasurable aspects. Discretion regarding the past is granted each spouse but no secrecy is promised for new events which may develop during the course of treatment. This is designed to prevent entrapment of the therapist in which he is defaulting on one patient by guarding the secrets of the other.

Physical examinations and laboratory studies follow. There are considerable advantages in having the physical examinations performed by the sex therapist. These are: seeing the bodies and the genitals as they are, rather than as they are described; observing patients' reactions to their own bodies, and to the doctor's examining them; learning each individual's autonomic response patterns to the stress of the examination; and discovering new clues to historical data. Patients are very reassured by the doctor's having examined parts of their bodies about which they are concerned. The physical examination augments basic trust and cements the therapeutic alliance.

A formal presentation is then made to the couple, summarizing the therapist's findings and recommendations, the probable origins of the difficulty and the contribution of each partner, the assessment of assets and liabilities, the outline of the projected course of treatment, provision of sexual and clinical information, and demonstration of principles of communication.

The first of two sensate-focus exercises is then described. The couple is instructed to undress in their bedroom with some light on. One is assigned to initiate playing with the partner's body *the way he or she always wanted to*. An attitude of playful exploration is encouraged. Genitals and breasts are off limits. The partner who is being played with is only to experience sensations and to protect the other from causing discomfort, since this is not his or her intention. After 15 or 20 minutes the couple is to exchange roles and repeat the procedure. If at the end of this experience either feels sexually aroused, he or she is encouraged to masturbate in the presence of the partner. The second sensate-focus exercise includes playing with the genitals of the partner following the same format. The couple is also instructed to examine each other's genitals. During this phase partners indicate to each other how they prefer to be touched, so that this can be included in the repertory of the other. Orogenital contact is encouraged as an option. The emphasis is placed on moment-to-moment pleasurable sensation rather than on goal-oriented achievement. The rate of progression of assignments is carefully tailored for each couple.

Mutual genital caressing follows. Intercourse is then added, usually in the female-astride position. Intercourse is usually delayed until both partners can participate in mutual touching or orogenital contact with full sexual responsiveness and orgasm. The couple is then instructed in various other suitable intercourse positions and therapy is tapered off. Couples may require special assistance in integrating their newfound gains into their everyday lives once therapy has been completed.

Case History. The 40-year-old wife had been seen by her current analytic therapist twice weekly for two two-year periods, separated by a four-year interval during which she was seen about a dozen times. She had seen several therapists previously. Her presenting complaints were inability to get along with her husband and to enjoy sex. The couple had three teen-aged children, and the wife had had a tubal ligation following an abortion 10 years earlier.

The wife had been born in France, her parents having emigrated from Hungary some years earlier. She had one brother 20 years her senior, who had already left home at the time of her birth. She was raised by governesses and saw little of her parents until moving to this country at age 8. Her mother was distant, demanding, and contentious, while her father was alternatively doting and sulking, depending on whether or not her behavior satisfied him. Sex was never mentioned explicitly. Still, at age 17, it came as no surprise to her when her father disapproved violently of her talking to boys. At age 20, while in college, she began seriously seeing the man who became her husband, whom she had known for many years. During the courtship she was sexually aggressive but her fiancé insisted on deferring sexual intercourse until after the wedding. The honeymoon was disappointing. She had never experienced orgasm during intercourse, and until recently, only rarely during manual or lingual manipulation of her clitoris by her husband. Masturbation was possible only by thigh squeezing. Attempts at manual masturbation produced severe anxiety and were always abandoned prior to orgasm.

The husband is a highly obsessive but sincerely committed professional, who developed ulcerative colitis at age 5 and had an ileostomy performed at age 16. At the time of his marriage, at age 22, he suffered a serious exacerbation of his ulcerative colitis, which lasted for two years. Symptoms abated after a laparotomy with lysis of adhesions. Reanastomosis at that time proved impossible. During the acute phase of his illness he visited a psychiatric clinic once weekly for a year. He has dealt with his ileostomy chiefly with denial. Very few people know that he has an ileostomy, and he leads an impressively active life. The patient denied any strong feelings concerning his ileostomy, although occasionally she dreamt of his expressing rage by spewing feces through the stoma. His disease had been well controlled for many years.

Their relationship was characterized by her slavish obedience and consequent resentment. The two of them conspired to elevate the husband to a position of moral perfection. Thus, they agreed that he served his clients more conscientiously than any other lawyer in the city. Of course, this necessitated long working hours. When he came home late, the wife was caught in a dilemma. He would righteously defend the demands of his work and she would be unable to express her desire for his presence or her resentment at being deprived of it. When she did complain, she received a rather elaborate lecture on ethical and moral values, which left her more angry and depressed. Her rage found expression in increasingly frequent, tantrumlike outbursts. His parents, who lived in Arizona, would visit during July and August. She would submit meekly to their demands, but her mounting rage would lead ultimately to an outburst, often involving physical threats to them, and would then subside with unbearable guilt and depression.

Her chronic rage and self-deprecation further interfered with her sexual enjoyment. She viewed orgasm as an achievement and every unfulfilling sexual experience as a failure. Although she enjoyed nongenital contact with her husband, she came to regard every overture on his part as leading to a confirmation of her lack of femininity. She was torn between her desire to avert such overtures and her wish to gratify her husband's legitimate and justifiable needs. She felt trapped in a cycle of rage and guilt.

Treatment was directed toward examining the roots of her defective self-esteem and her sexual inhibition. After two years she felt considerably more comfortable; and, although the explosive battles with her husband continued, they were shorter, less violent, separated by longer intervals, and followed by considerably less guilt and self-denigration. She had begun to perceive his role in perpetuating the situation and was relieved at not having to be the sole bearer of the burden of their difficulties. She stated her desire to stop treatment and in the ensuing four years was seen only infrequently, usually after a particularly violent blow up.

Four years later she reentered treatment, feeling she wanted to do something definitive to better her relationship with her husband; wanting to improve her sexual adaptation, which she had always been reluctant to discuss explicitly; and feeling she would do something about developing a career for herself now that her children were growing up. It became apparent that it would be necessary to involve her husband in any therapeutic approach. Since he refused to enter individual therapy, it was arranged that he accompany his wife once weekly. After an initial period of suspicious defensiveness, he responded gratifyingly, and together the couple was able to work through some of their destructive response patterns. Predictably enough, the wife derived further fuel for self-denigration from his improvement; her husband had changed radically in just a few months, whereas she had taken many years to make comparable progress. After a year, it was suggested that the husband discontinue regular visits and relinquish their therapy time to his wife, for work on her remaining difficulties. The husband himself was struck by the reluctance with which he retired from the conjoint sessions. He precipitated a few flare-ups in order to be seen again, and the relationship for the next year was remarkably smooth.

The wife's self-esteem had become more intact, and she began making plans to obtain training for a career. She felt that her therapeutic goals had all been achieved, save for sexual improvement. Although she talked much more freely about sex, there was little change in her attitude and response. At this point, one year following the end of the conjoint therapy, the suggestion was made that she and her husband enter sex therapy, while she remain in individual therapy.

COURSE OF CONCURRENT THERAPY

Following her individual visit with the sex therapist, the wife was quite pleased and regarded the project optimistically. During the second session, however, when she was seen with her husband, she felt that the therapist sided with him against her, and became angry. Although the analytic therapist was prepared for some competitive resentment when a colleague intruded on his therapeutic territory, even though he did so at his invitation, he was surprised by the intensity of his indignation when his patient reported that the sex therapist had been praising the virtues of her husband and wondering at her failure to respond to him. She reported that the sex therapist had suggested that she and her husband listen to the analytic tapes together. She felt that this would feed into her husband's need to control her and would kill the only vestige of privacy she had—that is, in her analytic therapy. At this point the two therapists met. It became apparent that the wife had been guilty of some distortion. For example, the sex therapist had suggested that the couple might replay tapes of their joint sessions, not those of her individual sessions. It was clear that she was unconsciously attempting to provoke a battle between the two therapists in much the same way as she had frequently divided her parents. When this was interpreted to her, she was able to begin to deal directly with the frightening prospect that she might in the near future become capable of and have to bear the responsibility for adult sexual responses.

After the meeting of the two therapists, the analytic therapist was able to deal with the wife's objections to the sex therapist in terms of her fear of the sexual activity she expected him to encourage. Her first response was to suffer an attack of acute anxiety while the sex therapist was describing the procedure for the initial sensate-focus exercise. She also felt quite guilty about the deprivation suffered by her husband due to the proscription of genital sex.

Though she continued consciously to be furious with the sex therapist and to be terrified of the exercises, she dreamt of the analytic therapist as a reliable but not very skillful driver of an old automobile, and at the same time dreamt that the sex therapist and his many assistants were actively and heroically keeping her house from falling apart.

After the next group meeting, the sex therapist gave the wife the tapes of his session, and she requested and was given the tapes of the analytic therapist. He was amazed at the next session to learn that she and her husband had listened to them together. She described this as a worthwhile experience, since her husband had responded sympathetically to the depression and angry frustration which had been so prominently expressed in them. She asked the analytic therapist to continue giving her his tapes, and he consented for the duration of the concurrent therapy.

During the second month of dual therapy, the patient attempted to masturbate digitally. Although it was necessary for her to keep her ankles crossed to avert anxiety, she was able for the first time to produce an orgasm in this way. She then fell asleep and dreamt of suffering paralysis of all limbs and dying. Her associations to this dream were to an episode at age 20, when she had a bitter quarrel with her mother about whether she would accompany her parents on an extended trip or stay home with her fiancé. Shortly after, her mother became weak and faint and a physican was called. In retrospect, she felt that these represented the first symptoms of the brain tumor which proved fatal to the mother. The analytic therapist was then told that the exercises had become much easier and more pleasurable, but the sex therapist consistently received a less optimistic picture.

The wife seemed to tolerate poorly what she and her husband regarded as good performance and once again became quite anxious about experiencing sexual pleasure, which she would avoid by retreating into obsessive thoughts. Her fury at the sex therapist was exacerbated, particularly when he responded to increased tension by suggesting that she take a week off from the exercises. The husband's support, while overtly consistent, was tempered by his repeated complaints at being deprived of intercourse, which fed the wife's guilt.

Some early associations were produced when the split in the transference, exemplified by her presenting herself as fragile to the sex therapist while describing significant improvement to the analytic therapist, was pointed out: She had been allergic to cow's milk in infancy and had required hypodermoclysis for nutrition, followed by feeding by a series of wet nurses. In relating this, she felt that these women were uninterested in her, had children of their own, and nursed her only for money. Thus, in her mind, early pleasurable experiences had been accompanied by communications concerning her unworthiness.

At this point in the therapy, she took a short vacation with her husband. During the few days they were away, she was more freely and responsively interested in sex than she ever had been. Her husband, however, much to her amazement, was unable to achieve a full erection. He was reluctant to acknowledge the significance of his flagging potency in the presence of his wife's new sexual responsiveness. He reported a dream to the sex therapist in which he was chased by knife- and gun-wielding Japanese warriors, an image he traced to looking at Japanese erotic art.

For the remainder of the conjoint therapy, the wife followed strides forward with regression and recrudescence of her inhibitory symptoms. During these periods her attitude toward the sex therapist was characterized by extreme contentiousness, which was interpreted as defensive. Her rage to some extent seemed to represent a displacement of her disappointment in her husband's unwillingness to deal with his contribution to the dysfunction.

When the sex therapist proposed ending his role in the treatment, the wife found all sorts of objections to him to justify her rage at his abandonment. Her vilification of him contrasted strikingly with her portrayal of him in her dreams, where he always emerged as sophisticated, skillful, and omniscient, often in contrast to the analytic therapist, who was seen as rather pedestrian and plodding.

Joint therapy was ended after four months. In the months following, the wife's conscious attitude to the sex therapist more closely approximated that implied in her dreams. Her gains appeared to be maintained and she spoke of him from time to time with fondness and great regard. Analytic therapy was terminated eight months after the end of joint therapy.

EVALUATION OF THE RESULTS OF TREATMENT

Evaluation interviews with the husband and wife were conducted six months following the end of sex therapy. The wife was orgastic by manual manipulation by the husband and in masturbation. Fear of excitement was no longer present. She consciously enjoyed intercourse and the frequency had increased markedly. There was much less emphasis on the importance of orgasm for self-esteem. She felt less fearful of her husband's reactions and criticism. The couple more openly shared their fantasies. The husband's potency disturbance disappeared. Though attributing most of her progress to her psychotherapy, and in spite of tensions connected with the sex therapy, she found the joint experience beneficial and did not think she could have achieved as much as she did without the sex therapy. Apparently there had been no important disruption in her relationship to her analytic therapist. Even her knowledge that the tapes of her sessions were being shared with an unseen group of psychiatrists did not produce discernible negative effects. The couple was later seen in a one-year follow-up visit by the sex therapist. He found that the gains they had made had been maintained. They seemed comparatively free from tension and happy in a work relationship they had established since she had taken a position in his law firm. The frequency of sexual relations had increased to three times a week. Sex had become a pleasurable and well-integrated part of their life together, rather than a source of conflict and recrimination. The wife reported experiencing orgasm in intercourse regularly, though requiring manual stimulation by her husband.

CONCLUSION

Our experience supports the notion that sex therapy and psychoanalytic psychotherapy can be conducted concurrently by two different therapists with greater benefit to the patients than by either therapy alone. There must be good communication between the two therapists and care must be taken early to explain to the patients the divergent methodologies involved. The study itself was helpful to both therapists in their work and did not have any discernible negative effects on the patients.

Most analysts do not have a working knowledge of sex therapy. They may perceive a given therapeutic maneuver as an error in judgment or as a countertransference reaction by the sex therapist. Thus, when in the early phases of treatment, the sex therapist pointed out to the wife that she seemingly had an eager and cooperative sexual partner in her husband, the patient and the analytic therapist reacted as if the sex therapist were taking sides with the husband rather than focusing on the status of the relationship. It was helpful to the analytic therapist to learn that in sex therapy one proceeds by identifying things as they are in the here-and-now.

Another important area of communication between the therapists concerned patient behavior in treatment. The wife dramatically split the transference, reacting to the sex therapist with much hostility and contentiousness, and denying all progress. The sex therapist's morale was maintained by the more optimistic communications reported by the analytic therapist. The sex therapist was also greatly helped by the analytic data that were reported to him by the analytic therapist. For example, he had been completely unaware of the anxiety attack that the wife experienced during the first sensate-focus instruction and her associations to it. These data enabled him to deal more effectively with her resistance, which represented her view of him and her husband as insufficiently caring figures. Another example involved the dream following the first orgastic response to digital stimulation, which clearly equated sexual responsiveness with murderous aggressive impulses toward her mother.

The analytic therapy benefited as well. As might be expected, a flood of dreams and striking associations came forth as her sexual inhibitions were challenged in the sex therapy, which provided fuel for the therapeutic work. The husband's role in perpetuating the couple's symptoms was more clearly delineated.

Our experience suggests a challenge to the well-entrenched idea among psychoanalytically oriented psychotherapists that treatment of a patient by more than one therapist at the same time is ineffective or even damaging. It is claimed that the transference will be diluted and that countertransference reactions will be directed toward the other therapist. In our case the transference was split in a dramatic way: the sex therapist represented the hostile, depriving mother, while the analytic therapist was endowed with the qualities of the loving, tolerant, but sexually repressive father. These representations developed despite our feeling that the analytic therapist was more similar personally to the mother and the sex therapist seemed to resemble the father. The nature of the two transferences, as might be predicted, reflected the patient's intrapsychic needs and the different behavior required of the two therapists. Forces promoting countertransference deflection, such as rivalry between the therapists, were minimized by the meticulous maintenance of open communications.

Dual therapy might have wider application. For example, in cases with severely conflicted partners in whom sexual inhibition is greatly overdetermined, it may be impossible for one therapist to deal with both the sex therapy instruction and encouragement, and a dispassionate examination of the intrapsychic determinants. The rather extreme resistance offered to sex therapy by our patient, we feel, would have forced her to discontinue had she not been able to resolve some of her conflicts in her analytic therapy. Also, had it not been for the specific assignment of sexual tasks in the sex therapy, her unconscious conflicts and resistances to adult sexual functioning could not have been demonstrated to her and worked through. Possibly other types of behavioral therapy could successfully be combined with psychoanalytic therapy, in which the behavioral therapy would serve as a structured and therapeutically controlled stimulus to the mobilization of repressed conflict, affect, and historical material.

Masters and Johnson, Flescher, and others have written of the value of various combinations of male and female therapists in resolving conflicts which could not adequately have been dealt with by a male or a female therapist alone. The basis for this idea has been that the gender of the therapist is an essential determinant of the nature of the transference neurosis. Our experience in this case, however, indicates that in concomitant treatment with two therapists of the same gender, a maternal-paternal transference split did in fact occur.

Most theories of psychotherapy lean heavily on the use of transference phenomena. We feel that our experience, in which the unique feature of the transference was that the observer and target therapists were both participants, provided an opportunity to observe objectively the emergence and evolution of transference reactions. Further application of this method might provide data extending our understanding of the nature of the psychotherapeutic process, as well as furnishing a more effective modality for treatment of sexual disorders refractory to conventional methods.

REFERENCES

Birk, L., and Brinkley-Birk, A. W. Psychoanalysis and behavior therapy, *Amer. J. Psychiatry* (1974) *131*:499-510. [See also, Chapter 9, this volume.]

Flescher, J. The "dual method" in analytic psychotherapy, in A. Esman (Ed.), *New Frontiers in Child Guidance*; Int. Univ. Press, 1958.

Flescher, J. Dual analysis, *Current Psychiatric Therapies* (1968) *8*:38-46.

Gullick, E., and Blanchard, E. The use of psychotherapy and behavior therapy in the treatment of an obsessional disorder: an experimental case study. *J. Nervous and Mental Dis.* (1973) *156*:427-431. [See also Chapter 16, this volume.]

Kaplan, H. S. *The New Sex Therapy*; Brunner/Mazel, 1974. [See also Chapter 25, this volume.]

Masters, W., and Johnson, V. *Human Sexual Inadequacy*; Little, Brown, 1970.

Woody, R. Integrated aversion therapy and psychotherapy: two sexual deviation case studies, *J. Sex. Res.* (1973) *9*:313-324.

19

Behavior Therapy— Integration with Dynamic Psychiatry

Lee Birk, M.D.

Utilizing two case reports as examples, Birk proposes that behavioral techniques can be integrated with interpersonal and dynamic psychotherapy with a resultant increase in efficiency in the therapeutic process.

When the therapist has several treatment options available, the need for choice requires greater precision in conceptualizing the mechanisms of symptom formation and maintenance. Behavioral techniques involve strategies specifically directed toward symptom removal. Loss of symptoms may serve the critically important function of helping to expose underlying conflicts and resistances, thus facilitating the process of psychotherapy.

Behavior Therapy— Integration with Dynamic Psychiatry

19

Lee Birk, M.D.

"Dynamic psychiatry" has evolved clinically through the efforts of physicians to help troubled patients, and derives largely from the ideas of Freud, Hartmann, Meyer, and Sullivan. Behavior therapy has developed from theory and experiments pertaining to learning. Unfortunately, positive results with behavior therapy have been used by some as ammunition to attack psychoanalytic theory and dynamic psychotherapy. This has exacerbated inherent difficulties in the synthesis of these two traditions, and slowed their integration at the practical level.

That psychotherapy has shortcomings is admitted even by its strongest proponents—lack of scientifically validated efficacy, need for long, costly treatment, frequent failure of "insight" alone in eliminating symptoms, and inapplicability of highly verbal methods to many patients. Behavior therapy has many achievements—better validated efficacy for certain disorders, brevity, high efficiency and low cost, and high success rate, especially with syndromes where anxiety is the salient maladaptive affect. Also, it has been successfully applied where conventional methods alone have yielded poor results (examples: the partial rehabilitation of autistic children, the management of chronic psychotics, and the treatment of sexual deviations and compulsive habits). However, behavior therapy is generally regarded as being less effective in dealing with such disorders as depression, acute psychoses, adolescent identity crises, or disorders of sexual identification. While some beginnings are now being made in applying behavioral principles to the treatment of certain depressive syndromes, as yet behavior therapy has not proved to be the treatment of choice for the kind of depression which stems primarily from pathological grief reactions. Also, in syndromes where guilt or anger (rather than anxiety) is the dominant affect, "pure" behavior therapy has not achieved outstanding success.

Reprinted by permission from *Behavior Therapy*, 1:522-526, 1970. Copyright 1970 by Academic Press, Inc.

Since the clinical problems patients present are frequently complex, it can be useful to combine the breadth and depth of a dynamic approach with the power and efficiency of relevant behavioral techniques. The notion that psychotherapy and behavior therapy are incompatible stems perhaps from the fact that few people are well trained in both traditions. Behavioral techniques can be the only or primary ingredient in treatment, or—if necessary—can be used as part of a total therapeutic approach. When used in the latter way, behavioral methods can be used to eliminate or reduce certain recalcitrant symptoms. Also, the techniques are often useful in forcing the clinician to sharpen his thinking about the patient and the mechanisms of the patient's symptoms and problems. Often, the availability of a technique capable of eliminating a symptom serves to catalyze psychotherapy, sometimes by permitting psychotherapeutic exploration of further areas and sometimes by highlighting resistances to treatment which might otherwise remain covert.

The following cases illustrate some of these points.

Case I.*The patient was a 20-year-old single man who entered psychotherapy because of increasing anxiety and depression after being judged medically unfit for military service because of persisting enuresis.

The patient's father, a career officer in the military, thought that the patient had outgrown this problem years ago, but his draft status brought to light the fact that he still wet the bed three to four times per week. His mother always protected him by changing the sheets and tactfully saying nothing. Just before beginning therapy he had become engaged to a nurse who was "very understanding" about his situation.

Although unsuccessful attempts at treatment in the past had included the "bell and blanket" conditioning technique of Mowrer, the therapist arranged for a behavioral consultation. It was felt that the previous unsuccessful attempt at conditioning therapy could reasonably only have been due to either or both of the following: (1) inappropriately combining the treatment method with fluid restriction, thus preventing the development of bladder distention as a conditioned stimulus; (2) failure to follow the conditioning procedure faithfully.

Although careful application of Mowrer's technique at first produced rapid success, the patient soon found himself not faithfully pursuing the prescribed behavioral regimen. This made his ambivalence about getting well obvious to him, and led, in turn, to the unmasking of his dependency needs and his passive-aggressive life-style. Thus, the conditioning procedure turned out to be a catalyst in the patient's psychotherapy. Because the referring therapist was both behaviorally and psychodynamically sophisticated and alert, he was able to recognize quickly and work through the practical obstacles. As a result, the patient was free from enuresis 3 weeks after beginning treatment with the conditioning apparatus.

The breakthrough in therapy came with the recurrent "accidental" disconnection of the conditioning apparatus by his mother in making his bed. This led him to wonder whether his mother was possibly trying to sabotage treatment by not reconnecting the apparatus, and eventually to his examining the fact of his own passive, dependent attitude

---

*This clinical material is from a case treated by a colleague, Dr. Richard Shader, associate director of psychiatry, Massachusetts Mental Health Center, by combined behavior therapy-psychotherapy.

in not making sure himself that it was reconnected. Following this, he began to examine his relationship with his fiancée from a similar vantage point. Also, he became aware of resentment toward both his parents, a resentment which previously he had rarely consciously acknowledged.

Sometimes behavior therapy and psychotherapy serve to catalyze each other, so that the two methods, used together, accomplish more than either applied alone. Case II provides such an illustration.

*Case II.** The patient, a 23-year-old homosexual, presented himself as a dangerously angry young man with a paranoid streak. During high school he had made a half-hearted attempt to poison an ex-lover and, prior to beginning therapy, he had killed seven pets violently. He had given each pet to his 15-year-old male lover; as soon as the boy grew attached to the pet the patient would murder it.

The patient was first seen individually for 6 hours, forming a strong relationship with the therapist. Then came 4 months of group psychotherapy by a male-female team, followed by anticipatory-avoidance conditioning, employing patient-selected erotic pictures of men, localized shocks as aversive stimuli, and "sexy" pictures of women as conditioned "relief" or "safety" stimuli. At the sixth session, he entered in a panic, saying that he had been "cruising" on the subway for 9 hours in a vain effort to become homosexually aroused. Virtually throughout the ensuing 2 hour emergency interview, he wept, at times violently, and poured out in concentrated form the feeling-facts of his homosexuality and its angry, narcissistic character. He spoke of one dream in which he made love to a man who "would have been me," had he ever been allowed by his mother to grow up as a man. In another dream, he rescued a dirty little old brown baby dumped in a trash can and covered with ashes: "Nobody loved the baby, but I loved it," he said, still weeping. Here the therapist said, "That baby is you, isn't it?" evoking several minutes of convulsive sobbing.

At the beginning of the interview, the patient tended to fuse the male therapist with his father and the female therapist with his mother. By the end of the session, he knew that both therapists were different from his parents and that both liked him. (This was unlike his mother, who had wanted him to be destroyed *in utero* by his abortionist grandmother, and his father who had "just stood by . . ." while his mother was alternately grossly seductive and violently cruel to him.)

The conditioning and/or his fantasies about the conditioning apparently produced a block in his ability to express his feelings homosexually and the resulting emergency interview was a pivotal point in his psychotherapy, which continued in group form for another year. He never felt the same about his homosexual activity, his therapists, or himself. There were only a few more homosexual episodes, all of which he described as "empty." In the course of his 79 treatment hours, he went from 6 to 0 on the Kinsey scale for homosexual adjustment (Kinsey, Pomeroy, and Martin, 1948), becoming a happily married man, obtaining high grades as a premedical student, and able to work effectively as a part-time laboratory technician.

Obviously, this was a patient with a large fund of unrecognized assets and it is difficult to extricate the relative roles played by expectation, suggestion, and fantasies about the meaning of the conditioning, or by identification, or by simple human acceptance by new kinds of objects, to name but a few possibilities.

*This case is from the author's research work in the treatment of homosexual men by combined behavior therapy-psychotherapy; a full case report is planned.

Discussion

Psychiatric patients suffer and seek help because of troublesome behaviors and especially because of painful "feelings." The latter can usefully be thought of as tremendously difficult-to-measure inner behaviors of the brain and viscera. Both troublesome behaviors and painful feelings can be initiated and maintained by internal consequences (thoughts and feelings) as well as by external ones (external stimuli). Psychiatry and clinical psychology, as developing applied sciences, cannot afford the luxury of excluding from their proper concern these inner stimuli merely because of their complexities and the practical difficulties in their measurement. When only external stimuli are taken into account, greater precision of measurement is possible but at the cost of ignoring relevant clinical data. Some clinicians try to justify their lack of concern with measurement by stressing the "humanity," "subtlety," and "enormous complexity" of the clinical problem. However, this does not excuse the clinician from being as rigorous as possible and bringing to bear relevant behavioral ethological, and anthropological methods of study. Only when the shadowy constructs of therapy are approached in this multifaceted way are they likely to become better defined, understood, and hence more useful.

Reference

Kinsey, A.C., Pomeroy, W. B. and Martin, C. E. *Sexual Behavior in the Human Male.* Philadelphia: Saunders, 1948.

20

Psychodynamic Behavior Therapy

I. Theory and Rationale

BEN W. FEATHER, M.D., PH.D.,
AND JOHN M. RHOADS, M.D.

The following two articles by Feather and Rhoads are of major importance because they constituted the first clinical demonstration of how psychoanalytic theory could be integrated with behavioral therapy. They must be considered together since the first describes the theory and rationale, and the second the technique, for the authors' innovative "psychodynamic behavior therapy." Other therapists had previously used the two approaches concurrently, complementarily, or alternatingly. Feather and Rhoads, however, ingeniously and creatively construct an integrated approach that they apply in the treatment of certain phobias, obsessions, and compulsions. They do this by applying the technique of systematic desensitization, not to a hierarchical series of imagined external phobic situations, as is done in conventional behavior therapy, but rather to fantasies involving the repressed, unacceptable inner impulses that lie behind the clinical symptomatology of their patients.

After reviewing both psychoanalytic and learning theory models of symptom formation, symptom maintenance, and the mechanisms of therapeutic change, the authors conclude that many of the concepts and much of the terminology in behavioral and psychoanalytic theory refer to similar phenomena and similar processes. Utilizing the model of phobias, they point out that unrealistic fears may arise either from classical conditioning or from intrapsychic conflict. In the latter instance, the causal conflict is less obvious and repression has obscured the connection between the causative factors and the phobia. They see the behavioral concept of generalization and the psychoanalytic concept of displacement as identical processes, occurring along semantic, symbolic, drive-, or affect-related dimensions. To the extent that a phobia is organized around drives or impulses, it could reasonably be presumed that therapeutic intervention at the level of the drive might generalize to all phobic behavior maintained by that drive. This becomes the basis for their methodology, namely, desensitization to drive-related imagery that causally relates to the avoidance behavior.

Psychodynamic Behavior Therapy

I. Theory and Rationale

BEN W. FEATHER, M.D., PH.D.,
AND JOHN M. RHOADS, M.D.

> *All science is a search for hidden likenesses*
> *(Bronowski, 1956)*

In medicine, the greater the number and variety of treatments advocated for a single disease, the greater the probability that the disease is not well understood and that none of the treatments are reliably effective. The same generalization would appear to apply to emotional disorders, for currently there is an almost unlimited number of therapies for psychoneuroses, each with its adherents claiming their method's superiority over other approaches, and each method indeed scoring some successes and some failures. Given our imperfect knowledge of etiology and our lack of a thoroughly reliable treatment for emotional disorders, such a variety of viewpoints could provide a healthy atmosphere for advancing our understanding of psychopathology. Unfortunately, however, there is a tendency for each "school" of therapy to crystallize prematurely and to begin to emphasize the theoretical and technical *differences* which presumably make it superior to other methods and to overlook or deny *similarities.*

Currently, the greatest schism is between the behavior therapies on the one hand and psychoanalysis and psychoanalytically oriented psychotherapies on the other. From the behaviorist's position, Eysenck asserts:

> Behavior therapy is an alternative type of treatment to psychotherapy; it is a superior type of treatment, both from the point of view of theoretical background and practical effectiveness; . . . in so far as psychotherapy is at all effective, it is so in virtue of certain principles which can be *derived from learning theory* . . . psychotherapy itself, when shorn of its inessential and irrelevant parts, can usefully be considered as a minor part of behavior therapy.[1]

Reprinted by permission from *Archives of General Psychiatry*, 26:496-502, June 1972. Copyright 1972 by the American Medical Association. This research was supported by Public Health Service Research Scientist Development Award No. K02-MH19523.

Writing in defense of a psychoanalytic position, Szasz declares:

> The difference between the effectiveness of behavior therapy and of psycho-
> analysis in the treatment of neuroses is not like the difference between
> penicillin and aspirin in the treatment of pneumonia. They are not competi-
> tive therapeutic methods whose relative value is a matter of medical judg-
> ment. Instead, the difference between them is more like that between closed
> and open societies, or between religious orthodoxy and scientific rationalism.
> Behavior therapy and psychoanalysis are essentially two rival systems of be-
> lief—one full of order, simplicity, and oppression; the other full of diversity,
> complexity, and freedom—whose relative value is a matter of moral judg-
> ment. Which state is more admirable, Sparta or Athens? Which man, Napo-
> leon or Camus?[2]

Rhetoric such as the above stimulates lively, often heated discussion but is not in the best scientific tradition of humility and open-minded inquiry as exemplified, for example, by Pavlov or Freud. There are some real as well as apparent differences between the two approaches, and the real differences should not be minimized or denied. Some of the apparent differences, however, become blurred or disappear altogether upon closer scrutiny, and it is the purpose of this communication to review some of the hidden similarities between a learning theory formu-lation and a psychoanalytic formulation of psychopathology, both at the theoretical and applied level.

A further goal is to show how certain elements of psychoanalytic theory and certain behavior therapy operations may be combined to provide a distinctive treatment method that promises to be quite effec-tive in selected cases. Both the discussion and the cases presented will be restricted for the most part to phobias, since the generality of the methods described has not been explored.

A Learning Theory Formulation of Phobias

During recent years, there has been a rapid growth in the develop-ment and application of psychotherapies based on conditioning and learning theories. These therapies have evolved from several different points of view and, today, represent a heterogeneous collection of tech-niques, all reliant, to some extent, on learning theory and often given the single label: "behavior therapy." Breger and McGaugh[3] distin-guished between three different positions, each of which has influenced current behavior therapy practice. These are: (1) Dollard and Miller,[4] as represented in their book; (2) the Wolpe-Eysenck position as represented in Wolpe's work[5]; Wolpe et al[6] and in the volume edited by Eysenck[7]; and (3) the Skinnerian position as seen in Krasner[8] and the work that ap-pears in the *Journal of Experimental Analysis Behavior*.

Learning theorists Dollard and Miller made an impressive attempt

to translate psychoanalytic concepts into Hullian learning theory terminology. Their work still provides a useful bridge between psychoanalysis and learning theory but, while it stimulated a great deal of laboratory research, no distinctive therapy technique has evolved from it.

While there has been a rapid proliferation of behavior therapy techniques which often appear quite unrelated to one another, two main
streams of theory and practice can be identified. One of these is based
on operant conditioning, or the systematic application of punishments
and rewards in order to alter behavior in desired directions. The other
behavioral approach, and the one to be considered here, relies heavily
on classical or Pavlovian conditioning theory for its explanatory concepts.

An early example of a deliberately conditioned fear action in a
human subject was reported by Watson and Rayner.[9] By frightening
their subject with a loud noise while a white rat was present, a fear
reaction to the white rat and similar furry objects was conditioned. They
suggested that the conditioned fear might be alleviated by feeding the
child in the presence of the feared object. This method was later applied
by Mary Cover Jones,[10] who successfully treated a child with fear of a
white rat and similar objects by systematically feeding the child while he
was near the feared object.

While these examples are of historical interest, it was not until the
1940s that a systematic attempt to apply learning and conditioning principles to the treatment of psychoneuroses was made. Wolpe[5] observed
certain parallels between neuroses in human patients and experimental
neuroses in animals. His ideas were stimulated in part by experiments
by Masserman,[11] who found that cats that had been made neurotic by
being shocked in a small cage could be cured if they could be induced to
feed in the experimental cage in which the neuroses had been produced.
From a series of animal experiments conducted in 1947, Wolpe[5,12] concluded that the neurotic behavior in the animals was indeed caused by
the intense electrical shocks in a confined cage; that the neurotic behavior was elicited by exposing the animal to similar cages; and that
there was a generalization such that the more similar the cage was to the
one in which the animal was shocked, the more intense was the neurotic
behavior.

Wolpe drew a very close parallel between what he and others had
observed in experimental neuroses in animals, on the one hand, and
human phobias on the other. He states,

> All human neuroses are produced as animal neuroses are, by situations
> which evoke high intensities of anxiety. In animals, anxiety of the requisite
> intensity can be built up as a response to previously neutral stimuli in one of
> three ways. The animal can be (1) subjected to difficult discriminations on the
> Pavlovian model, (2) exposed to a relatively small number of severe noxious

stimuli, or (3) exposed to a relatively large number of small noxious stimuli. . . .[5]

Neurotic anxiety presumably is conditioned and there results a state in which a previously neutral stimulus tends to elicit anxiety. The neutral stimulus, which becomes the conditioned stimulus for anxiety, is any stimulus in the environment at the time of the initial conditioning. In time, there may be generalization of the anxiety to other stimuli, which either are physically similar to the initial stimulus or come to be treated similarly by the mechanism of mediated generalization.

Wolpe's emphasis clearly is on the possibility of any pattern of environmental stimuli which are present during an initial evocation of anxiety becoming the phobic object. This might be called an "accidental conditioning" theory of phobias. In other words, if sufficient anxiety is aroused in a person, whatever stimuli happen to be in the environment at the time will become the eliciting stimuli for the phobia. This formulation requires the minimum explanatory concepts: (1) classical conditioning of an anxiety response, wherein a previously neutral stimulus comes to elicit anxiety and (2) generalization of the conditioned anxiety response to other stimuli which are similar to the conditioned stimulus.

For the treatment of phobias, Wolpe advanced a counterconditioning hypothesis which he called the "reciprocal inhibition principle,"[5] an extrapolation from Sherrington's neurological "reciprocal inhibition."[13] According to this principle, stimuli which tend to elicit anxiety will lose their potential to do so if a response antagonistic to anxiety can be elicited in the presence of the anxiety-evoking stimuli. Wolpe and others have used a variety of behaviors such as assertive responses and sexual responses which presumably inhibit anxiety, but the typical behavior employed is muscle relaxation produced by a modification of Jacobson's[14] progressive relaxation training.

Wolpe soon gave up attempts to juxtapose the actual phobia-related stimuli with relaxation and began to ask phobic patients to imagine such stimuli. This made the method much more flexible but, as will be discussed later, removed nearly all similarities between the therapy operations and the laboratory experiments upon which they purportedly are based. Thus, systematic desensitization has come to consist of the anxiety-inhibiting response of muscle relaxation juxtaposed with the suggestion of anxiety-eliciting stimuli presented in a hierarchical order from least to most anxiety-evoking. Breger and McGaugh note that the use of the terms *stimulus* and *response* is

> . . . only remotely allegorical to the traditional use of these terms in psychology. The "imagination of a scene" is hardly an objectively defined stimulus, nor is something as general as "relaxation" a specifiable or clearly observable response. . . . counterconditioning is no more objective, no more controlled, and no more scientific than classical psychoanalysis, hypnotherapy, or treatment with tranquilizers.[3]

Another criticism raised is that the particular learning principles employed are outmoded and unable to account for evidence from laboratory studies of learning, let alone the complexities of the psychotherapy situation. Kimble[15] has shown, for example, that a subject's attitude toward an experiment is an important factor in determining the level of classical conditioning achieved. Breger and McGaugh also observe that in actuality behavior therapists *behave* in a way that is inconsistent with their own position. Many of the published cases of Wolpe, Lazarus, and others are described in terms of interpersonal conflicts and complex cognitive strategies rather than in terms of stimuli and responses. Similarly, in the extensive case literature on systematic desensitization, many examples can be found of suggestions for improving interpersonal relationships, supportive statements and reassurance, guilt-relieving comments, and other familiar techniques of supportive psychotherapy.

There is a growing consensus that systematic desensitization is an effective treatment for phobic symptoms, and the literature on outcome studies has been reviewed by Paul.[16] There is much less agreement, however, that whatever efficacy behavior therapy might have is related to the impressive background of theory and experiments upon which it purportedly is based. Breger and McGaugh, for example, find practically no relationship between modern learning theory and current practices of behavior therapy.

A Psychoanalytic Formulation of Phobias

Phobias have had a prominent place in the psychoanalytic literature for many years. As early as 1895, Freud[17] emphasized the pervasive role of anxiety in phobias and contrasted them with obsessions in which other emotional states, such as anger and doubt, appeared to be more central. In the classic case of Little Hans, he emphasized the similarity between phobias and hysteria.[18]

Freud saw the simplest compromise between a drive and the defense against it as consisting of experiencing the anxiety that caused the defense to become manifest, while the reason for the anxiety is repressed. Anxiety-hysteria, in which the fear that motivated the defense is still manifest, is the simplest psychoneurosis and the neurotic reactions in children often have this characteristic.

In all other neuroses, however, the anxiety has been elaborated further. Freud's original formulation of the phobia was that it is an attempt to deal with anxiety by substitution and displacement. The connection between the feared situation and the original instinctual conflict has become concealed. The substitute fear, as Freud formulated it, ''on the one hand has certain associative connections with an idea which was rejected; while on the other hand, because of the remoteness of that idea, it escapes repression."[19] The phobic individual then experiences anxiety in situations in which it is often quite difficult to relate it to the specific conflict.

Freud's original psychodynamic formulation of the phobia as representing an attempt to escape from an internal dangerous impulse or its consequences by avoiding a specific external condition which, by substitution and displacement, represents the impulse, has changed very little over the years. The minimal inferred mechanisms are three: (1) conflict, (2) repression, and (3) displacement.

In spite of Freud's straightforward simplicity in describing the essential phobic mechanism, actual cases rarely seem so simple. Fenichel pointed out that

> due to repression, phobias frequently have an indefinite, nebulous content, comparable in their lack of clarity to the manifest content of dreams; it often takes a great deal of analytic work to ascertain precisely what the patient is afraid of. In some cases, the content of the fear had at one time been clear and definite, but later in the course of the neurosis, it became vague and indefinite. The forces of repression continue to wage war on the symptom as an offshoot of the repressed. Thus, an understanding of the complicated or vague symptom of long standing may frequently be attained by determining the circumstances of its first appearance.[20]

There is a seeming paradox here, in that phobias are taken as the simplest demonstration of how symptoms arise and provide a paradigm of all other neuroses in which the anxiety may not be manifest, while many writers have emphasized the complexities encountered in unraveling the intricate relationships between initial conflicts and phobic symptoms. Freud,[21] however, in *The Introductory Lectures*, provided a key when he noted the similarity between phobias and dreams. He observed that the manifest content of phobias for the specific object or situation which elicits phobic anxiety is comparable to the manifest content of dreams; in each case, the manifest content is a facade behind which is concealed the latent thoughts that connect the displaced object (or dream imagery) to the initial conflict. Freud's relating the overt content of the phobia to the manifest content of dreams influenced Fenichel[20,22] to pay particular attention to certain recurring details in phobias and to interpret these details according to the rules for dream interpretation.

Lewin, pursuing the dream-phobia parallel further, describes the relationship more explicitly:

> The phobic facade is built up like the manifest content of a dream. There are, of course, simple dreams with little or no distortion and comparable anxieties that may or may not justify the appellation, phobia (Freud, 1926). But the regular predominance of displacement as a source of distortion in phobias indicated that, as in dream formation, the conscious and preconscious ideas that instigate the anxiety are linked with unconscious, libidinal, and aggressive impulses, and that the latent thoughts of the phobia, those that deter-

mine the facade were subjected to the primary process. Evidently, the manifest text of the phobias, influenced by this dip into the unconscious and the primary process, shows not only the effect of displacement, but of other id processes as well, such as condensation, disregard of time and consistency, etc.[23]

Many psychoanalysts since Freud have elaborated upon the complexity of phobic symptom formation in individual cases. Helene Deutsch,[24] for example, emphasized the role of aggressive and exhibitionistic impulses in the etiology of agoraphobia. She also called attention to the role of the choice of companion in agoraphobic patients and concluded that "the characteristic feature of agoraphobia is that between the subject and the object against whom the hostile tendencies are directed, an identification takes place under conditions inherent in the Oedipus constellation." Miller's[25] analysis of a case of street fear provides an example of the overdetermination or multiple etiology of phobic symptoms in which several of the elements described above were identified. He also called attention to the tendency of the phobic individual not only to withdraw from activities directly related to the phobic situation, but to restrict activity and function generally and to experience difficulty in verbalizing and receiving insight.

Rangell's analysis of a doll phobia also emphasized the complex overdetermination of phobic symptoms. In an introductory overview of his case, he comments:

> The phobic symptom was greatly over-determined, which accounted for its tenacity and long duration. The doll can be pictured as the hub of the wheel. From the hub, there radiate outwards numerous spokes, each representing an origin, a motive, a cause, or an historical determinant feeding into the hub doll. The various spokes also have interconnecting links, in irregular fashion, joining the various parts together into a network.[26]

Thus far, we have considered only, and in limited detail, the more salient features of phobic symptom formation as viewed by psychoanalysis. The central features are conflicts over internal impulses, repression, and displacement. The specific conflicts involved are as varied as the life experience of the individual and the displacement may be to any object or situation in the environment. Thus, while mechanisms involved are usually fairly limited, the clinical picture as it evolves in the psychoanalysis of a given case may be quite complex. Some writers have emphasized the similarity between phobic symptom formation and the manifest content of dreams, while Lief[27] has observed that *one* type of selection of the phobic object may be based on the association of sensory cues, contiguous in time with a critical attack of fear. This latter mechanism, discussed in a later section, will be recognized as identical to one learning theory formulation of phobias.

It is beyond the scope of this communication to discuss in detail psychoanalytic therapy of phobias; however, certain observations on therapy made by various writers deserve comment. Many analysts have noted the tenacity with which phobic patients hold on to their symptoms and the necessity for modifying a basically interpretive technique to effect a cure. The most familiar example is Freud's[28] discovery that interpretation alone did not bring about a change in the symptom and that it was necessary for the analyst to intervene actively at some point and induce the patient deliberately to expose himself to the fearful situation. This was the first "parameter" or noninterpretive technique introduced into psychoanalysis and is a technique which, in one way or another, has been employed by therapists of nearly all persuasions.

Weiss[29] noted that agoraphobias are extremely resistant to therapy and observed that some cases are analyzed for as long as 10 or 15 years with slight or no improvement and the patient may remain agoraphobic for life. Miller,[25] as mentioned earlier, has called attention to the frequent difficulty in verbalizing or receiving insight in phobic patients, while in one case,[30] he was able to effect a symptomatic cure of a phobia of flying in a pilot, quite rapidly, by interpreting material elicited during sodium pentothal interviews, within the context of a warm, permissive therapeutic relationship.

Salzman,[31] in an article on obsessions and phobias, advocated several innovative therapeutic techniques. He believed that it was necessary that the treatment differ radically from classical psychoanalytical technique and, in addition to repeated interpretation, recommended encouragement to action and "active assistance in stimulating new adventures for the patient." He observed that "it is a commonplace that while the patient may have adequate insight into the origin, symbolism, and function of his phobia, he is still unable to risk the initial venture into the heretofore out of bounds area of living," and felt that the bulk of the problem after some insight is achieved is to assist the phobic patient to enter those areas of living that he has avoided. He suggests using the leverage afforded by positive transference in encouraging the patient and at time physically accompanying the patient into the phobic area. Others who have modified psychoanalytic therapy for phobic patients are Tucker[32] and Ivey,[33] both of whom recommend using supportive and directive techniques in addition to interpretation.

Some Relationships between Learning Theory and Psychoanalytic Psychotherapy

Thus far only one learning and one psychoanalytic approach to phobias have been discussed. Over the past three decades a number of articles have been published on the relationship between learning theory and various aspects of conventional psychotherapy. They have ranged from simply attempts to point out that (1) neuroses are learned and (2) psychotherapy is a process of relearning, to more detailed analyses of specific theories and practices and to specific suggestions for modifications of conventional therapies.

Alexander[34] views the problem in psychotherapy as consisting in finding an adequate interpersonal relation between therapist and patient. Initially, this attempt is frustrated because the patient applies feeling and behavior patterns which were formed in his past and do not apply either to the current therapeutic situation or to his life situation. During treatment, the patient unlearns the old patterns and learns the new ones. Alexander sees this relearning as following the same learning principles studied by experimental psychologists and believes that the essential process is the acquisition of "emotional insight."

Marmor[35,36] has written extensively on similarities among various schools of psychotherapy and psychoanalysis and tends to view the psychotherapeutic process in general as a learning process. The fundamental problem in psychotherapy, according to Marmor, is "how best to enable or cause a patient to give up certain acquired patterns of thought, feeling, or behavior in favor of others which are considered more 'mature,' 'adaptive,' 'productive,' or 'self-realizing.' " If the learning theorist is a member of the stimulus-response school, he structures this task as an effort to teach the patient new habit patterns; if he belongs to the cognitive school, his task is to teach the patient new patterns of perception and new cognitive insights.

Marmor points out that the mere acquisition of intellectual or even emotional insight does not result in immediate change in the neurotic pattern, but that effort must be given to overcome the patient's tendency to cling tenaciously to his previous behavior patterns and to enable him to generalize his insight to all similar situations. These two tasks comprise essentially what is involved in the psychoanalytic concept of working through. Marmor sees working through as a kind of operant conditioning in which the therapist's overt or covert approval and disapproval act as subtle rewards and punishments.

That reward is much more efficient than punishment in altering behavior is a generally accepted learning principle. Marmor applies this principle to psychoanalysis, pointing out that punishment suppresses other responses in addition to the one punished and suggests that in analytic language punishment would lead to ego restriction while reward would lead to expansion of ego function. The therapist thus should be alert to the patient who "sees" punishment and criticism where it does not exist (especially in the transference) and should point this out repeatedly and explicitly to him. Punishment is equally ego restricting whether it is real or imagined.

Shoben,[37,38] in viewing psychotherapy as a problem in learning theory, observed four factors that appear to be common to all schools of psychotherapy: (1) all schools of psychotherapy can with some justice claim cures; (2) (neurotic) patients tend to present a similar problem, in that one of their primary motivations is anxiety and much of their symptomatic behavior is maintained on the basis of anxiety reduction; (3) the goal common to most psychotherapies is the modification of underlying anxiety; and (4) all types of psychotherapy employ some form of therapeutic relationship and conversational content. The common problem characterizing neurotic patients, then, is anxiety and maladaptive behaviors which temporarily reduce anxiety. The goal of psychotherapy, according to Shoben, "is to eliminate the anxiety and thereby to do away with the symptomatic, persistent, nonintegrative behavior." To accomplish this goal most therapists converse with the patient about his anxiety and the situations calling it forth both currently and historically. This formulation is equally compatible with both psychoanalytic theory and the classical conditioning formulation of the learning and unlearning of neurotic behavior; neither approach, in other words, deals exclusively with the overt behavioral symptoms but each attempts to modify the underlying anxiety which maintains the symptomatic behavior. One notes that this formulation is not compatible with aversive conditioning therapy which makes no attempt to reduce anxiety, but rather directly punishes undesirable overt behavior.

The question may be raised, then, why does talking about anxiety-provoking memories and cues with a therapist bring about a lasting change in the anxiety and its consequent neurotic behavior? Shoben suggests that, if neurotic anxiety is produced by the repression of some unextinguished response, it should follow that the anxiety can be reduced in one of two ways—either by the elicitation of unreinforced responses, thus leading to the extinction; or by the connecting of different affects to response tendencies which have been repressed. In either case, the first step in therapy would be to bring into consciousness that which has been repressed. When the patient is able to verbalize the repressed tendencies associated with his anxiety, he sees or demonstrates insight. This should not be equated with cure, regardless of how important it is as a step toward recovery. Merely being able to talk about anxiety cues does not necessarily make them any less threatening. Extinction or counterconditioning is still necessary.

Shoben prefers a counterconditioning hypothesis to simple extinction through nonreinforcement to account for anxiety reduction. His view on how counterconditioning may occur in psychotherapy is similar to Marmor's in that he emphasizes the overt and covert rewards inherent in the therapeutic relationship.

The earliest and most thoughtful attempt to relate psychoanalysis to learning theory was Thomas French's[39] classical paper on psychoanalysis and the experimental work of Pavlov. At the simplest level the Pavlovian concept of conditioning and the psychoanalytic concept of the association of ideas are shown to be nearly identical. Less obvious, but nevertheless important, is the parallel between inhibition in Pavlovian theory and repression in psychoanalysis. Both interfere with the occurrence of a response, and both mechanisms entail the assumption that absent reactions remain available if inhibition or repression is removed.

French made a convincing argument that the establishment of the normal object choice at the time of puberty is equivalent to a process of differentiation in Pavlov's sense. Further, he noted that when a normal love object is thwarted, for example, by death, there is a tendency to regress to the generalized infantile object and to react with all women after the pattern learned toward the mother. This is an example of the disappearance of differentiation resulting from an increase in the strength of an underlying drive. The concepts of both disciplines suggest that reality functioning of the ego depends on conflict, but that the conflict must not be so strong as to preclude the development and maintenance of differentiations. It can be argued that the task of the therapist is to aid the patient in achieving realistic differentiations and that in order to do so he must reawaken the conflicts in an intensity sufficiently low to permit differentiation to occur.

French pursues the reciprocal relationship between generalization and differentiation further in analysis of primary and secondary processes. Let us take a simple example: A hungry man dreams of food. This may mean that when hunger was present before, the sight of food was followed by food itself, and that hunger now evokes a conditioned image of food. In psychoanalytic terms, this would be called "primary process." Psychoanalytic theory goes further and holds that conditioned images have a reward value similar to the imagined object. Pavlovian theory would predict that conditioned images of this type would be subject to the laws of differentiation; i.e., not being followed by real food, they would be extinguished. Thus would develop the distinction between wish and reality which, in part, is what is meant by secondary process.

When discrimination between conditioned images (wishful fantasy) and reality is difficult, distinctions between the real and the unreal become blurred, as in the unconscious. In Pavlovian terms, the unconscious originates in the conditioning of responses to drive states. This conditioning may lead to a situation where a drive calls up the image of a satisfying object (primary process). Adequate differentiation would lead to accurate discrimination between such images and reality (secondary process); but Pavlov demonstrated that discriminations involving very high levels of excitation and inhibition may be difficult or impossible. In such a situation, the individual does not adequately distinguish between wish and reality. Thus, there are parallels between Freudian and Pavlovian theories which suggest that something as complex as the unconscious may fruitfully be approached from either frame of reference. For further discussions of French's paper, the reader is referred to articles by Kubie[40] and Kimble.[41] The former is written from the point of view of a psychoanalyst and the latter from the point of view of a learning theorist.

A Rationale for Psychodynamic Behavior Therapy

It will be recalled that at the most basic, conceptual level a conditioning model and a psychoanalytic model of phobias have several common features. The conditioning model entails (1) the classical conditioning of an anxiety and (2) generalization of the conditioned anxiety response to other stimuli which are similar to the conditioned stimuli. The psychoanalytic model involves (1) conflict, (2) repression, and (3) displacement. In either instance the proposed mechanisms are inferred rather than directly observable.

In the case of classical conditioning of an anxiety response, it is infrequent that the therapist (behavioral or analytic) can elicit an unequivocal history of accidental conditioning. More frequently, patients tell of developing fear of situations that once were either neutral or, more typically, outright attractive. The latter case, fear and avoidance of a previously attractive situation, clearly can be seen as a conflict.

Nevertheless, there are cases which seem to fit the classical conditioning model. The most straightforward example might be a man who fears driving after being injured in an automobile accident. This kind of phobia is quite different from another one in which a woman develops a fear of driving immediately after a vivid fantasy of leaving her husband and driving to another town to meet a lover. Unrealistic fears of phobic magnitude may arise either from classical conditioning or out of conflict in the psychoanalytic sense. These two kinds of phobias differ, however, in that in the former the apparent cause is obvious, both to the patient and therapist, while in the latter the apparent cause (conflict over impulses) can be elicited only by careful, skillful interviewing. The major difference, then, is that when a conflict is causal, repression ensues and the connections between the initially causative factors and the current phobia are obscured. If conflict is not involved, as in the man who was accidentally injured in an automobile, there is no need for repression and the patient can state clearly the circumstances of the beginning of his fear. This kind of phobia is seen much less frequently than the former. More typical is the patient who is fearful in certain situations and has no idea why he is.

So far we have suggested that phobias may arise as a result of either accidental conditioning or conflict; that in the former repression does not occur or is minimal and that in the latter repression is the rule. Let us examine the remaining mechanism of generalization and displacement. Wolpe has emphasized generalization along the dimension of physical similarities of environmental cues. (The fear-conditioned cat is fearful in all cages that are similar to the one in which it was conditioned.) This concept of primary stimulus generalization might account for why the man who fears driving after an accident is fearful of driving all cars and not just the one in which he was injured. It would not account for why the lady who wished and feared to meet a lover not only cannot drive, but also cannot leave her house. However, there are a number of dimensions along which a learned response, such as anxiety, may generalize. Except for primary stimulus generalization, all other kinds of generalization refer to dimensions that are internal rather than environmentally determined and thus are unique to the individual and his present and past experiences. Generalization and displacement then may be viewed as identical processes.

Displacement or mediated generalization may occur along semantic or symbolic dimensions or may occur along dimensions of drive or affect. Fenichel,[22] Miller,[30] and others have emphasized symbolic displacement, while French's synthesis suggests that drives, serving as conditioned stimuli, might assume crucial importance. To the extent that phobias may be organized around drives or impulses, some important therapeutic implications follow. For example, in cases of multiple phobias in the same individual, the feared objects or situations often seem unrelated either by symbolism or by physical similarities. If the seemingly different feared situations all represent occasions for a specific drive to be heightened, then a parsimonious explanation of multiple phobias is at hand. Otherwise, one would have to postulate multiple etiologies, such as a series of unrelated, accidentally conditioning events.

An important practical implication of this point of view is that successful intervention at the level of the drive should generalize to all of the phobias that are maintained by that drive. In operational terms, one might apply the behavior therapist's technique to systematic desensitization to the drive-related imagery underlying the avoidance behavior rather than to images of the environmental stimuli being avoided. One would then expect modification of all the drive-related phobias.

If matters were as simple as the above formulation suggests, then why do phobias not extinguish by simple nonreinforcement? The psychoanalytic concept of repetition compulsion is sometimes called upon to explain the persistence of symptoms over long periods of time. Among psychoanalysts there is no general agreement about the validity of the concept, and its heuristic value is questionable since, essentially, it is an untestable hypothesis. An explanation might be found in French's discussion of differentiation in Pavlovian terms of reality testing in the psychoanalytic sense. If a conflict (drive or impulse and defense against it) is sufficiently intense, the individual fails to discriminate between the impulse and its execution, the wish from the deed. Thus, reality testing is impaired. The same idea, stated in Pavlovian terms, is that, if excitation and inhibition are sufficiently intense, the organism fails to form an adequate differentiation. The phobic patient who avoids those situations that intensify his impulses can be thought of as failing to differentiate his wishes from his actions, his thoughts from his deeds.

In a subsequent communication we will describe and discuss the clinical application of psychodynamic behavior therapy to a number of patients.

REFERENCES

1. Eysenck HJ: *Behaviour Therapy and the Neuroses*. Oxford, England, Pergamon Press, 1960.
2. Szasz TS: Behavior therapy and psychoanalysis. *Med Opin Rev* 2:24-29, 1967.
3. Breger L, McGaugh JL: Critique and reformulation of "learning theory" approaches to psychotherapy and neurosis. *Psychol Bull* 63:338-358, 1965. [See also Chapter 4, this volume.]
4. Dollard J, Miller NE: *Personality and Psychotherapy. An Analysis in Terms of Learning, Thinking, and Culture*. Toronto, McGraw-Hill Co Canada Ltd, 1950.
5. Wolpe J: *Psychotherapy by Reciprocal Inhibition*. Stanford, Calif, Stanford University Press, 1958.
6. Wolpe J, Salter A, Reyna LJ: *Conditioning Therapies: The Challenge in Psychotherapy*. New York, Holt, Rinehart & Winston, 1964.
7. Wolpe J: Reciprocal inhibition as the main basis of psychotherapeutic effects, in Eysenck HJ (ed): *Behaviour Therapy and the Neuroses*. New York, Pergamon Press, 1960, pp 88-113.
8. Krasner L: The therapist as a social reinforcement machine, in Strupp HH (ed): *Second Research Conference on Psychotherapy*. Chapel Hill, NC, American Psychological Association, 1961.
9. Watson JB, Rayner P: Conditioned emotional reactions. *J Exp Psychol* 3:1-14, 1920.
10. Jones MC: A laboratory study of fear. The case of Peter. *J Genet Psychol* 31:308-316, 1924.
11. Masserman JH: *Behaviour and Neurosis*. Chicago, University of Chicago Press, 1943.
12. Wolpe J: Experimental neurosis as learned behavior. *Brit J Psychol* 43:243-268, 1952.
13. Sherrington CS: *The Integrative Action of the Nervous System*. New Haven, Conn, Yale University Press, 1906.
14. Jacobson E: *Progressive Relaxation*. Chicago, University of Chicago Press, 1929.
15. Kimble G: Thomas M. French on the relationship between psychoanalysis and the

experimental work of Pavlov, in Kimble G (ed): *Foundations of Conditioning and Learning*. New York, Appleton-Century-Crofts, 1967, pp 581-586.

16. Paul GL: Outcome of systematic desensitization: I. Background, procedures, and uncontrolled reports of individual treatment, in Franks CM (ed): *Behavior Therapy: Appraisal and Status*. New York, McGraw-Hill Book Co Inc, 1969, pp 63-159.

17. Freud S: *The Standard Edition of the Complete Psychological Works of Sigmund Freud*. J Strachey (trans), London, Hogarth Press Ltd, 1962, vol 3 (1895), pp 71-87.

18. Freud S: Analysis of a phobia in a five-year-old boy (1909), in *The Standard Edition of the Complete Psychological Works of Sigmund Freud*. J Strachey (trans), London, Hogarth Press Ltd, 1955, vol 10, pp 5-153.

19. Freud S: The unconscious (1915), in *Sigmund Freud Collected Papers*. J Riviere (trans), New York, Basic Books Inc Publishers, 1959, vol 4, pp 98-136.

20. Fenichel O: *The Psychoanalytic Theory of Neuroses*. New York, WW Norton & Co Inc Publishers, 1945.

21. Freud S: *Introductory Lectures on Psychoanalysis*. London, Hogarth Press Ltd, 1917, vol 15 and 16.

22. Fenichel O: Remarks on the common phobias. *Psychoanal Quart* 13:313-326, 1944.

23. Lewin BD: Phobic symptoms and dream interpretation. *Psychoanal Quart* 52:295-322, 1952.

24. Deutsch H: The genesis of agoraphobia. *Int J Psychoanal* 10:51-69, 1929.

25. Miller ML: On street fear. *Int J Psychoanal* 34:232-240, 1953.

26. Rangell L: The analysis of a doll phobia. *Int J Psychoanal* 33:43-53, 1952.

27. Lief HI: Sensory association in the selection of phobic objects. *Psychiatry* 18:331-338, 1955.

28. Freud S: Turnings in the ways of psychoanalytic therapy (1919), in *Sigmund Freud Collected Papers*. J Riviere (trans), New York, Basic Books Inc Publishers, 1959, vol 2.

29. Weiss E: *Agoraphobia in the Light of Ego Psychology*. New York, Grune and Stratton Inc, 1964.

30. Miller ML: Psychotherapy of a phobia in a pilot. *Bull Menninger Clin* 10:145-153, 1946.

31. Salzman L: Obsessions and phobias. *Contemp Psychoanal* 2:1-15, 1965.

32. Tucker W: Diagnosis and treatment of the phobic reaction. *Amer J Psychiat* 825-830, 1956.

33. Ivey EP: Recent advances in the psychiatric diagnosis and treatment of phobias. *Amer J Psychother* 13:36-50, 1959.

34. Alexander F: The dynamics of psychotherapy in the light of learning theory. *Amer J Psychiat* 120:440-448, 1963. [See also Chapter 1, this volume.]

35. Marmor J: Psychoanalytic therapy as an educational process: Common denominators in the therapeutic approaches of different psychoanalytic "schools." *Sci Psychoanal* 5:286-299, 1962.

36. Marmor J: Theories of learning and the psychotherapeutic process. *Brit J Psychiat* 112:363-366, 1966.

37. Shoben EJ Jr: A learning-theory interpretation of psychotherapy. *Harvard Educ Rev* 18:129-145, 1948.

38. Shoben EJ Jr: Psychotherapy as a problem in learning theory. *Psychol Bull* 46:366-392, 1949.

39. French TM: Interrelations between psychoanalysis and the experimental work of Pavlov. *Amer J Psychiat* 12:1165-1203, 1933.

40. Kubie LS: Relation of the conditioned reflex to psychoanalytic technic. *Arch Neurol Psychiat* 32:1137-1142, 1934.

41. Kimble GA: *Foundations of Conditioning and Learning*. New York, Appleton-Century-Crofts, 1967.

Psychodynamic Behavior Therapy

II. Clinical Aspects

BEN W. FEATHER, M.D., PH.D.,
AND JOHN M. RHOADS, M.D.

This second paper by Feather and Rhoads elaborates their treatment methodology. The first step quite naturally consists of eliciting information about psychological conflicts related to the specific symptoms. Next, after training the patient in muscle relaxation, desensitization is employed utilizing fantasies directly related to the etiological conflicts and unacceptable impulses. The authors suggest that patients resolve their conflicts about these unacceptable impulses through gaining the ability to make an adequate differentiation between the reality of their actions and the fantasy of their impulses. This of course has wide potential implications for the treatment of other disorders of behavior. They also raise an intriguing question as to whether the therapeutic effects of systematic desensitization techniques result from "helping patients to form more accurate discriminations between fantasy and reality" or from the "desensitization" process itself.

Does such an integrated approach necessarily offer any improvement over conventional behavior therapy, inasmuch as the latter may also effectively remove the symptom in such cases? There are two answers. First, as the authors indicate, there are cases in which the conventional hierarchy of imagined external situations simply does not work, where getting to the repressed inner impulses may prove more effective. Second, and more importantly, the addition of insight into the connection between the repressed impulses and the anxiety gives the patient "a tool that he can . . . apply to new situations." Thus, although insight in itself may not be essential for a therapeutic result to occur, it contributes to the patient's ability to cope more effectively with subsequent stresses.

Psychodynamic Behavior Therapy

II. Clinical Aspects

BEN W. FEATHER, M.D., PH.D.,
AND JOHN M. RHOADS, M.D.

In a previous paper[1] we compared learning theory and psychoanalytic approaches to the understanding of certain phobias, obsessions, and compulsions, and described the rationale for an innovative therapy. The cases presented here illustrate the rationale for and the technique of psychodynamic behavior therapy. Like most therapeutic innovations, this has evolved from clinical experience and has been shaped as much by therapeutic necessity and trial and error as by theory, with modifications of systematic desensitization in some instances preceding any theory-derived rationale.

Most of the patients were preselected in that they were referred by other psychiatrists (usually psychoanalysts) specifically for behavior therapy for phobias, obsessions, and compulsions. Two to five interviews were spent taking a psychiatric history. There are some differences in emphasis from the usual such history: We obtain a more detailed symptom history, and give somewhat less emphasis to early childhood experiences. "Psychological mindedness" or ability to achieve insight is not considered essential and, in fact, may be an indication to consider other treatments. Psychological mindedness in the therapist is essential. In the initial interviews the goal is to uncover the conflict underlying the phobia or phobias, and all sources of information such as dreams, fantasies, slips of tongue, and symptomatic acts are utilized. Inferences from this information are not interpreted to the patient.

We have found directed fantasies to be an invaluable technique in discovering the nature of conflicts underlying phobic symptoms. Patients are asked, "What is the worst possible thing you can imagine happening?" in whatever the situation is that he fears. The first re-

Reprinted by permission from *Archives of General Psychiatry*, 26:503-511, June 1972. Copyright 1972 by the American Medical Association. This study was supported by Research Scientist Development Award K02-MH19523 from the Public Health Service.

sponse usually has to do with "going to pieces," "losing control," or "becoming totally paralyzed." When this is pursued further and he is asked to imagine just how he would go to pieces and lose control, his fantasies usually take the form of carrying out some violent or socially taboo behavior. For example, in 30 cases of speech phobia, nearly one-half the patients fantasized such violent acts as kicking the lectern over, shouting obscenities at the audience, or physically attacking the audience; the rest fantasized exhibiting themselves by undressing, urinating, masturbating, etc. Five young men had the fantasy of their pants falling down.[2] Often the patient will quickly reassure the therapist (or himself?) that he would not really do such a thing.

The patient's ability to regress in the service of the ego is a valuable asset. Some patients cannot permit themselves to fantasize just how they might lose control, but are able to imagine how "someone else who has the same problem" might act. Specifically guided imagery similar to that suggested by Leuner[3] may be used for patients who have difficulty allowing themselves to fantasize. The frequency and intensity with which some patients insist that they "really aren't like that" suggests defective discrimination between fantasy and reality and the need for external reassurance and validation by the therapist.

If the history reveals that a conflict underlies the phobia or phobias, the patient is trained in Wolpe's modification of Jacobson's muscle relaxation technique.[4] Usually the major part of one or two sessions is devoted to relaxation training and the patient is asked to practice relaxation at home for 15 minutes twice daily. At this point, a hierarchy consisting of graded fantasies of enacting the relevant impulses is constructed collaboratively with the patient. Care must be taken to assure that the fantasies are the patient's and not the therapist's. This constitutes a gray area, for the therapist reinforces some fantasies and not others.

The next step is to have the patient imagine these fantasy scenes, beginning with those which elicit the least anxiety and gradually moving on up the hierarchy to the most threatening imaginary scenes. The highest item on the hierarchy often is the same fantasy elicited earlier by the question, "What is the worst thing you can imagine happening?"

Concurrently with the systematic desensitization carried out in the office, usually once or twice weekly, the patient is required to begin confronting the phobic situation in real life in progressive "doses" that can be tolerated with little or no anxiety. Treatment is not terminated as successful until the patient can reenter those areas of life experience that were out of limits, with little or no anxiety.

Several modifications of this approach have been tried, such as modifying the hierarchy of scenes as new fantasy material emerges during the session, or abandoning the rigid, hierarchic order altogether. Another modification has been a dual therapist approach. This consists of one therapist carrying out systematic desensitization, while the other concerns himself with studying the patient's reaction to behavior therapy and the behavior therapist. This approach was introduced as an investigative tool and has revealed important instances of transference reactions and resistances.[5]

Case Studies

Case 1. Mr. A. was a 39-year-old mechanical engineer at an air force base involved in testing experimental airplanes. Ten years prior to his hospital admission he developed a fear of driving his car. Eventually he had to give up driving altogether and had to bicycle to and from work. For 16 years he held a responsible job involving handling classified information. For 10 years he had become increasingly fearful of accidentally disclosing secrets, and developed obsessive thoughts and compulsive rituals to prevent doing so. He had to be the last to leave his office each day, had to check all wastebaskets, and double-check the locks on file cabinets. Nevertheless, he was so obsessed with fears that he had to stop writing all personal letters and payment of bills. Always shy, he cut off his few social contacts lest he disclose the undisclosable.

For seven years he saw a psychoanalyst three times a week, but his illness worsened. He then took a medical leave of absence, admitted himself to a university hospital, and was treated with 25 electric shock treatments and occupational therapy. This led to confusion, memory loss, and the ability to make leather belts and billfolds. While there, he read an article about lobotomies and referred himself to Duke Hospital to obtain one.

He was totally incapacitated. He had a compulsion to pick up and examine every tiny scrap of paper he saw to make sure that it did not contain secrets he had disclosed. Cigarette filters had to be carefully unrolled and minutely examined. Dressing required up to 1½ hours each morning as he had to search each pocket painstakingly to make sure it did not contain classified information. The swallowing of his pills required 15 minutes or more. He avoided swinging doors whenever possible, and if he could not he had to check behind the door he had just passed through.

He was moderately depressed and chronically anxious. He was distrustful of psychiatrists, but demanded that his brain be operated on.

The relationship among his many symptoms gradually emerged. He had been angry at his mother while driving her in his car two days before her death. Her death preceded the onset of his driving phobia by about six months. The phobia began immediately after reading a newspaper account of an accident which clearly could not have involved him, but which made him feel compelled to drive to the scene of the accident and talk to the police to assure himself that he had not caused it. After that he would always circle back around the block he had just covered. A 3-mile trip thus became a 12-mile series of loops. While driving he constantly watched the rear-view mirror for the bodies of pedestrians that he might have hit. The wonder is that he did not kill somebody.

He was angry at his boss because a co-worker had been promoted before he was. His fear of disclosing secrets followed a revenge fantasy of deliberately giving away secret information.

His fear of swinging doors was related to the fear that the door might swing back and strike someone behind him, killing or mutilating them.

His pill-taking ritual was related to the fear that he might inadvertently overlook one of his pills, which might be taken by another patient who might then die.

For each of his phobias, obsessions, and compulsions there was a related fantasy of death and destruction; thus, much of his behavior seemed designed to safeguard against his carrying out such mayhem. The element common to all his symptoms was a hostile, destructive impulse embellished by fantasy and defended against by his compulsions. Behavior therapy was begun.

His most disabling symptom—picking up pieces of paper—was dealt with first. It was reasoned that this compulsive act had at one time been anxiety-reducing and was, therefore, strongly reinforced. If the symptom could be made aversive or could be followed by aversive consequences, it would be extinguished.

As it happened, Mr. A did not feel compelled to pick up paper in areas he had never been in before. So it was insisted that he begin picking up every scrap he saw wherever it was. He was required to bring his collection to the therapist's office each day. As the number of shopping bags full of scrap paper increased, so did his anger. His task was made more aversive by maids and janitors who jeered at him for doing the work they had been doing. As his requests to be relieved of his work became frantic, he was allowed to stop picking up paper first in one hallway and then another. Within two weeks he no longer picked up paper, and no longer felt anxious when he saw scraps of paper in the hallway.

Coincident with the above phase of treatment, he was taught muscle relaxation and a hierarchy for his driving phobias was constructed. The dimension of this hierarchy was the number of pedestrians and their distance from the street in which he was driving. The lowest item on the hierarchy was driving a car in an empty parking lot. The highest item was driving his car in the downtown rush-hour traffic with many people crossing the street.

Despite exposures to the lower items on the hierarchy, he was never able to get over being anxious if there were a pedestrian in sight. When questioned as to exactly what he was thinking when he became anxious, he reported that he imagined accidentally running over someone and killing him. When relaxed again, he was asked to imagine the scene again, but this time to imagine that he *deliberately* ran over someone. He rebelled at the idea, and asked if the therapist were trying to make some kind of monster out of him. He was assured that he was not being told to run over people, but only to imagine it, which he was already doing. Further, he was asked to embellish the imaginary scene of running over someone in any way that he wished, and to imagine that he was thoroughly enjoying the act. The scene was repeated a number of times during the session and each time, after a minute of imagery, he was asked to report exactly what he had imagined. His fantasies became more and more bloodcurdling as he imagined running up on the sidewalk to hit pedestrians, driving through large crowds of people, and turning on the windshield wipers to remove the blood. On the second presentation of the scene he began to smile, and on the third and subsequent scenes he laughed aloud. At the end of the session his manner changed, and he said he felt guilty over being so hostile. It was repeatedly emphasized to him that there is a vast difference between fantasies and acts. He had no more difficulty in imaging driving the car, so he was instructed to rent a car and begin actual driving practice. Within a period of two weeks he progressed from driving in an empty parking lot to driving anywhere in the city and to taking trips across the state on weekends.

Concurrently with the treatment of his driving phobia, another therapist under our supervision was attempting systematic desensitization for his fear of writing. There was little success using a conventional hierarchy until it was discovered that his fantasies invariably went to revealing secret information. He was then asked to imagine *deliberately* disclosing all the secrets of his company by emptying all the file cabinets into the street. There was an almost immediate remission in his writing phobia, and he was instructed to begin writing at least six letters per day, which he did with little difficulty.

The pill-taking ritual, dressing ritual, and avoidance of swinging doors subsided and disappeared without any direct treatment or mention of them.

At the end of two months' hospitalization and 40 behavior therapy sessions, he was asymptomatic and returned to work. Follow-up visits at six months and one year showed that the therapeutic effect had generalized to other areas of his life. He had taken up golf, which he had avoided for fear he might hit someone with the ball. He was more active socially. He had married. He stated that he was functioning better in every area of his life than he had for over 10 years.

Comment. The psychopathological disturbance consisted of a mixture of phobic, obsessive, and compulsive symptoms, with the compulsive features predominating. The avoidance behavior, as well as his compulsive rituals, had a common denominator: they either prevented him from acting on unacceptable impulses, or they undid the damage he might have done if he had "accidentally" acted on an impulse. Failure to discriminate between reality on the one hand and his impulses and their associated fantasies on the other was striking. He acted *as if* he really had caused a wreck or revealed secret information. While he could discriminate fantasy from reality at an intellectual level, his behavior was directed more by emotions than by cognition, and at the emotional level reality testing failed. The practical advantages of understanding the psychodynamic factors underlying symptoms seem clear in this case. Systematic desensitization applied in the customary way, i.e., to an anxiety hierarchy of environmental cues, had no effect. When his fantasies were directed more toward his impulses, i.e., by having him imagine *deliberately* carrying out what he had imagined would happen accidentally, there were dramatic changes.

The favorable results in this case suggest that, when behavior therapy is applied to the central conflict underlying several symptoms, generalization of therapeutic effect will occur. Desensitization was applied to two phobias—driving and writing—and a form of impulsive therapy to the compulsion to pick up paper, yet other dynamically related symptoms disappeared. Not only was the anxiety hierarchy abandoned, but the content of the imagined scenes was guided in part by the therapist's knowledge of the conflicts involved and in part by the patient's associative and imaginative processes.

At first the patient's attitude toward the behavior therapist was quite negative. It changed gradually to positive after a lengthy period of marked ambivalence. He carried out the aversive assignments with scrupulous attention to detail while protesting vigorously that the treatment could not possibly help him. While maintaining a facade of resistance and rebellion, he began to arrive earlier and earlier for his appointments, had difficulty leaving the office at the end of sessions, and called the therapist in his office and at home demanding extra appointments. The observer therapist also noted these changes and observed the development of what appeared to be a passive dependent transference attitude toward the behavior therapist. The behavior therapist helped the patient extricate himself from this passive dependent relationship by gradually shifting his stance from that of an authoritarian God-like or father-like figure to a less active, more neutral, and somewhat benign figure. Early in treatment the behavior therapist set rigid requirements for the patient and insisted that they be met. Later in the course of treatment the patient himself was involved in setting goals at his own pace.

The therapist deliberately used the leverage afforded by his relationship with the patient to exert pressure toward behavioral change. It would not be accurate to call this technique utilization of the transference. Since the therapist was deliberately dogmatic, authoritarian, and rigid early in the treatment, the patient's attitudes, first of negativity and resentment, then ambivalence, and later passive dependency, were realistic to the situation rather than transferences from earlier relationships.

Case 2. Dr. B was a 37-year-old physiologist who had been in supportive psychotherapy for several years for recurrent anxiety attacks. During the course of treatment he disclosed that he had a fear of flying, though earlier in life he had been a navy pilot. Over a three-year period his anxiety reached the point where he avoided flying altogether. This was a great inconvenience to him because he had to attend a number of professional meetings and his fear necessitated losing too much time on other means of transportation. Also, his fear interfered with visits to his mistress who lived far enough away so that he could visit her only by flying. He was referred for behavior therapy for the flying phobia.

After the initial interview he admitted to other severe phobias. He could feel comfortable in an audience only if he sat in the back row next to an exit. This phobia was especially inconvenient because he was partially deaf.

He managed to get through his classes or talks by taking heavy doses of tranquilizers.

He was terrified of cocktail parties, and often had to leave them because of his anxiety. He had begun to avoid parties and had withdrawn from most social contacts.

A detailed symptom history with emphasis upon the fantasies associated with his phobias was obtained. The worst thing he could imagine happening in an airplane was that he would go berserk, lose control, strike other passengers, and urinate and defecate. He did not fear dying in a crash but feared what he might do if the plane encountered any difficulty.

While attending a chamber music recital shortly before therapy began, he thought about jumping up, waving his arms, and shouting obscenities at the audience. He fantasized the hostile looks his older male colleagues would give him. Though he recognized it as ridiculous, he had to leave in the middle of the performance in a state of great anxiety. For years he had had the recurring fantasy of attending a concert at Carnegie Hall, sitting in the second row from the front, and disrupting the performance by vomiting all over the man in front of him, stepping on people as he left his seat, and distracting everyone's attention from the music as he fled from the hall.

At cocktail parties his anxiety focused on "doing something stupid" such as spilling a drink over several people. This fantasy was preceded by anger and annoyance at people at the party. He thought how stupid his colleagues were, how inane their chatter was, and how he would like to tell them so. His public speaking anxiety was greatest when the content of his talk was designed to demolish someone else's ideas.

Though his recurring fantasies had the common theme of hostile aggression, he saw no connection between them. Rather, he felt that the explanation in each feared situation was that he might become so tense that he could not control his body movements. He "inadvertently" demonstrated this for the therapist by "clumsily" knocking the telephone off his desk.

As he planned to attend lectures in the near future we decided to treat that phobia first. He was taught muscle relaxation and took to it readily, removing his shoes and coat and loosening his tie while commenting about how comfortable the couch was and how good he felt. When he achieved a state of apparent deep relaxation, he was asked to imagine sitting in a large audience and doing whatever came to his mind. After about a minute he was asked to report what he had imagined.

He had fantasized sitting in the middle of the lecture room next to the slide projector while a colleague he disliked was giving a talk. He was annoyed by the noise of the slide projector. He was asked to repeat the scene a total of six times during this session and each time told to imagine vividly and with pleasure whatever occurred to him. In each successive fantasy he became increasingly angry until finally he imagined knocking over the slide projector, toppling it onto the man sitting next to it, and jumping up and down on it, demolishing it and the lecture. Throughout this session he remained deeply relaxed and reported no anxiety.

He was asked to practice relaxation once each day at home and to try sitting in the middle of an audience before returning. At his next visit he reported that he had sat in the middle of an audience at a concert and was less anxious. He was again asked to imagine the audience situation, and the most violent thing he imagined was blowing his nose loudly. When this change was commented on, he said that for some reason he felt a lot "tamer." He was asked to sit in the front row of an audience before returning for his next appointment. When he returned he said that for the first time in several years he could sit comfortably anywhere he wanted and added that he had taken an airplane trip the week before and had experienced practically no anxiety. He broke off treatment at this point. He was seen for follow-up interviews one and two years later and was found to be free of all phobic symptoms (though not of his characterological problems). There was no evidence of symptom substitution.

Comment. Dr. B was seen eight times but only 2½ sessions were devoted to systematic desensitization. A symptom history was obtained in the first 2½ sessions, and relaxation training was initiated at the end of the third session. Following his enthusiastic acceptance of lying on the couch and relaxing, he missed two appointments—each time calling an hour or two after his appointment time to find out when he should come.

During the fourth session he broke down and cried most of the hour. He returned for two sessions of systematic desensitization before breaking off entirely.

Based on his behavior with the behavior therapist, as well as on information previously obtained by the observer therapist, it seems likely that intense dependency needs had been reactivated by lying on the couch and receiving instructions in relaxation. He vacillated between giving in to the temptation to regress (e.g., session 4) and resisting.

The most striking feature of the case was the rapid symptomatic relief and generalization of the therapeutic effect. We suggest that these effects occurred because systematic desensitization was applied not to imagery of environmental cues, as is customary, but to imagery of enacting unacceptable impulses; these hostile aggressive impulses were common to all his phobias, and it appeared that systematic desensitization in one area generalized to the others.

Case 3. Mrs. C, a 41-year-old housewife, was referred for behavior therapy. She had a four-year history of a severe washing compulsion related to the fear of contamination by cockroaches. Although she had not seen a cockroach for nearly one year, her preoccupation with looking for them, scrubbing areas of the house where they "might have been," and washing her hands and arms had reached the point where she was spending 12 to 18 hours per day in compulsive rituals, had lost 4.5 kg (10 lb) from frantic exertion, and had a bleeding dermatitis of both hands and arms.

Her illness had begun four years earlier, coincident with two important life events: her mother was slowly dying in a nursing home, and the patient became unexpectedly pregnant. She was anxious and depressed at the discovery of the unwanted fourth pregnancy.

At the onset of her illness, she was living with her family where her husband was a seminary student. She had never seen a cockroach in or near their home, but recalled that she had seen them previously in the adjacent state to which they moved the following year. Despite the absence of real cockroaches, she became obsessed with the idea that she might find them and began compulsive hand washing.

After they moved, she did indeed find cockroaches, and soon her life became organized around this and related compulsions, even though the exterminator visited weekly. After one year, they moved to a new rectory. In the new rectory there were no cockroaches but the symptoms increased. Her husband occasionally had business in the old rectory, and each time he returned the patient insisted that he undress at the door, put his clothes in a special bag to be sent to the laundry, and wash all the doorknobs that he might touch.

The contamination fear generalized to objects that might have been touched by her husband, who might have touched something in the old rectory, which might have been touched by a cockroach. All activities of the family were organized around her illness. Any member of the family who might be contaminated had to wipe off doorknobs, light switches, books, chairs, etc., after touching them. She dropped all social contacts, and spent the entire day until 2 A.M. scrubbing away the omnipresent contamination. Since no cockroaches were present in the home after they moved, most of the contamination seemed to emanate from her husband, who still had occasional contact with the rectory where cockroaches previously had been seen.

Concurrently with the discovery of her pregnancy four years earlier, and with the onset of obsessions and compulsions, she developed a strong feeling of revulsion for her husband. Not only were sexual relations out of the question, but being touched by him or even seeing him led to a feeling of disgust. In four years, intercourse had occurred only once, and for the past year there literally had been no physical contact with her husband. She attempted to explain this on the basis of fear of pregnancy. When this fear was confronted, she said that she was too preoccupied with cockroaches and cleaning things to bother with sex.

Because her preoccupation with cockroaches began in the absence of cockroaches, it was inferred that they must symbolize something else she wished to avoid. Since the feeling of disgust for her husband was identical to her feeling of disgust at the sight of a cockroach, especially when she could see "his feelers sticking up and wiggling at me," it was hypothesized that her more central conflict was sexual, and that the avoidance had been displaced to cockroaches. It was decided to desensitize her to her husband rather than to cockroaches. If the hypothesis were correct, one would expect any therapeutic effect to generalize to the cockroach obsession and washing compulsions.

First, her husband was instructed to stop carrying out his wife's compulsions. He and the children were no longer to change clothes and wipe doorknobs and light switches to ease her burden of scrubbing. He was delighted; she was enraged. She complained bitterly that she would have to stay up all night to assure that nothing was contaminated. By the time of her next visit she had indeed stayed up two nights scrubbing the house, and angrily and tearfully demanded that she be given some relief. A schedule of times—initially six hours per day—that she could scrub was established and all her compulsive activity had to be restricted to those times. Throughout the course of her treatment the permitted scrubbing time was gradually reduced until it reached the level of one hour three days per week.

Next she was taught muscle relaxation and an attempt was made to construct a desensitization hierarchy around the theme of physical contact with her husband. Intercourse was easily the highest item, but it was difficult to find any scene involving her husband that did not elicit intense disgust. Even to imagine looking at a photograph of her husband across the room elicited immediate strong disgust. A neutral scene, a snow-covered mountain, had to be used as the first scene of hierarchy. The rest of the hierarchy consisted of imaginary scenes, first looking at photographs of her husband, then directly at her husband in the distance, then touching him with her hand, imagining sequentially the stages of foreplay they had engaged in before her illness, and finally imagining intercourse and orgasm. The hierarchy had to be altered from session to session when certain scenes could not be imagined without discomfort. One scene in which she was to imagine her husband fondling her breasts repeatedly elicited disgust until she volunteered that she had been imagining that her husband's hands were dirty. She was told to imagine that his hands were clean, and she was then able to imagine the scene comfortably.

By the eighth session of desensitization, she could comfortably imagine all the scenes in the hierarchy up to and including mutual genital manipulations. She then was instructed to begin carrying out the scenes in reality, starting with the ones lowest on the hierarchy and moving on to subsequent ones only when she felt completely free of discomfort. Enacting the scenes in real life proved much easier for her than imagining them in the office. At first both she and her husband approached the homework with unfeeling, mechanical rigidity. But the mutual sexual stimulation soon became pleasurable, and she began to ask when they could progress to having intercourse. The scrupulosity with which previously she had avoided "contamination" was still reflected in her scrupulous attention to carrying out instructions to the letter.

In the 20th session it was learned that while the letter of the law was being obeyed, the spirit was not. She tearfully confessed that while she had restricted the scrubbing to the permitted hours, this had been made possible in part by using paper towels to touch various items in the house. She expected to be severely criticized. She was told merely to stop using the paper towels. We were both relieved when she found that she could do this.

By the 25th session she had had intercourse with orgasms, something she had never had before. She insisted on restricting sexual relations to five days immediately before and after her periods because of her wish to avoid pregnancy and her inability to find a suitable contraceptive.

At the termination of treatment, she wished to retain one hour three days per week when she could scrub things if she felt like it, and this was agreed to. She no longer thought about cockroaches or contamination except during the ritualized scrubbing time, but insisted that if she saw one she would feel as bad as ever. As her symptoms receded, she had increased time and energy. For the first time in years, she became interested in her husband and his church work and involved herself in church and community activities. She regained weight, dressed more attractively, and regained a level of functioning comparable to her premorbid state.

She was seen for a follow-up interview after six months by the behavior therapist and the referring therapist. The referring therapist made the following notes:

". . . I asked her about roaches and she replied, 'I mind them as much but I see very few. When I do see them I feel bad and I clean the area just as I used to. Well, that is not quite right, as then I might not even have touched the area—too contaminated to even go near. On the other hand, I no longer dread that I *might* see one—in fact I now expect not to see one where I used to expect to see one.' "

Both the patient and her husband had requested approval for a vas deferens ligation for the husband at the beginning of treatment. The sterilizing operation was not recommended initially because of the neurotic component of her avoidance of intercourse. After the six-month follow-up, her remaining fears of unwanted pregnancy seemed realistic and her husband was then seen by her referring psychiatrist for an evaluation prior to the procedure. He found no contraindication and the operation was performed.

At two-year follow-up the effect of her treatment was more evident than at termination or at the six-month follow-up. She had not seen a cockroach for the past several months and the last one she had seen was simply removed and only the immediate area was wiped up. She said that her reaction to it was not much different from what it would have been prior to her illness. She had done no compulsive cleaning for the past six months, and had abandoned even her allotted cleaning time.

There was continuing improvement in her relationship with her husband. They were having pleasurable sexual relations on the average of twice each week.

Comment. This case illustrates the application of the operations of systematic desensitization to a conflict thought to underlie an obsessive compulsive neurosis. We believe the preoccupation with avoiding cockroaches and the scrubbing of areas where they might have been represented a symbolic displacement of her wish to avoid sex. Her avoidance of sex appeared to have two components: the realistic fear of pregnancy and a neurotic avoidance of intercourse, even at times when she could not have conceived, such as during her last pregnancy. It could be argued that she had two separate and unrelated areas of psychopathological disturbance: frigidity and a cockroach obsession. The identity of affects, i.e., the same disgust associated with her husband and with cockroaches, suggests, however, that the two areas were related psychodynamically. Further evidence for such a relationship is the ease with which the obsessive and compulsive symptoms receded and finally disappeared with little direct therapeutic attention paid to them.

Case 4. Mr. D, a 23-year-old senior medical student, referred himself for treatment for a severe public-speaking phobia. He had had no difficulty giving talks in high school and college but soon after entering medical school found it difficult to talk before groups of any size. For a while he was able to get through brief case presentations at a patient's bedside to groups of six or fewer people, but he was extremely anxious on these occasions, and had begun to avoid public speaking whenever possible. Though considered one of the brighter students in his class, he was considering dropping out of medical school because of the anxiety.

A few weeks before he entered therapy, he had had an acute anxiety attack while trying to present a case to a group of about 20 staff members. He was able to say only a sentence or two before he panicked and collapsed. A cardiologist found his pulse rate to be 180 beats per minute, and told him that he had paroxysmal auricular tachycardia. The patient's own diagnosis was that he had a speech phobia rather than a heart disease and he requested psychiatric treatment.

In the initial interviews, he was tense, anxious, and angry. He sat forward stiffly in his chair and spat out answers through clenched teeth in a staccato manner. In spite of his angry demeanor, he denied ever feeling any anger. He was asked to pay very close attention throughout the ensuing days to any feelings of anger or annoyance he might have and to write them down and bring the list on the subsequent visit. He came back emptyhanded, still insisting that he was never angry. He then began relating incidents in which he thought other people would have gotten angry. Again he was asked to pay close attention to his own feelings and to bring a written list of events that annoyed him. For the third session he brought two pages of notes concerning things which had angered him. He spent the entire hour recounting how enraged he had felt during the past week. The central theme was having his knowledge, authority, status, or prestige questioned directly or indirectly in any manner. A resident who had pointed out an error in his work-up of a patient and a nurse who had addressed him as mister had enraged him, and he had fantasies of verbally and physically attacking them. He could not understand why these things had not bothered him before.

There was a pattern to his public-speaking phobia. When he knew in advance that he would have to present something at a conference, he would bury himself in the library, look up every reference to the topic, and try to anticipate every question or criticism in order to prepare an answer for it. He noticed a direct relationship between the amount of preparation he did and the degree of anxiety he experienced at a presentation.

Another trigger for anxiety was to ask questions in a lecture. When he asked questions to gain information, he felt no anxiety; but when, as was his wont, he asked questions to demonstrate his superior knowledge, he became acutely anxious. Interpersonal situations involving older men, or those where the possibility of having his knowledge or authority questioned arose, also led to anxiety attacks.

For years he had had almost daily severe headaches and bruxism. Both symptoms were due to the constant tension in his neck and face muscles. When he commented on an anger-provoking situation with, "You might as well grit your teeth and bear it," it was suggested that it might be better to relax his masseter muscles and bear it.

Over the next three sessions, he was taught muscle relaxation and, as one might anticipate, he carried out the assigned home exercises religiously. Within three weeks his headaches and bruxism disappeared altogether.

In the seventh session he reported that he had been able to present a case to a small conference with only moderate anxiety. This improvement occurred *prior* to desensitization.

Desensitization was carried out over the next five sessions. An anxiety hierarchy was not constructed; rather, he was asked to imagine as vividly as possible standing up and giving a talk to groups that he might expect to have to address. He was asked to imagine the content of the talk he was giving and to report his fantasies in detail after every imaginary scene. His fantasies almost invariably involved expressing hostility by putting down everyone in the audience. At times, these fantasies made him too anxious to proceed and he would then change the content to less conflictual scenes.

By the 12th treatment session, he had given talks to groups of up to 50 staff members and had experienced very little anxiety. He had stopped his overpreparation for talks. He was much less anxious in interpersonal and social situations. He commented that he seemed to have developed a sense of humor about things which had previously made him either anxious or furious. For the first time since the onset of his phobia he was able to concentrate on what a lecturer was saying, as he was no longer obsessing about how he would feel if it were he giving the lecture. These fantasies vacillated between imagining that he would give a far better lecture on the one hand and panic on the other.

Therapy was discontinued by mutual agreement after the 20th session. A six-month follow-up revealed that he had had no more speech anxiety even though on several occasions he had spoken to groups of 100 or more.

Comment. This case illustrates the use of a patient's spontaneous fantasies of enacting unacceptable impulses. It could be argued that he would have recovered just as quickly if conventional systematic desensitization had been used. It is interesting to note, however, that improvement began *before* any desensitization, i.e., juxtaposition of muscle relaxation and fantasy, had occurred. It is tempting to speculate that his ventilation of anger was the main therapeutic agent. It would be informative to attempt this technique without the use of muscle relaxation. This case, like previous ones, demonstrates generalization of the therapeutic effect to symptoms that were not directly dealt with in the treatment.

COMMENT

Two cases of obsessive compulsive neurosis, one case of multiple phobias, and one of a single phobia have been discussed. During the course of treating these cases, as well as others not reported here, a therapeutic technique was developed that would appear to hold some promise for future application to a variety of clinical problems.

The technique, stated most simply, consists of eliciting information about psychological conflicts related to the specific symptoms, such as phobias, obsessions, and compulsions. No assumption is made that such conflicts are always present or are always identifiable, if present. In these four cases, the nature of the conflict had to do with unacceptable impulses and attempts to inhibit them. Additionally, there was difficulty in discriminating between fantasy and reality.

Once a conflict that underlies one or, more frequently, a number of symptoms has been identified, the patient is taught muscle relaxation and then is directed to fantasize *deliberately* carrying out the impulses which are involved in conflict, while relaxed. In addition, an attempt may be made to substitute a pleasurable affect for the anxiety associated with such fantasies. Some patients require frequent reassurance that they are not being urged to act out their impulses, and this discrimination repeatedly is reinforced. After anxiety is reduced, patients are required to reenter those situations which had occasioned anxiety. They are *not* told to carry out socially or personally unacceptable impulses. They are *not* urged to be more aggressive, assertive, sexual, or more of whatever expression was inhibited. In this regard the technique differs radically from Wolpe's[4] assertive training in which patients are urged to be more assertive in their interpersonal relationships. We believe that, once the intensity of the conflict has been reduced, the patient is in a better position than the therapist to decide what behavior is acceptable and appropriate for him in his environment. We do not assume that increasing assertiveness is always therapeutic. In this respect, the treatment is closer to psychoanalysis than to behavior therapy in its basic assumptions and aims.

How does psychodynamic behavior therapy differ from and how is it similar to psychoanalysis or psychoanalytically oriented psychotherapy on the one hand and systematic desensitization on the other? It should be clear that the techniques described here are quite different from the usual techniques of psychoanalysis. In psychoanalysis there is no clearcut distinction between analysis as investigation or information-seeking and analysis as a therapeutic technique. These two functions are interwoven throughout the course of psychoanalysis. Put differently, the analyst does not divide treatment into distinct fact-finding and fact-utilization phases. The techniques described here do rest on such a dichotomy. The initial sessions are devoted to obtaining information sufficient to make a limited psychodynamic formulation of the current symptoms. Only during this phase do the therapist's activities resemble psychoanalysis. Attention is paid to all behaviors that might indicate the operation of unconscious mechanisms. Once a limited psychodynamic formulation has been made, the emphasis shifts from information gathering to the active process of desensitization described earlier.

Resistance operated in each of the cases presented here, as well as in other patients we have treated with this method. Behavioral evidence for resistance has included frequent forgetting of appointments, arriving late, and failing to carry out therapeutic assignments such as relaxation exercises at home. In two cases resistance led to premature termination of treatment even though some symptomatic relief was achieved. The problem of resistance encountered in behavior therapy is discussed elsewhere in some detail by Rhoads and Feather.[5]

Transference and countertransference both occur, but transference when present is utilized as leverage for behavioral change rather than interpreted. Strictly speaking, interpretations are not utilized at all. There is, however, an intriguing possibility that desensitization and effective interpretations operate in a similar fashion. To illustrate, let us take the case of Dr. B, who had the fantasy of jumping up in a large gathering and shouting obscenities. A minimal interpretation to him might have been, "It would appear that you were quite angry at somebody." Repeated interpretations made over a period of time, relating his hostile impulses to his anxiety specific to those impulses, might be expected eventually to reduce the anxiety associated with such impulses. As a result of the therapist's nonpunitive attitude, he gradually would have formed a discrimination: he would have learned that it is not dangerous to think such things and that there is a difference between thinking them and doing them. Perhaps something very similar happened when the therapist simply told him to imagine vividly enacting these impulses while relaxing. In either case, the discrimination between fantasy and reality by the ego is reinforced.

Given a possible similarity of the therapeutic mechanisms of interpretation and desensitization, there remain two rather striking differences. The first difference is that for interpretations to be effective they have to be accepted. If interpretations are not accepted and yet are thought to be correct and relevant, resistance is operating and must be dealt with. This source of resistance was circumvented in the case of Dr. B, who in the face of rather strong evidence did not see himself as angry or hostile and who saw no connection between his impulses and his anxiety. This might be considered a therapeutic plus for desensitization, except for the fact that its value is offset by a second difference between interpretations and desensitization. The difference is that if the patient never learns intellectually the connection between his impulses and his anxiety, i.e., if he has learned nothing new about himself, he has not been given a tool that he can use in the future and apply to new situations. To the extent that insight can be effective prophylactically, it should be superior to desensitization.

It is suggested by the above line of reasoning and by the clinical examples that desensitization operates by conflict resolution. French[6] has shown that conflict can be described in either Pavlovian or Freudian terms, that the behavioral referents are identical, and that the mechanisms involved are either identical or quite similar. In order to say that a conflict has been resolved, either partially or completely, one must show evidence that either the intensity of impulses or the intensity of inhibition against them has been reduced, or both. The cases presented all provide evidence that inhibitions were reduced in intensity, and the fact that there were no increases in impulsive behavior would suggest that conflicts were resolved primarily through assisting patients to make differentiations between reality and fantasy.

There are many references to symptom substitution in the behavior therapy literature.[7-11] These authors typically point out that symptom substitution rarely occurs following systematic desensitization and then claim that the absence of symptom substitution represents a failure of psychoanalytic prediction. What is implied and sometimes stated explicitly,[7,11] but never documented, is that learning theory predicts that symptom substitution should not follow symptomatic treatment and that psychoanalytic theory predicts that it should. Neither statement appears to be true. Franks, while perpetrating the myth that psychoanalytic theory predicts symptom substitution, does point out that maladaptive behavior after treatment is not necessarily inconsistent with a behavioral model. He notes that "if one maladaptive behavior is successfully extinguished, a child may resort to another to gain his ends, and then to another—all parts of that individual's hierarchical repertoire of maladaptive behavior."[8] Thus, one author, writing from a learning theory point of view makes no specific prediction concerning symptom substitution.

We have been unable to find anywhere in the psychoanalytic litera-ture the prediction that symptom substitution is inevitable or even likely to occur following psychoanalytic or nonpsychoanalytic treatment. Perhaps the most thoughtful discussion of symptom substitution is found in Weitzman's[12] paper on behavior therapy and psychotherapy. Arguing from the theoretical position of psychoanalysis, he finds no reason to predict the inevitability of symptom substitution and gives a cogent discussion of why such an outcome should not be expected.

In any event, the issue cannot be resolved at the theoretical level. Neither learning theory nor psychoanalytic theory is precise enough to make such predictions. To the extent that there is a problem, it is an empirical one, and it seems to have been resolved: what appears to be symptom substitution is rare following any form of treatment and its incidence is no higher in systematic desensitization than in any other therapy.

In the years immediately following World War I the Hungarian psy-choanalyst Sandor Ferenczi[13-17] published a series of papers on a varia-tion he termed "active therapy." Frustrated by "the comfortable but tor-pid quiet of a stagnating analysis" in certain obsessional patients, Ferenczi utilized such devices as the issuance of orders and prohibitions to the patient. These were intended to interrupt habitual abnormal pathways of discharge, such as certain tics, urethral and anal habits, mannerisms, and postures. He utilized forced fantasies both in patients who daydreamed as a resistance and in those who rarely daydreamed. He insisted that those patients with a poor fantasy life must make up a fantasy about the presumably repressed affect. One patient was in-structed to fantasize something aggressive about the analyst, while a phobic, obsessive woman had to sing a song during the hour, thereby bringing out her exhibitionistic and onanistic drives. Ferenczi insisted that these had to be conducted within the context of psychoanalysis, and could be used only under certain special circumstances where difficul-ties had arisen. He justified his method by referring frequently to Freud's advice, that after a certain time one must call upon anxiety hys-terics to face rather than avoid situations which induced anxiety. When Ferenczi pushed his method to interacting physically with patients, a psychoanalytic storm broke over his head, and he retracted much of what he had written, and ceased to practice it.

Glover,[18] in his critique of Ferenczi's method, felt that there were many dangers inherent in it, though he did approve of the technical variation of forced fantasies. In a reference to the matter of symptom substitution, Glover was concerned primarily with whether the symptoms were really depleted of libido, or whether they were shelters behind which the ego hid from problems of new adaptation. Glover renamed active therapy "analytically guided interference," stated that it differed in principle from customary analysis, and warned against the risk of the therapist playing the part of the superego by issuing injunctions and prohibitions lest he behave in the same way as "the non-analytical therapeutist who pins his faith on exhortation, persuasion, guidance or therapeutic pedagogy." We do not consider our method to be psychoanalysis or a variant thereof but rather an application of psychoanalytic theory to the practice of behavior therapy.

How is a psychodynamic approach to behavior therapy similar to and how does it differ from conventional systematic desensitization? In addition to the theoretical and background similarities discussed earlier, certain operations are similar. Both employ a detailed symptom-oriented history. Both approaches use muscle relaxation, although we do not assume that relaxation reciprocally inhibits anxiety. Relaxation may operate by inhibiting anxiety or it may operate by providing an optimal setting for eliciting drive-related fantasies, thus aiding in their differentiation from reality. Another possibility is that relaxation contributes little or nothing to desensitization.

Both approaches use directed imagery but in this regard the techniques differ markedly. Guided by the "accidental conditioning" theory of learned anxiety, the conventional behavior therapist looks to the environment for the conditioned anxiety cues and tends to disregard internal impulses and their related imagery. Further, he assumes that when a patient is told to imagine a certain scene in an anxiety hierarchy the patient does just that. This naïveté appears to be a carry-over from laboratory learning experiments where it was often erroneously assumed that what the experimenter defined as the conditioned stimulus would be attended to by the subject selectively and exclusively. This is sometimes not the case even in animal experiments and rarely is it the case in human experiments.

In the context of behavior therapy, "presenting a stimulus" and "asking a patient to imagine a scene" are very different operations. Weitzman questioned patients about their imagery after each of approximately 200 desensitization sessions. He reports:

> Without exception, when closely questioned, patients reported a flow of visual imagery. The initiating scene, once visualized, shifted and changed its form. Moreover, these transformations took place continuously and, when the imagining was terminated by the therapist, had produced images which were quite removed in their content from the intended stimulus. These con-

tents and the transformations they exhibit compel a characterization as a form of spontaneous and apparently autonomous fantasy familiar to many dynamically oriented therapists.[12]

Beck, encouraged by the successful use of fantasies in systematic desensitization, has made a useful exploration of the use both of spontaneous and induced fantasies in psychotherapy. Spontaneous fantasies were found to be a help in more clearly delineating patients' problems, and structured or guided fantasies were found to facilitate a realistic appraisal of external problems. His use of induced fantasies is quite similar to the techniques described in the cases presented here. His interpretation of the mechanism by which induced fantasies exert a therapeutic effect also is similar to our own. He believes:

> Rehearsals in fantasy produce a cognitive restructuring. With each voluntary repetition of the fantasy, the patient is enabled to discriminate more sharply between real dangers and purely imagery or remote dangers. As he is able to appraise the fantasy more realistically, the threat and the accompanying anxiety are reduced. He no longer expects disastrous consequences from entering innocuous situations that he had previously conceptualized as dangerous.[19]

It has been suggested that the therapeutic effects of conventional psychotherapy result from the *incidental* deconditioning that may occur. An equally valid suggestion is that the therapeutic effect of systematic desensitization results from helping patients to form more accurate discriminations between fantasy and reality. This hypothesis would seem to be an especially interesting one for psychoanalytic investigators to pursue.

In conclusion, a rationale for a psychoanalytic contribution to behavior therapy has been described. Case material has been presented to illustrate the application of some psychoanalytic principles to behavior therapy. The number of cases treated by this approach is still small, and generalizations must be limited; no claims of superiority over other therapeutic techniques are made. Rather, an attempt has been made to show common ground between psychoanalysis and behavior therapy at both a theoretical and an applied level, in the hope that others will be stimulated to study these intriguing, but all too often hidden, similarities.

References

1. Feather BW, Rhoads JM: Psychodynamic behavior therapy: I. Theory and rationale. *Arch Gen Psychiat* 26:496-502, 1972. [See also Chapter 20, this volume.]
2. Van Egeren L, Feather BW, Hein P: Desensitization of phobias: Some psychophysiological propositions. *Psychophysiology* 8:213-228.
3. Leuner H: Guided affective imagery. *Amer J Psychother* 23:4-22, 1969.
4. Wolpe J: *The Practice of Behavior Therapy*. New York, Pergamon Press, 1969.

5. Rhoads JM, Feather BW: Transference and resistance observed in behavior therapy. *Brit J Med Psychol 45*:99-103.
6. French TM: Interrelations between psychoanalysis and the experimental work of Pavlov. *Amer J Psychiat 12*:1165-1203, 1933.
7. Eysenck HJ: Learning theory and behavior therapy. *J Ment Sci 105*:67, 1959.
8. Franks CM: *Behavior Therapy: Appraisal and Status*. New York, McGraw-Hill Book Co Inc, 1969.
9. Paul GL: Outcome of systematic desensitization: I. Background, procedures, and uncontrolled reports of individual treatment, in Franks CM (ed): *Behavior Therapy: Appraisal and Status*. New York, McGraw-Hill Book Co Inc, 1969, pp 63-159.
10. Wolpe J, Lazarus A: *Behavior Therapy Techniques*. New York, Pergamon Press, 1966.
11. Yates AJ: Symptoms and symptom substitution. *Psychol Rev 65*:371-374, 1958.
12. Weitzman B: Behavior therapy and psychotherapy. *Psychol Rev 74*:300-317, 1967. [See also Chapter 7, this volume.]
13. Ferenczi S: On the technique of psychoanalysis (1919), in Rickman J (ed): *Further Contributions to the Theory and Technique of Psycho-Analysis*. New York, Basic Books Inc Publishers, 1952, vol 2, pp 177-189.
14. Ferenczi S: Technical difficulties in the analysis of a case of hysteria (1919), in Rickman J (ed): *Further Contributions to the Theory and Technique of Psycho-Analysis*. New York, Basic Books Inc Publishers, 1952, vol 2, pp 190-197.
15. Ferenczi S: The further development of an active therapy in psychoanalysis (1919), in Rickman J (ed): *Further Contributions to the Theory and Technique of Psycho-Analysis*. New York, Basic Books Inc Publishers, 1952, vol 2, pp 198-217.
16. Ferenczi S: Contra-indications to the "active" psycho-analytic technique (1925), in Rickman J (ed): *Further Contributions to the Theory and Technique of Psycho-Analysis*. New York, Basic Books Inc Publishers, 1952, vol 2, pp 218-230.
17. Ferenczi S: Psycho-analysis of sexual habits (1925), in Rickman J (ed): *Further Contributions to the Theory and Technique of Psycho-Analysis*. New York, Basic Books Inc Publishers, 1952, vol 2, pp 259-297.
18. Glover E: *The Technique of Psycho-Analysis*. New York, International Universities Press Inc, 1958.
19. Beck AT: Role of fantasies in psychotherapy and psychopathology. *J Nerv Ment Dis 150*:1, 1970.

The Use of Assertive Training and Psychodynamic Insight in the Treatment of Migraine Headache

22

A Case Study

Peter Lambley, Ph.D.

This paper reports a single case study in an A/B/C experimental design, in the successful treatment of a woman who suffered from severe migraine headaches.

Operating on the assumption that this disorder has psychodynamic, behavioral, and neurological elements which are mutually interactive, a treatment program was initiated using assertion training, followed by helping the patient to achieve psychodynamic insight into her migraine-related conflicts. While the assertion training significantly reduced the frequency of headaches, the ultimate reduction in both frequency and severity followed the second or dynamic phase of treatment.

Physiological responses in the body occur in response to psychological conflict, and these responses may become conditioned to psychological stimuli. The behavioral treatment of such psychophysiological responses, including work with biofeedback methodologies, has been an important area of recent clinical research. It is likely that this will ultimately prove to be an important area for the amalgamation of psychodynamic and behavioral approaches.

The Use of Assertive Training and Psychodynamic Insight in the Treatment of Migraine Headache

A Case Study

PETER LAMBLEY, PH.D.

Despite developments made in recent years in drug treatments and behavior and psychotherapies, many people who suffer from migraine headaches receive little alleviation of their symptoms. Standard methods of treatment include the use of pharmacological techniques for reducing the severity of the symptoms[4] and a variety of psychodynamic techniques which attempt to unearth and ventilate underlying conflicts in the patient's personality, particularly conflicts over the expression of feelings of repressed hostility or guilt[6].

Both of these treatment methods have drawbacks. In the case of drug treatment, severe side effects frequently prevent the use of the most efficacious drugs in certain patients, whereas in psychotherapy, patients are not always able to make use of cognitive insights to modify the autonomic, learned patterns of behavior that govern the precipitation of migraine attacks.

In the last decade, behavior therapeutic methods have been applied to the treatment of the disorder in the hope that these may overcome some of the problems of the older methods. These techniques focus on getting the patient to control aspects of his autonomic environment and so alleviate debilitating symptoms. Sargant et al.[13] and Wickramaskera[16], for example, have reported success using a temperature training method, in which the patient is trained to increase the temperature in his hands, while Lutker[7] conditioned relaxation in a young student to the feelings of tension occurring prior to a migraine attack. Other work has been reported by Mitchell and Mitchell[9] and by Dengrove.[3] Mitchell and Mitchell tested the efficacy of several behavioral techniques in various combinations and found combined desensitization and asser-

From *Journal of Nervous and Mental Disease*, 163:61-64, 1976, The Williams & Wilkins Co. Reproduced by permission.

tive training to have the best effects (see also [12]). Dengrove, a bioenergetic practitioner, attempted to broaden his patients' perception and experiences of underlying feelings of anger by getting them to express their feelings directly. This set of techniques has been of use in aborting migraine attacks.[10]

There has been a tendency, however, in the literature for advocates of each school to argue that only their approach offers the best remedy, and this may well have had a lot to do with the fact that not enough patients are helped sufficiently despite the claims of effectiveness made by the proponents of each orientation. This theoretical reductionism to aspects of psychological, neurological, or behavioral functioning does not allow for the mutual interaction that occurs between these multiple aspects of organism functioning to be accounted for.[2,5]

Migraine is essentially a psychosomatic condition, and as such, it involves functioning of somatic and psychological systems in close integration. Treatment methods that use only aspects of this integrated whole may not succeed as well as those that treat multidimensional functioning. From this point of view, it would appear necessary for the methods derived from several viewpoints to be integrated into a workable treatment program in order that a full recovery be permitted. A nonreductionistic systems approach is described by Von Bertalanffy,[15] and its applications in psychiatry are reviewed by Meir.[8] In this epistemology, the focus of study is the *structure* of behavior, the code that operates behind the observed raw data of functioning.[11,14]

The ability of the clinician to uncover the form of this structure and then alter it therapeutically depends to a large extent on the nature of the data available through his interaction with the patient. Considerations of the relevant dimensions of patient functioning and inferring the necessary isomorphic structure of the interrelationships between the available data facilitate a more comprehensive approach to an integral somatopsychic therapeutic operation.

In this paper, the value of such an approach is demonstrated in a patient who suffered from several migraine attacks over a long period of time. Both behavioral and psychodynamic data were of use in the full treatment of the patient's condition; either applied alone achieved only partial success. The treatment program was carried out along single case experimental lines as described by Barlow and Hersen[1] using an A/B/BC design.*

---

*In this design, base rates are first taken (phase A), treatment method 1 is applied, and the effect on base rates noted (phase B); then treatment method 2 is applied alongside method 1 (phase BC). This allows a comparison to be made between the effects of each method. Theoretically the procedure should then be reversed, but ethically this is not always possible.

Case Study

The patient, a 38-year-old married woman, suffered from incapacitating migraine attacks from the age of 16. Medication had been of some use in the early phases of the disorder, but in the years prior to her seeking treatment, had lessened in impact. Her marriage was fairly stable and secure with no overt psychopathology evident. She had no severe medical problems and was a highly intelligent and well-read individual. Case history data revealed several areas of possible psychodynamic conflict with specific people such as her mother and her husband. Behavioral analysis indicated that she was unable to cope with day-to-day altercations with shopkeepers, policemen, doctors, etc., in that she was not able to assert herself in an argument or debate. She also tended to avoid possible points of friction with people in general, preferring to put on a good face rather than risk confrontation. Intense anxiety was experienced in each such situation.

Etiologically, it appeared that her mother had enforced a high achievement-oriented cultural milieu at home, with the emphasis on the appearance and maintenance of prestige; extreme forms of emotional expression whether negative or positive were not tolerated. She married into a family that maintained a similar tradition, and although she considered her life to be happy, this happiness was marred by frequent migraine attacks that interfered with family arrangements.

Treatment and Results

Base rate measures were taken during a 1-month waiting period prior to the commencement of treatment (phase A). The patient was asked to grade the severity of her migraine attacks on a 5-point scale; she was also asked to record every attack. After these rates were taken, she was questioned about any possible relationship between the occurrence of a migraine attack and her experience of anxiety whether situationally or cognitively induced. There appeared to be no clear-cut correlation but any such relationship may have been obscured by the fact that she had an average of three attacks a week and experienced some anxiety every day.

It was hypothesized that the patient had avoided experiencing anxiety in situations despite the fact that she was often angered by these situations, simply because she had never been taught to express herself assertively and because of the negative reinforcement afforded such expression.

Treatment of choice then for this case was assertive training and behavior rehearsal to enable her anger and related feelings to be expressed in appropriate contexts. Each conflict area was delineated and assertive behaviors planned; her husband agreed to cooperate in this phase, and the patient thus received reinforcement and encouragement for the expression of affect in such situations (phase B).

The patient continued to record intensity and frequency of her migraine attacks and the effects of assertive training can be seen clearly in Figure 1. The frequency of attacks dropped considerably but intensity only slightly.

It was felt that treatment up to that stage had only been partially successful and that further intervention was necessary. The woman had been taught what to do when confronted with conflict but not how to ensure that the conflict did not occur in the first place. It was decided in this final stage to develop her insights into the reasons for the conflict and thus enable her to develop full self-control of her migraine attacks (phase BC).

The patient, as is normal in psychosomatic conditions, was very slow to develop workable insights, primarily because she had never been allowed to develop a mode of thinking that focused on these inner conflicts. Cognition and attention span had previously been focused on a narrow range of socially relevant stimuli and public interaction from an early age. The development of a new pattern required that her conversations and interactions with significant persons in her environment change accordingly in order that external referents be paired with her new insights, and it was in this area that problems occurred. Her husband proved unwilling to cooperate here since he considered public debate about inner conflict unseemly, and this led to the patient experiencing considerable resentment toward him, for both his present attitude and his past behavior. She was able to understand the relationship between this resentment and her migraine, and when confronted with this, her husband was able to cooperate more appropriately.

Following this, she was able to elaborate further on this insight and began to develop an integration between her cognitive and behavioral processes that was able to prevent her migraine attacks. As Figure 2 shows, there was a decrease in intensity of attacks in the first 4 weeks and, thereafter, a gradual decrease in frequency and intensity over the next 3 months.

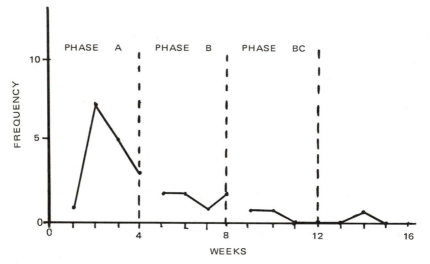

FIGURE 1. Average weekly frequency of migraine attacks.

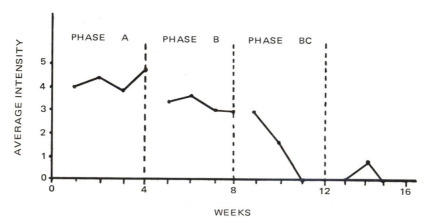

FIGURE 2. Average weekly intensity of migraine attacks.

At 9-month follow-up after treatment had discontinued, the patient had been completely free of severe attacks for 5 months and reported an occasional migraine-type headache of low intensity that disappeared overnight. She was still experiencing conflict with the development of more adaptable behavior and insight, but appeared to be sufficiently motivated to persist with her attempts. She also reported that her relationship with her husband was more disturbed than previously, which upset her, but she felt that this was preferable to her migraine attacks.

CONCLUSION

The structure of the problem appeared to be concentrated around the experiencing of sustained physiological arousal without the patient being able to express it. Over time, this anger-arousal reaction had become linked to anxiety about the consequences of its expression, and a physiological reaction to this conflict developed with important, secondary, psychosocial gains (incapacitation, medical attention, withdrawal from both conflict and stimulus situation). Treatment succeeded because the manifestations of this structure were modified in an integrated manner so that the effects gained at one level (assertive training) could be built upon and supported by modifications made at a related level (psychosocial insight).

If one postulates that the migraine-supporting system within a patient comprises somatic, behavioral, and psychological interacting subsystems, then the structure of the disorder is in itself none of these subsystems alone, but the interrelational code embedded in these subsystems. Accordingly, after examination of system functioning, the most appropriate subsystem is selected for working with first. In the case described above, this was a behavioral subsystem; in other cases, drug treatment or psychotherapeutic interventions of differing natures may well be appropriate. Once an inroad is made into modifying this subsystem, the effects of the changes in this subsystem have to be integrated with the developments in other areas.

It was clear in the case presented here that assertive training had the physiological effect of providing a pain-inhibiting anger-arousal outlet that allowed some relief to be obtained from pain, but that this effect, to achieve its fullest efficacy, had to be integrated with the patient's higher order cognitive functioning for the development of psychodynamic insight.

REFERENCES

1. Barlow, D. H., and Hersen, M. Single-case experimental designs. *Arch. Gen. Psychiatry*, 29: 319-325, 1973.
2. Bellak, L., and Berneman, M. A. A systematic view of depression. *Am. J. Psychother.*, 25: 385-393, 1971.

3. Dengrov, E. Behavior therapy of headache. *Am. Soc. Psychosom. Med. Dent.*, *15:* 41-48, 1968.

4. Freedman, A. P. Headache. In Freedman, A. M., and Kaplan, H. I., Eds. *Comprehensive Textbook of Psychiatry,* pp. 1110-1113. Williams & Wilkins, Baltimore, 1967.

5. Lachenmeyer, C. W. The reduction of psychology to physiology: A new interpretation. *J. Gen. Psychol.*, *86:* 39-53, 1972.

6. Lippman, C. W. Recurrent dreams in migraine: An aid to diagnosis. *J. Nerv. Ment. Dis.*, *120:* 273-276, 1954.

7. Lutker, E. R. Treatment of migraine headache by conditioned relaxation: A case study. *Behav. Ther.*, *2:* 592-593, 1971.

8. Meir, A. Z. General systems theory. *Arch. Gen. Psychiatry*, *2:* 302-310, 1969.

9. Mitchell, K. R., and Mitchell, D. M. Migraine: An exploratory treatment application of programmed behavior therapy techniques. *J. Psychosom. Res.*, *15:* 139-154, 1971.

10. Palmer, R. D. Desensitization of the fear of expressing one's own inhibited aggression. In Rubin, R., Fensterheim, M., Henderson, J. D., and Ullman, L. P., Eds. *Advances in Behavior Therapy*, pp. 241-253. Academic Press, New York, 1973.

11. Pribram, K. H. *On Neurological Knowing* (Mimeograph). Stanford University, Stanford, 1968.

12. Price, K. P. The application of behavior therapy to the treatment of psychosomatic disorders: Retrospect and prospect. *Psychotherapy*, *11:* 138-155, 1974.

13. Sargant, J. D., Green, E. E., and Walters, E. D. Preliminary report on the use of autogenic feedback training in the treatment of migraine and tension headaches. *Psychosom. Med.*, *35:* 129-135, 1973.

14. Sperry, R. W. Mind, brain, humans and values. In Alema, G., Bollea, G., Floris, V., *et al. Brain and Mind Problems*, pp. 286-298. Il Peniero Scientifico, Rome, 1968.

15. Von Bertalanffy, L. The mind-body problem: A new view. *Psychosom. Med.*, *26:* 29-45, 1964.

16. Wickramaskera, I. E. Temperature feedback for the control of migraine. *J. Behav. Ther. Exp. Psychiatry*, *4:* 343-345, 1973.

Intensive Group Therapy

23

An Effective Behavioral-Psychoanalytic Method

LEE BIRK, M.D.

There is a wealth of literature reporting on the clinical usefulness of psychodynamic group psychotherapy, particularly with patients for whom social interaction represents either an important problem area or an effective vehicle for the exploration of significant psychodynamic conflicts.

This paper reports on an experience with intensive group psychotherapy designed to test the hypothesis that a synergistic effect would result from combining a psychoanalytic and a behavioral format. Patients were selected whose previous treatment had been largely ineffective, and they showed remarkable gains over an 18-month period. Careful attention to behavioral diagnosis allowed the therapist to select several target behaviors which were central to each patient's maladaptive patterns. These behaviors were systematically identified, interrupted, and subjected to the punishment/reinforcement techniques of behavior therapy. At the same time the associative group process was used to uncover the historic and dynamic meanings of these behaviors. In this fashion, insight and group processes were added to the therapeutic forces leading toward change.

This paper is valuable at three levels. First, it is an important addition to the technical literature on group psychotherapy. Second, it is a demonstration that the dynamically sophisticated behaviorist, or the behaviorally sophisticated analytic therapist, will possess a flexibility which allows the format of treatment to be adapted to patient needs in an effective fashion. Third, it shows that a synergistic effect can result when two seemingly antithetical techniques are used simultaneously in a well-thought-out plan of group intervention. This is consistent with the experiences reported for individual psychotherapy.

Intensive Group Therapy

An Effective
Behavioral-Psychoanalytic Method

LEE BIRK, M.D.

Group therapy is valued by psychoanalytically oriented therapists for many well-recognized reasons.[1] Among these is the fact that the variety of group members effects a multiplicity of transferences—rich, vivid, and easily interpretable—rather than a single mixed transference experience focused solely on the person of the therapist. Also, material introduced by one member may both reflect a core conflict for him and simultaneously elicit examination of parallel, although often more subtle, conflicts in other members, with the result that the resonant response to shared experience often takes the form of therapeutic cognitive comparisons. A third reason is that a cohesive group creates a naturally empathetic atmosphere, supportive of painful affects and the emergence of dreaded personal secrets that, against the backdrop of a group of listeners who are nonprofessional yet for the most part nonjudgmental, can be faced squarely, with less avoidance and more therapeutic benefit than in individual therapy. Finally, peer interpretation, especially when aspects of the conflict are ego-syntonic, provides essential and powerful leverage in many otherwise unmotivating clinical settings.

Psychoanalysts have long recognized the clinical value of an intensive therapeutic effort carried on five days a week over many months. The incorporation of the analytic hour into the patient's daily life supplies an impetus to thorough and subtle examination of the key issues and conflicts within his life context; it also fosters a valuable sense of mission and immersion in the task of insight-based change.

It was my belief that a five-day-a-week format for group therapy would combine the intense-focusing advantages of psychoanalysis with those accruing from the multiphasic reality testing apposite to the group

From *American Journal of Psychiatry*, 131:11-16, January 1974. Copyright 1974 by the American Psychiatric Association. Reprinted by permission. The author wishes to thank Dr. Ann Brinkley for her assistance in designing the patient evaluation scale and in writing the theoretical parts of the paper.

experience. For a group to meet five times a week substantially reduces the crisis or severity criterion by which therapy group members tend to judge their own and others' use of group time. On a once-a-week basis, groups tend to adopt a crisis-first scheme for allotting time to themes under discussion with the conspicuous result that other issues—mere feelings, for example—may assume an exaggerated, artificial intensity in order to justify their presentation to the group. Or they may be suppressed altogether under the mistaken but pressing assumption that regardless of their felt personal urgency, some problems—again, feelings are the best example—would fail to measure up to the group's threshold value with respect to seriousness or general interest. For example, a typical remark in groups meeting less frequently is the excuse: "Well, I just thought that would be too boring to waste everyone's time on."

This paper reports on the first 18 months of experience with an intensive five-day-a-week group formed expressly to test what was predicted to be the synergistic effects of combining these previously separate formats. It was also my explicit purpose to combine the historically uncombined tools of psychoanalysis and behavior therapy; these have, by conscious design, become the mainstays of my approach to group leadership.

Group therapy, unlike individual therapy, shifts its emphasis from an almost exclusive focus on retrospective narration to a concentration on, and examination of, observable social interaction.[2] The feelings engendered by the social interactional situations within the group do, of course, lead associatively to welcome and useful material, both from the recent past (similar feelings and situations in the patient's current life outside the group) and from the remote past. Both kinds of relevant associations are reinforced and encouraged—those from the remote past especially so, since this often leads to useful cognitive insights about how and why and from whom a particular behavior was learned developmentally.

As is well known by behavior therapists, the most effective and efficient method for eliminating maladaptive behavior is to isolate it *in vivo*: to point it out, label it, and punish it while at the same time systematically reinforcing alternative, increasingly adaptive modes of behavior.[3] Within a group setting maladaptive social behaviors easily become conspicuous target symptoms. As the other group members begin to understand and imitate the therapist's actions, these target behaviors become especially responsive to group interactional pressures. (Previously these target behaviors served exclusively as defenses, maintained by negative reinforcement—that is, by the contingent avoidance or reduction of painful feelings.) Interrupting these behavioral patterns by punishment (mere exposure or negative comment) and focusing on them elicits a feeling linked to the behavior and leads to group examination of the analytic origins of the particular feeling-behavior liaison—an insight in the psychoanalytic sense that serves to potentiate behavioral change. It is not uncommon for the therapist to use analytically oriented questions to help interrupt a target response. For example, "There you go again, slapping hell out of your leg! That must really hurt! Why do you always do that?"

One of the key elements in my approach to intensive group therapy is individualized behavioral diagnosis. For each patient in the group the therapist arrives at a precise, fine-grained description of one or two pivotal maladaptive behaviors actually operative and observable within the group. When these target behaviors are interrupted and thus exposed, the associative group process works to uncover the meaning underlying them—that is, the basic, faulty world-view/feeling-disorder in the context of which the behaviors appear to make sense. If the choice of key target maladaptive behaviors is a correct one (correct behavioral diagnosis), if the punishment is sufficient to interrupt and suppress the habitual maladaptive pattern, and if the chosen alternative reinforced behavior is truly more adaptive in the real world outside the group, the new behavior will permanently replace the old. In behavioral terms, this happens because the new behavior successfully competes with the old behavior inasmuch as it "works better" and brings more reinforcement.

The Patients

For the charter members of this intensive group,* the author chose eight people who might be called analytic failures: they had been exposed to psychoanalytic and psychotherapeutic procedures over a long period of time without either subjectively satisfying results or appreciable, objectively manifest behavioral change. These patients—all of them analytically sophisticated individuals—are described in terms of the particular maladaptive social behavior of each. At the outset, all were guarded about what more they might expect to gain from still further therapy; six of the eight were particularly skeptical about the idea of a group format.

Table 1 gives the patients' age, sex, and type and duration of previous therapy. Further details concerning the patients follow herewith:

Patient 1 was a 56-year-old unmarried Ph.D. scientist, a hearty and deeply likable man. When the group began, however, he was very isolated from people, unable to experience real closeness and warmth, extremely inhibited sexually, and beset by deep feelings of masculine inferiority. He did credit his previous therapy with enabling him to finish the work for his Ph.D., but he remained very troubled, especially in terms of his

*Identifying clues have been minimized and actual names changed in order to protect each patient's anonymity. The group began with three members and gradually expanded to eight.

TABLE 1. Patients' Age, Sex, and History of Previous Therapy

			Number of previous therapists	Maximum continuity with one therapist (years)	Previous therapy		
Patient	Age	Sex			Type	Years	Total hours
1*	56	M	1	7	Individual	7	300
2†	46	M	3	7	Psychoanalysis	15	3,500
3	26	M	2	2	Psychoanalysis	2	300
					Individual	1	
4	27	F	4	1.5	Individual	3	250
5†	28	F	4	7	Individual	7	550
					Synanon	1.5	
6	40	M	7	7	Individual	15.5	2,100
					Group	4	
7	48	F	5	8	Individual	12	550
8	20	M	5	5	Individual	7.5	750
Mean			4	5.6		9.3	1,038

*One hospitalization.
†Three hospitalizations.

relationships with women. He had had a complicated relationship with a woman lasting several years that very briefly (for a period of about two months) had involved intercourse, but this was undertaken with such great feelings of tension and strain that no ejaculation and very little real pleasure resulted. Although the relationship dragged on and on, with periodic, emotionally painful contacts, the patient had not actually had intercourse with this woman or any other woman for more than five years prior to the beginning of the group. He reported having to use beating fantasies to produce enough sexual excitation to make masturbation or intercourse possible. On those rare occasions when he had had intercourse, it was made possible only by his imagining a young woman being beaten by a man. In these fantasies, the patient identified with the helpless woman being beaten.

For this man, there were two target behavioral symptoms: the first was his striking use of self-ridicule. For example, he would painfully slap his leg or call himself "little Joey" instead of expressing the feelings of inferiority, sadness, futility, and nihilism that evidently troubled him. The second was his habit of offering suggestions or opinions in a self-defeating, calculatedly dissonant and alienated way, which had the effect of further alienating him from other group members.

The treatment of these behaviors followed a typical course: After the behavioral diagnosis was made, in which self-ridicule, for example, was established as a target behavior, the first step was to begin punishing target responses by interpreting each abruptly, thus actually interrupting the full response. By consistently blocking his stereotyped acting-out behavior in this way, his underlying feelings of inferiority and nihilism were eventually revealed and directly expressed. As the patient began to express his feelings directly, the therapist reinforced each appropriate

expression by means of sympathetically put questions, positive comments, and interpretations. The therapist's interventions thus served
the dual function of reinforcing the patient's expressing these feelings
directly and of helping him analyze them. In this way he was able to
learn how and to what extent his self-concept had been falsely and ad-
versely affected by his early developmental learning experiences. This
patient, like a good analysand, inevitably began to make use of this con-
tingency-potentiated cognitive learning. He would catch himself responding to situations with a particular feeling-state—inferiority in this
case—and would successfully interrupt this root feeling response by imposing an alternative response, reminding himself of the false origins of
the feeling. As one would predict, the other group members, following
the therapist's example and their own perceptions, began to use the
same punishment-reinforcement contingencies and to make effective interpretations of their own.

Patient 2 was a 46-year-old university professor in one of the social sciences. He suffered from severe recurring depressions—three of them requiring hospital admission—apparently in spite of his being a veteran of three analyses lasting a total of 15 years. He had
written half a dozen successful books and was generally very well regarded in his field.
During his first analysis this patient had worked out his inhibitions about sexual intercourse and had had a series of affairs prior to entering the group. He was unable, however,
to make a lasting commitment to a woman or to overcome his chronic and periodically very
severe depression.

For him the target maladaptive behavior was his socially detached
concentration on depressed feelings "inside" in the service of excluding
people (versus sharing with people).

Patient 3 was a 26-year-old professional man. In his analysis he had grappled unsuccessfully with a profound fear of women. Although during his earlier treatment he had
been able to have intercourse on several occasions, he had been unable to resolve his
obsessional concerns about whether, when, and how to hold hands with or put his arm
around the women he (with much dread) forced himself to date.

The target maladaptive behavior for him was his habit of suppres-
sing feelings of resentment over not being treated fairly (of being ignored, of being cheated, of not being given enough), to the point where
these finally erupted as strong anger, after which he would be overcome
with guilt and would criticize himself harshly both for his outburst and
for his inability to be more generous.

Patient 4 was a 27-year-old artist/roving graduate student who was severely depressed
and suicidally preoccupied at the time she joined the group. When she began she complained, "Somehow I don't feel real; I feel like a nonperson. . . ."

The target behavior for her was her persistent use of tears and confusion to avoid expressing anger and to ward off appropriate feedback
and criticism from others.

Patient 5 was a 28-year-old woman—a highly intelligent but unstable and irresponsible college graduate with a master's degree in counseling. She had been addicted to heroin and had spent seven years in individual psychotherapy plus a year and a half in Synanon. She spoke positively about her previous therapy as "the only thing that kept me alive," but when she entered the group she was nonetheless seriously depressed and self-destructive; she talked actively of killing herself "unless things get better." She was not then addicted to heroin but was shooting it several times a week.

For her the target behavior was her use of angry, provoking behaviors and/or seductiveness to avoid discussion of real conflicts and feelings.

Patient 6 was a 40-year-old physicist whose presenting problems were social isolation, an extreme lack of self-confidence, sexual and social immaturity, and inability to urinate except at home and in a few other "safe" places. Prior to his entering the group his therapy had been largely unsuccessful.

The target maladaptive behaviors for him were the habitual meekness and delicacy in his expressive style, and his passivity, manifested particularly by his hesitancy about bringing up his own pressing concerns and a low initiative in thinking about his own concerns in an action-oriented way.

Patient 7 was a 48-year-old executive secretary, unhappily divorced, perpetually discontent and angry. She was also in individual therapy with another therapist at the time she joined the group and she continued her work with him while in the group.

The target behaviors for her were dropping her voice to inaudibility near the end of sentences and at moments of maximal feeling (apparently in order to perpetuate the parentally derived feeling of never being understood) and using questions of fact, or interposing theoretical, structural, or administrative issues, to reduce the full emotional impact of sensing other people's feelings.

Patient 8 was a 20-year-old, bright graduate student, the son of two professional parents and the veteran of seven and one-half years of signally unsuccessful therapy. During his college career he had made several suicidal gestures (by cutting his arms with a razor blade and by ingesting drugs). His overwhelmingly intense anger convinced several psychiatrists who saw him in consultation that he had in fact become a genuine suicidal/homicidal risk. He complained with vitriolic bitterness both of his "complete lack of success with women" and of his mother's hatred for him. He claimed that his mother in a fit of temper had attempted to kill him when he was a child.

The target maladaptive behaviors for him were talking so softly as to be inaudible, especially when angry, and expressing his concerns in stark, exaggerated black-and-white terms in the service of demonstrating "my situation is impossible and people are impossible."

RESULTS AFTER 18 MONTHS OF INTENSIVE GROUP THERAPY

Table 2, which deals with Patient 5, illustrates the general rating scale I designed to measure subjective and behavioral change—change that is not limited to the narrowly defined target maladaptive behaviors.

Table 3 shows the amount of change in the behavioral target symptom(s) for each patient, and also the total amount of change (total points improvement) in the 20 items of the general change ratings. The ratings of change in behavioral target symptoms represent the mean of nine separate evaluations—one by the therapist and one by each of the eight patients in the group, including a self-evaluation by each patient. The general change ratings represent the mean of the patient's self-rating and the therapist's rating. Seven of the eight patients experienced a significant positive change in their life situations.

At the end of the 18-month period Patient 1, the scientist with the beating fantasies who had not slept with a woman for five years, was sleeping with a woman whom he hoped to marry. His relationship with her was a tender and loving one and the previous beating fantasies were no longer a part of his sexual life. In a group meeting Patient 2 said about him: "When Joe came into this group I didn't like him at all; he was so tight and rigid I just couldn't stand him. Now he says things like 'I deserved it!' and 'fuck' and I really am fond of him; I respect him and deeply like him."

Patient 2, the depressed professor, was no longer depressed. Moreover, he was living with a woman whom he hoped to marry. Patient 3 had said to him: "In my mind you have completely dumped this behavior, absolutely and completely—it's incredible!" About himself, this patient said: "Those [depressed] feelings have the quality of having happened in a previous life!"

Patient 3, the young professional who was afraid of women, was living with a woman. He said about himself—and he rated himself lower than any of the other eight of us rated him in terms of change—

> I do agree that in many areas of my life I am much less sensitive to this issue than I used to be. I'm much less easily hurt and I'm much less easily infuriated. I have a lot more understanding of how I do react. This business with the birthday cake*—I knew how I would have reacted two years ago, and I knew I wasn't *feeling* the same way as I would have. I feel that what has changed in me is that I used to feel that I had just nothing and it really hurt me that someone else would get something and I wouldn't, but I don't *feel* that I have nothing any more; I mean, I feel that I have a lot, and it doesn't really hurt me that much when someone else gets something. I was happy to celebrate happy birthday with Sidney.

*Patient 2 (Sidney) and Patient 3 (Dick) happened to have the same birthday. Patient 4, not knowing this, brought a birthday cake to the group but the cake said only "Happy Birthday Sidney." The group duly celebrated with Sidney and it was only at the end of the hour that someone revealed it was also Dick's birthday.

TABLE 2. Ratings for Patient 5 on General Rating Scale*

| | | Ratings after 1.2 years in group | | |
| | Before-group | | | |
Item	self-rating	Self	Present therapist	Previous therapist
Depression	1	4	3.5	3
Suicidal feeling	1	4	5.5	3
Guilt	1	4.5	3	3.5
Anxiety	1	4	3	3
Anger	1	4	4	5
Self-defeating behavior	1	3	4.5	4
Self-destructive behavior	1	5.5	3	4
Drug dependency	1	5.5	4.5	–
Assertiveness (anger)	4.5	4.5	4	5.5
Assertiveness (warmth)	2	5	5	–
Fun	3	5	5	5
Friends	4	5	4	5
Enjoyment of work	4	4	4.5	4.5
Relations with men	4	4	4	4
Relations with women	5	5	4	5.5
Sexual pleasure	3.5	4	4	6
Quality of heterosexual attachment	1	3	2	3
General effectiveness	2	4	4	4
Self-esteem	2	3	4	3
Self-realization	2	3	3	3
Total	45	84†		

*Scale: 1 = extremely severe: 6 = no problem at all.
†Total change in self-rating was 39; taking intensity-frequency data into account, the total change was 44.

TABLE 3. Change in Target Behaviors and General Ratings

Patient	Years of previous therapy	Years of intensive group	Change in target symptom(s)*	Change in general rating scale
1	7	1.6	5.0	41
			4.8	
2	15	1.6	5.3	62
3	3	1.4	4.6	47
4	3	1.3	5.2	52
5	7	1.2	5.3	44
6	19.5	1.3	2.7	5
			3.1	
7	12	0.8	4.8	−5
			3.5	
8	7.5	0.6	4.0	25
			3.5	
Mean	9.3	1.2	4.3	34

*Based on the mean of nine ratings; maximum change = 6.0.

Patient 4, the confused roving graduate student who felt "like a nonperson" was no longer chronically depressed or suicidally preoccupied. She reported that she did feel like a person, but a person in the middle of therapy, with some remaining serious conflicts to work out. For the past nine months she had been working as a high school teacher and was considering a career as a psychotherapist.

Patient 5, the heroin-shooting, suicidally depressed, irresponsible young woman, had not taken heroin at all for more than a year and, by specific invitation, was applying for a job as a college mental health service psychotherapist. She said about herself: "I feel I have changed enormously. . . ." Patient 2 said about her: "I think Rachel has changed more than any other member of the group. . . ."

Patient 6, the meek physicist, had to be considered a treatment failure at the 18-month follow-up. Part of the reason was believed to lie in the technical difficulties and psychodynamic problems involved in punishing and interrupting this patient's passivity. His passivity was not a sharply defined, discrete response occurring at a clearly delineated time; rather, it amounted to an absence of appropriate initiating responses over a considerable period. Moreover, there was an additional psychodynamic problem: remarks by the therapist and others that one might expect to be punishing were in fact demonstrated to be empirically reinforcing because of the passive-aggressive anger underlying his passivity.

In view of these factors the revised treatment plan depended primarily on *ignoring* (extinguishing) this patient's passivity, while reinforcing all active departures from it. Also, it was forcefully pointed out to him that on his current passive curve he would be in his late 90s before he finished his treatment! On the hopeful side it should be said, however, that this patient's bottom-of-the-class standing in the group (made more obvious by the data collection for this paper) was a cognition that was profoundly and atypically disturbing to him.

Patient 7, the angry executive secretary, was considered a treatment success and likely to be an even greater treatment success in spite of her low general change scores since these reflected an immediate postcrisis situation. She in fact changed very considerably, especially in terms of how she presented herself to other people. Also, she succeeded in cutting herself off from a very destructive and chronic affair. She was working toward a career involving more responsibility and independence, perhaps in the field of hospital management.

Patient 8, the bright but deeply bitter student who at the outset of treatment was unwilling to believe he could expect anything of importance from therapy and who said that going to graduate school and becoming a professional was the only thing worth living for, has recently decided to delay his entrance to graduate school. Going to graduate school would necessarily involve his going to another city; he decided to postpone this for one year in order to finish his therapy in the group. He now has a girl friend with whom he is having sexual relations, and he has changed quite considerably, even though he has been in the group for only about seven months.

Conclusions

The facts presented in this paper—that is, the patient evaluations of subjective feeling changes or their behavioral manifestations in real-life settings—strongly support the efficacy of intensive group therapy conducted on the basis of behavioral and psychoanalytic principles. The changes in the behavioral styles and lives of difficult patients were evidently related to the positive effects of this combination of formats and conceptual-methodological frameworks.

In lieu of more formal concluding remarks, it is more in keeping with the informal, often provocative, spirit engendered by the group experience to close with the words of one of the group's initially most skeptical members:

> When I was in analysis with Dr. X. for seven years—he's a very, very rigid Freudian—five minutes would go by and I would say nothing and he would say nothing, and then I would talk and he would go "Hmmm." Not all the time—frequently he would talk at length and I would talk. . . . He was a very, very aloof figure for me. I was afraid of him. Everything was extremely formal. His office was extremely formal . . . and [pause] I didn't feel warm toward him, and I didn't feel he felt warm toward me.
>
> Now in this group I genuinely feel caring about each one of you, and I feel that you feel caring about me. Now what this does for me is that it enormously increases my *trust*. I trust you all. . . . I don't believe any one of you would screw me, or intentionally give me bad advice . . . or try to hurt me in any way. I mean, I believe all of you care about me and would try to help me if you could.
>
> That's the first thing.
>
> The second thing is, you do get many points of view.
>
> The third thing is, I learn a lot from watching [what others in the group say] because so much of it strikes me as absurd and unrealistic and not in line with reality. I learn from the problems of other people, and the discussion of these problems. . . .
>
> I just feel that Dr. Birk is with *us*, whereas Dr. X., in a very fancy Freudian way, was with theory.

Two of this patient's three former analysts were also people whom he did trust. In different ways both of these two helped him: the first analyst helped him overcome his sexual inhibitions, and the third helped him pull out of a serious and severe depressive spiral that began and was getting worse during his treatment with his second analyst. The reason the quotation is cited is to point out that the group atmosphere, even with all its explicit emphasis on target behaviors, punishment, and reinforcement, was one this patient singled out as promoting special and deep trust.

These may not be hard data, but they are nevertheless relevant to the prognosis for the effectiveness of intensive group therapy.

References

1. Guttmacher J, Birk L: Group therapy: what specific therapeutic advantages? *Compr Psychiatry* 12:546-556, 1971
2. Shapiro D, Birk L: Group therapy in experimental perspective. *Int J Group Psychother* 17:211-224, 1967
3. Birk L, Stolz S, Brady JP, et al: *Behavior Therapy in Psychiatry*, Task Force Report no 5. Washington, DC, American Psychiatric Association, 1973

24

A Study of Treatment Needs Following Sex Therapy

ALEXANDER N. LEVAY, M.D.,
AND ARLENE KAGLE, PH.D.

The initial reports of sex therapy, utilizing a Masters and Johnson approach, tended to be somewhat overly optimistic. Subsequent experience has indicated that while the therapy is very effective with a majority of patients suffering from sexual dysfunction, there is nevertheless a significant group who either fail to resolve their difficulties or do so only to find their symptoms ultimately returning.

Levay and Kagle studied a group of such patients and found that half could profit from a second brief trial of sex therapy, while the other half required the addition of long-term psychotherapy in order to resolve or alleviate severe underlying intrapsychic and interpersonal conflicts or marital discord. Their experience suggests that psychoanalytically oriented individual and conjoint therapy can make a significant contribution to the resolution of problems which fail to respond, or only partially respond, to a trial of sex therapy.

A Study of Treatment Needs Following Sex Therapy

24

ALEXANDER N. LEVAY, M.D.
AND ARLENE KAGLE, PH.D.

Since the publication of *Human Sexual Inadequacy*[1] the Masters and Johnson method of rapid treatment of sexual disorders has become widely practiced and acclaimed. Several modifications of the basic technique have been introduced, notably Schumacher's variation of the duration and intensity of treatment (personal communication from S. Schumacher) and Kaplan's departure from dual therapy teams to single therapists.[2] Follow-up studies of these therapies so far have indicated that short-term treatment is highly efficacious and efficient and that gains made are essentially maintained for as long as five years.[1,2] Although published studies indicate that approximately 80% of all patients experienced symptom reversal and that few of these relapse, our experience suggests a more cautious judgment and calls for a more complex and comprehensive assessment of treatment results. In particular there is a need for detailed study of long-term symptom reversal and improvement.

This paper will attempt to evaluate the effectiveness of treatment by describing and analyzing the results of the treatment of 19 of 45 couples who were originally seen for classical two-week Masters and Johnson therapy[1] and returned on their own initiative for additional treatment with one of us (A.N.L.) because their sexual adjustment had deteriorated or failed to progress. The first phase of treatment was conducted by a dual sex cotherapy team of psychiatrists who had received formal training in sex therapy at the Reproductive Biology Research Foundation in St. Louis. The second phase of treatment consisted of individual or conjoint therapy or both as indicated by the needs of the couple and was conducted by A.N.L. alone or by referral.

From *American Journal of Psychiatry*, 134:970-973, 1977. Copyright 1977 by the American Psychiatric Association. Reprinted by permission. The authors wish to thank Virginia Lozzi, M.D., associate in clinical psychiatry, Columbia University College of Physicians and Surgeons, cotherapist for all 45 cases described in this paper.

Method

Phase 1

Between June 1971 and June 1973, 45 couples referred by themselves or their physicians/therapists for sex therapy were seen for 2 weeks in Masters and Johnson intensive sex therapy. Criteria for acceptance into treatment included (1) presence of a sexual dysfunction, (2) willingness to work out the problem as a couple, (3) motivation to work out the problem for one's own sexual functioning and pleasure, (4) the absence of prohibitive psychopathology and/or intramarital conflict, and (5) the absence of overwhelming reality or organic factors. All patients were private patients, mostly of upper-middle-class background, and ranged in age from 19 to 69 years. Presenting problems included all the categories of sexual dysfunction reported by Masters and Johnson in a comparable distribution. After the 2-week treatment period couples were seen for follow-up at least twice, at 2 weeks and 2 months. In addition they were asked to return for a 1-year follow-up. Only 4 couples did so; 3 are among the 19 reported here.

Of the original 45 couples, 10 cases were judged to be unimproved or deteriorated. In all the remaining 35 cases there was some degree of improvement or complete symptom reversal after the 2-week treatment period. Others in the field have reported similar results.[1,2]

Phase 2

After the termination of the original 2-week treatment period, 19 of the 35 improved couples (54%) returned of their own volition for further therapy with A.N.L. These couples left short-term treatment at all stages of improvement. In all cases the couples described a deterioration of sexual functioning or a failure to progress in the period following treatment as their reasons for seeking additional help.

During this second phase of treatment couples divided into one of two distinct treatment groups. Eight couples were seen in short-term follow-up treatment, which consisted of additional sex therapy. This first group was characterized by the ability to progress as a couple out of treatment. In each case the deterioration or lack of further progress was accessible to treatment within 10 sessions or less. The other 11 couples failed to respond to a second course of sex therapy and were seen either together or individually for more extensive and traditional psychotherapy. This second group was notable in that in every case there was moderate to severe underlying psychopathology and/or unconscious conflict, which required additional therapy exceeding 50 treatment hours.

Results

Since becoming sexually functional is structured as a step-by-step process in sex therapy, we have chosen to subdivide improvement into five major stages plus a sixth category for individuals who are totally dysfunctional: stage 0, nonfunctional—no sexual desire, arousal, or sensation; stage 1, the identification of pleasurable sexual sensations along with discernible arousal, i.e., erection for the man and lubrication for the woman; stage 2a, the ability to experience sustained arousal and orgasm by self-stimulation; stage 2b, the ability to experience sustained arousal and orgasm by self-stimulation in the presence of one's partner; stage 3, the ability to experience sustained arousal and orgasm by manual or oral stimulation by one's partner; stage 4, the ability to function satisfactorily and experience orgasm in intercourse; stage 5, the ability to integrate stage 4 level of sexual functioning into one's normal life routine on a regular basis.

All 19 couples were evaluated according to these stages at four different points: before treatment, after phase 1 treatment, before phase 2 treatment, and after phase 2 treatment. In terms of sexual functioning the initial level did not prove to be a predictor of long-term treatment outcome, with the possible exception of a tendency for couples consisting of a sexually functional man married to an anorgasmic woman to require long-term additional treatment. There was also a trend which suggested that couples in which both partners could masturbate to orgasm before treatment had a simpler course of therapy. However, these findings may be an artifact of the small sample size.

An analysis of outcome performed after phase 1 and also before phase 2 and the results after phase 2 therapy were also not useful in determining whether a couple would require short- or long-term additional treatment. Thus, it seems clear that it is not possible to depend on the level of sexual functioning alone in developing a treatment plan for couples requesting sex therapy. What is predictive is the degree of psychopathology: moderate to severe underlying conflicts or marital discord were present in all couples who required long-term additional therapy.

Discussion

Experience in the second phase of treatment (and with some 300 couples seen subsequently in modified sex therapy) indicates that for many couples the treatment format has to be individually tailored and integrated with one or more of the psychotherapies in order to bring about lasting results. Although the treatment of choice for some couples is sex therapy alone, others need additional help. Similar conclusions have been reported in the literature, notably by Kaplan and Sager.[2-5]

Reasons for Return

We have subdivided the reasons for return to treatment by these 19 couples into the following categories that we feel are relevant to all couples seeking sex therapy:

1. *Treatment Overload.* Some of the patients who returned had experienced sex therapy as too intensive and overwhelming. Two-week treatment had not allowed for the necessary assimilation and working through of basic concepts and new behaviors. As a result these couples were left with a combination of residual problems and uncertainty about treatment direction and goals that did not allow them to grow on their own or resulted in a relapse. Altering the rate and duration of treatment so that the assignment of tasks was more in harmony with the couple's ability to participate resulted in successful utilization of therapy.

2. *Severity of Symptom(s).* When the presenting sexual dysfunction was severe and of long duration, the course of sex therapy was often, of necessity, extended. Even with a highly motivated and therapeutically adept individual, it is often asking too much to expect that all the developmental steps and assimilative tasks necessary to become fully sexual can be accomplished in a two-week period. Several couples returned for treatment primarily because they needed to have additional treatment time to work through these required stages. Needless to say, the situation is further compounded when both partners suffer from a dysfunction or when a spouse becomes dysfunctional near the end of treatment as a direct consequence of his/her mate's improvement. Given additional time, however, most couples can resolve these unforeseen problems.

3. *Presence of Psychopathology.* Other problems occur if, in addition to the sexual dysfunction, psychopathology is present in one or both spouses. As was seen in the second group of couples who returned, unconscious, unresolved conflicts, various psychiatric syndromes, or emotional immaturity gravely influenced the course of treatment. In cases in which severe pathology is present, albeit latent, the sex therapy can activate conflict, symptom formation, and even full-blown psychotic episodes. Similar experiences have been reported by Kaplan and Kohl[6] and Meyer and associates.[7]

Treatment procedures can be seen as a series of diagnostic tests in which the therapeutic tasks bring out relevant problems with great intensity and clarity. For instance, the need to maintain a parent-child relationship is brought into focus when a couple is asked to interact on a reciprocal basis. Similarly, anxiety reactions have been experienced following a first orgasm by individuals who have clearly exceeded both their superego limitations and ego ideal expectations.

If psychopathology is present in one or both partners, one of three outcomes is possible. For some people the successful completion of a specific sexual task, combined with the powerful emotional backlash reaction that often occurs, somehow serves as a corrective emotional experience and leads to profound insight into the dynamics of the sexual dysfunction. From then on resolution of the unconscious conflict and integration of the newly found sexual gains take place with surprising ease and rapidity. It is important for the therapist not to mistake these dramatic events for an incipient decompensation of the individual or failure of treatment but to support fully and facilitate this process to a successful termination.

Unfortunately this does not occur often. Instead, even without a breakthrough the emotional backlash to the sex therapy is of such magnitude and severity that it requires the temporary or prolonged suspension of this phase of treatment while the intra- or interpsychic problems can be worked out. It helps if during individual or joint treatment the therapist is prepared to reintroduce the spouse and/or the sex therapy as soon as sufficient progress has been made. It is important that neither the patients nor the sex therapist sees this as a failure but, rather, understands that the sex therapy helped focus on problem areas that required work before further sexual progress could be made.

The third possible outcome in cases involving psychopathology is a successful and seemingly uneventful course of sex therapy. This occurs when the dynamic underpinnings of the sexual problem are bypassed without resolution because of the very favorable conditions that sex therapy provides, including therapist support, expected superego relief, and a "honeymoon" atmosphere. All of these provide an ideal setting for a "flight into health" type of symptom reversal. These couples subsequently relapse and require an extensive therapeutic intervention similar to the couples already discussed, but they have the advantage of having already experienced what their sexual lives and marital relationship could be like once they work out their problems.

As we have already pointed out, the effect of such pathology on the course of treatment should not be overlooked or minimized. Although some claims have been made that psychopathology can be successfully bypassed in sex therapy, our experience in long-term follow-up indicates that stable results are only accomplished when and if the relevant intra- or interpsychic problems are resolved or at least reduced. This finding reinforces the importance of competence in diagnosis and broad training in psychotherapy in order to adequately treat sexual dysfunctions.

It is interesting to speculate about the 15 improved couples and the 10 treatment failures who did not return for the 1-year follow-up or additional therapy. Although it is not surprising that the latter group did not reenter a therapy they did not find helpful, we are looking forward to the results of a follow-up study of the entire sample in order to determine their subsequent course of therapy, if any, and their present state of sexual functioning.

Problem Areas

Finally we would like to comment on three factors that have been present alone or in combination in all of the 11 couples who required extensive further therapy. In fact it is useful for treatment purposes to categorize individuals seen for sex therapy not only in terms of presenting sexual diagnosis but also in terms of these factors, since they seem to play a key role in perpetuating sexual dysfunction. We see these as impairments in specific ego functions and have labeled them as problems in the areas of pleasure, intimacy, and cooperation.

Pleasure dysfunctions are primarily associated with an inability or difficulty in identifying, experiencing, and/or enjoying pleasurable sensation, i.e., difficulty in having sex for oneself. Pleasure dysfunctions often respond well to standard sex therapy, at least initially, since the treatment offers techniques for dealing with the lack of attention (low arousal) or overattention (spectatoring) often associated with this condition and also provides superego relief. However, when sexual activity is no longer monitored by the therapists, patients often regress or relapse.

Intimacy dysfunctions are primarily associated with inability or difficulty in experiencing and/or enjoying closeness, binding, and union with another person. Such individuals often find it hard to carry out the prescribed activities of sex therapy that focus on the mutual aspects of sexuality. Here difficulty is associated with having sex with another person. Again short-term treatment provides techniques for dealing with these blocks, but when the couple's intimacy is no longer supported as well as diluted in treatment by the therapists, relapse is likely to follow.

Many variants and varieties of marital discord are subsumed under the label of cooperative dysfunctions. The primary aspect of this factor, however, is an inability to collaborate, act as a team, or agree on common goals, priorities, or values. Although pleasure and intimacy dysfunctions can be unilateral, cooperative disorders almost invariably involve both spouses. Often what underlies this condition is a need by both partners to compete with or deprive each other, usually accompanied by other manifestations of transferential rage and retaliation. Giving to the partner sexually, or in other ways, is experienced as a loss or defeat. This can be described as a difficulty with sex for another person. Consequently, during sex therapy, pleasuring the partner is seen as self-negating, and treatment often becomes stalled when the task involves reciprocity. For these couples conjoint therapy is often essential before any meaningful sex therapy can get under way.

When these dysfunctions are found in combinations, treatment is much more difficult and time-consuming. In our experience, stage 5 sexual functioning is impossible until all these areas of difficulty are worked through to a considerable extent.

CONCLUSIONS

Sex therapy is a powerful, effective, and efficient therapy. However, it is not a panacea. Work with 19 couples who returned for additional treatment following traditional short-term sex therapy served to highlight the types of residual problems that necessitated additional treatment. The presence of the type of psychopathology that blocked progression or maintenance of gains in sex therapy proved to be a differentiating factor between the 8 couples who required only short-term intervention and the 11 couples who required long-term additional therapy.

It is useful for treatment purposes to categorize patients not only in terms of presenting sexual diagnosis but also in terms of the types of psychopathology (of pleasure, intimacy, and cooperation) that interfere with progression in sex therapy. We have found that these dysfunctions need to be worked through if sex therapy is to have lasting effects. When these factors are present in combination or alone, sex therapy is a helpful but insufficient means for successful resolution.

Our experience indicates that sex therapy has to be further modified in order to maximize and stabilize gains for each couple. The treatment format needs to be open-ended; flexible in the rate and sequence of task assignments; and, when indicated, coordinated or integrated with other psychotherapies, principally psychoanalytic psychotherapy and conjoint therapy.

REFERENCES

1. Masters W, Johnson V: *Human Sexual Inadequacy*. Boston, Little, Brown and Co, 1970
2. Kaplan HS: *The New Sex Therapy*. New York, Brunner/Mazel, 1974 [See also Chapter 25, this volume.]
3. Sager CJ: Sexual dysfunctions and marital discord, in *The New Sex Therapy*. Edited by Kaplan HS. New York, Brunner/Mazel, 1974, pp 501-516
4. Sager CJ: The couples model in the treatment of sexual dysfunctions in the single person, in *Sexuality and Psychoanalysis*. Edited by Adelson ET. New York, Brunner/Mazel, 1975, pp 124-142

5. Sager CJ: The role of sex therapy in marital therapy. *Am J Psychiatry* 133:555-558, 1976
6. Kaplan HS, Kohl R: Adverse reactions to the rapid treatment of sexual disorders. *Psychosomatics* 13:185-190, 1972
7. Meyer JK, Schmidt C Jr, Lucas M, et al: Short-term treatment of sexual problems: interim report. *Am J Psychiatry* 132:172-176, 1975

The New Sex Therapy

Basic Principles of Sex Therapy

HELEN SINGER KAPLAN, M.D., PH.D.

The following chapter from Helen Singer Kaplan's superb book, The New Sex Therapy, *illustrates the basic principles which underlie her approach to the treatment of patients with sexual dysfunctions utilizing a method which is both dynamically and behaviorally sophisticated. Her approach is flexible, combining conjoint and individual psychotherapy with the systematic prescription of sexual experiences. In this sense it uses a "behavioral" methodology, guided by the therapist's sensitive awareness to the underlying psychodynamic conflicts and processes involved in the development of symptoms, the meaning of these symptoms relative to the couple's interpersonal relatedness, and the response to therapeutic intervention.*

As presented by Dr. Kaplan, sex therapy is a form of psychotherapy in which guided sexual experiences are crucial to treatment but constitute only one aspect of the therapeutic process. The treatment goals are closer to those of behavioral therapists, namely, the relief of the patient's sexual symptoms rather than the resolution of underlying psychodynamic conflicts. This does not mean that such conflicts are ignored. Indeed, they are carefully monitored and attended to when they result in resistance or serve as an obstacle to carrying out the carefully prescribed sexual experiences designed to eliminate the patient's sexual symptoms.

The New Sex Therapy

Basic Principles of Sex Therapy

HELEN SINGER KAPLAN, M.D., PH.D.

25

Sex therapy differs from other forms of treatment for sexual dysfunctions in two respects: *first, its goals are essentially limited to the relief of the patient's sexual symptom and second, it departs from traditional techniques by employing a combination of prescribed sexual experiences and psychotherapy.*

SYMPTOM RELIEF

Sex therapists differ somewhat in how they define their therapeutic goals. All focus on improving sexual functioning; however, some espouse somewhat broader objectives and also include improvement of the couple's communication and in their general relationship in the therapeutic end point. However, the primary objective of all sex therapy is to relieve the patient's sexual dysfunction. All therapeutic interventions, the tasks, psychotherapy, couples therapy, etc., are ultimately at the service of this goal. This admittedly limited objective distinguishes the new sex therapy from the other modalities of treatment such as psychoanalysis and marital therapy. Psychoanalysts and marital therapists also treat patients whose chief complaint is sexual dysfunction. However, they feel that sexual problems are invariably expressions of underlying conflicts and/or destructive interpersonal transactions. The main aim of analytic and marital therapy extends beyond relief of the patients' sexual problems and includes the resolution of broader intrapsychic and interpersonal difficulties. Thus psychoanalysts and marital therapists do not treat the sexual symptom in isolation from other problems. Nor is the sexual symptom treated directly. The immediately operating, "here and now" causes of the sexual disability are not modified in psychotherapy and marital therapy. Instead the therapeutic emphasis is on resolv-

Reprinted by permission from *The New Sex Therapy*, Brunner/Mazel, New York, 1974, Chapter 11, pp. 187-200.

ing the sexually distressed patient's deeper intrapsychic or interpersonal difficulties. Improvement of sexual symptoms which may occur during the course of therapy is regarded as a product of the resolution of more basic personality problems and/or changes in pathological marital dynamics. For these persons the psychotherapist does not terminate treatment when the patient's impotence improves or the woman experiences orgasm. Treatment is concluded only when therapist and patient feel that basic unconscious conflicts which derive from childhood and/or the fundamental sources of marital discord have been resolved.

In contrast, while the many remote and deeper intrapsychic and interpersonal influences which may underlie some sexual symptoms are recognized and respected, the initial site of therapeutic intervention is the modification of the immediate causes and defenses against sexuality. The remoter structure of the problem is dealt with in sex therapy only to the extent that it is necessary to relieve the sexual target symptom and also to insure that the disability will not recur. Psychodynamic and transactional material is interpreted and neurotic behavior is modified, but only if they are directly operative in impairing the patient's sexual functioning or if they offer obstacles to the progress of treatment.

Sex therapy is considered completed when the couple's sexual difficulty is relieved. This is not to say, of course, that treatment is terminated as soon as the patient manages to have intercourse on one or two occasions. Treatment is ended, however, when the dysfunction is relieved and when the factors which were directly responsible for the problem have been identified and resolved sufficiently to warrant the assumption that the patient's sexual functioning is reasonably permanent and stable. The case below illustrates treatment governed by the limited objective of relieving the sexual symptom, and also the manner in which we generally handle related deeper intrapsychic and marital problems in sex therapy.

CASE 8: SYMPTOMATIC TREATMENT OF PREMATURE EJACULATION

It was apparent at the initial interview with the young couple that the husband who was seeking help for his severe premature ejaculation harbored a good deal of unconscious hostility toward his wife. He seemed to be angry at her yet at the same time also quite dependent on her. He also seemed to be afraid that he would lose her and be abandoned by her if he did not "perform." He seemed totally unaware of any of these feelings.

It is highly probable that these conflicts had their roots in the husband's childhood interactions with his mother. It is also possible that these unconscious processes played a role in the genesis of his problem. A psychoanalyst faced with this case would probably attempt to resolve the patient's oedipal conflicts and help him gain insight into the unconscious sources of his anger at women and his fear of abandonment by maternal figures, with the hope that he would thereby gain ejaculatory competence.

A marriage counselor, on the other hand, would try to identify and resolve the transactional causes of the problem, i.e., the hostilities between the couple which very possibly might be reinforcing the husband's prematurity. And this approach has validity, for it was clear that this couple had marital problems. The wife was afraid on some level of awareness that if the husband were to function well sexually, he would abandon her for a more attractive woman. Her insecurity had an adversive effect on their sexual system and probably contributed to the problem of prematurity. The marriage counselor or interpersonally oriented therapist would therefore attempt to resolve these destructive marital interactions as his first order of business.

In contrast, the sex therapist's initial objective is to modify the immediate cause of prematurity. Presumably the immediate pathogenic factor in this disorder which must be modified is the man's lack of awareness of the erotic sensations premonitory to orgasm. Thus, during the first therapeutic session, the patient and his wife are instructed in the Semans procedure, which is an effective means of teaching ejaculatory control by behavioral methods, which do not produce insight into intrapsychic or interpersonal dynamics. He will instruct the wife to stimulate her husband's penis and the patient to focus his attention on the premonitory cues to orgasm. However, if interventions are limited to the prescription of such behavioral tasks most patients will not gain ejaculatory control. On the contrary, the sex therapist must be an extremely skilled psychotherapist and couples therapist if he is to be successful. However, he employs those skills in order to implement the top priority objective, namely, the relief of the sexual target symptom. Thus again psychodynamic and/or transactional material, the deeper causes of the sexual symptom, must be dealt with skillfully and effectively, but we do so only insofar as these present obstacles to the couple's sexual functioning and/or give rise to resistances to carrying out the essential therapeutic tasks.

Treatment. In this case, treatment initially proceeded without obstacles so that after four sessions Mr. A. was able to exert good ejaculatory control in the female superior position. However, at this point treatment reached an impasse. The couple managed to avoid sex for the whole week. He complained that he was extremely involved with business and could not find the time to devote to the sexual tasks. His wife was irritable and tired and did not pursue the issue. In other words, treatment had mobilized resistances which took the form of avoidance of doing the sexually therapeutic task. Treatment cannot succeed unless the couple carries out these tasks and therefore these resistances must be resolved before therapy can proceed. Therapeutic emphasis was therefore shifted away from the behavioral aspect of treatment, and focused now on clarifying and resolving the husband's hostility and also the wife's anxieties, which seemed to have been mobilized by his improvement. Apart from fostering the husband's ejaculatory control, this also afforded the therapist the opportunity to work with important marital and personal problems. In this case sufficient insight and resolution were achieved in the next few sessions by confronting the couple with their avoidance of the sexual tasks, and by an active interpretation of the unconscious conflicts which had given rise to their resistances, to enable the husband to achieve excellent ejaculatory control.

Treatment was terminated when Mr. A's ejaculatory control seemed stable, although, of course, many problems remained unsolved. Relief of the sexual dysfunction is the usual termination criterion in sex therapy unless it becomes clear that severe marital difficulties or neurotic conflicts preclude satisfactory sexual functioning despite the patient's good ejaculatory control, or unless the couple wishes further treatment for other problems which have come to light in the course of sex therapy.

Can sexual functioning really be corrected with any degree of permanence by such direct intervention which is essentially limited to modifying surface causes without resolving underlying difficulties? Can sexual symptoms be treated in relative isolation? Can the conflicts be circumvented? Traditional psychiatric theories would predict that such an approach could not be effective; however, evidence of the efficacy for sex therapy is mounting rapidly. For example, 98% to 100% of premature ejaculators can achieve good sexual functioning within a few weeks if they carry out the sensory training procedure properly. The prognosis for other dysfunctions is not as excellent. Nevertheless, an extremely high proportion of sexually dysfunctional patients, approximately 80%, can be relieved of their symptoms by sex therapy which limits intervention to modifying the immediate obstacles to sexual functioning, without concomitant changes in basic personality structure or of the fundamental dynamics of the marital relationship.

As was illustrated in the case, to a certain extent conflicts are resolved, of course, and the quality of marital interaction and communication modified in the course of treatment. However, sex therapy addresses itself primarily to the specific immediate conflict and the specifically sexual aspects of the relationship which are directly impairing sexual functioning in the "here and now." We intervene directly to remove the specific immediate obstacles to sexual functioning and so we modify the couple's constrictive sexual system, thus allowing their sexuality to develop freely. Immediately, operating conflicts which impair the sexual response are resolved by the experiential methods of sex therapy. However, the remote causes, the unconscious conflicts which have created the obstacles to sexual functioning in the first place, may or may not have to be resolved to protect the patient's sexual responses from their influence.

Both clinical observation and common sense support the validity of limited goals and the task-specific intervention approach of sex therapy.

First, many patients with sexual problems seem to be free of other difficulties, and certainly these persons require treatment of the specific sexual problem only. On the other hand, there are many people who have serious oedipal conflicts, castration anxieties, and neurotic personalities, and whose marital relationships are highly destructive, and nonetheless they enjoy excellent sexual functioning. Obviously, although such difficulties *may*, and often do, cause sexual dysfunctions, they do *not* invariably do so. Everyone's unconscious oedipal guilt does not lead to inhibition of ejaculation or impotence. Mechanisms must exist whereby good sexual functioning can coexist with emotional conflicts and marital difficulties. There must be naturally occurring bypass mechanisms or modifying factors or defenses which protect the delicate sexual functions from the destructive influences of neurosis and disruptive marriages. In a sense, brief treatment of sexual dysfunctions attempts to accomplish such bypass or circumvention or defense erection when this is necessary. For again, while many patients have isolated sexual problems, often the sexual symptom appears enmeshed in more extensive psychopathology. In such cases, the therapist first attempts to circumvent or lay aside the neurotic problem as much as is possible and works directly to improve sexual functioning. Only if such limited intervention is not successful are we prepared to work on a deeper level and to help the patient to resolve deeper intrapsychic conflicts and transactional difficulties which are perpetuating his symptom.

Thus, although I recognized that Mr. A's premature ejaculation was probably related to his unconscious hostility toward women, I did not interpret this as long as it did not present a specific obstacle to therapy. I did so only when the husband's hostility gave rise to resistances which interfered with treatment. It may be speculated that the husband's ambivalence toward his wife made him reluctant to "give" her good sex at this point. His unconscious conflicts surrounding women impeded his gaining ejaculatory continence by motivating him to arrange his work schedule so that he could not "find time" to perform the prescribed exercises. When this became apparent, he was confronted with his avoidance of the exercises and the presumed unconscious reasons for his behavior were actively interpreted. However, no such interpretations were offered during the initial phase of treatment; at that stage, the wife was merely instructed to repeatedly stimulate her husband's penis and stop just before he was reaching orgasm. The patient was admonished not to think about his wife during this experience, or about past sexual failures, or to let himself be distracted by any other thoughts, but to focus his attention exclusively on his genital sensations as he experienced mounting excitement and impending orgasm.

The experience of repeatedly focusing his attention on the genital sensations of coming close to orgasm while he is engaged with his partner seems to be the essential cure-producing agent, the "active ingredient" in the treatment of premature ejaculation, and the therapist employs his skills to create the secure sexual ambience which is necessary to get the couple to engage in this experience.

Sometimes virtually no resistances are mobilized by this procedure. More commonly, as was illustrated in this case, obstacles arise which can be worked through within the brief treatment format. At other times, neuroses and marital difficulties give rise to virtually insurmountable obstacles which tax the therapeutic skills of even the most gifted therapist.

The obstacles take many forms: the patient may start to obsess during the experience and so fail to focus his attention on his erotic sensations; he might fail to follow the directions and employ some rationalization to obscure his real anxiety; or resistances might be mobilized in the wife who may discourage him from performing the prescribed exercises or find other ways to sabotage the treatment. Evidence of such obstacles signals the therapist that the success of therapy is contingent upon the resolution of intrapsychic or marital problems. The goals of treatment are then extended to include resolution of the conflicts which give rise to such resistances. The successful management of these obstacles to treatment progress constitutes the essence of the psychotherapeutic sessions.

TECHNIQUE

This case also illustrates the important technical difference between sex therapy and traditional treatment, namely, the synergy between the sexual tasks and the psychotherapeutic process. In other forms of psychotherapy the therapeutic process occurs in the therapist's office. In traditional treatment, based on the psychoanalytic model, the therapist never intervenes directly in the patient's life, except perhaps to admonish him against self-destructively "acting out" his conflicts and resistances. He generally refrains from making specific suggestions, and certainly never assigns tasks. In fact, any direct behavioral prescriptions are regarded as "manipulating" the patient, an approach which is considered by many authorities to be contraindicated in psychoanalytic therapy. Instead the psychoanalyst relies exclusively on the events which transpire within the therapeutic sessions, particularly on the patient-therapist relationship, to obtain his results. Marital therapists who generally employ conjoint sessions, in which the husband and wife and therapist participate to resolve marital discord, also consider the couple's experiences during the office visit as the primary therapeutic force. Similarly, behavior therapists who also treat sexual dysfunctions use various techniques which are designed to extinguish the fears and inhibitions which impair the patient's sexual response. These are generally administered in the therapist's office under his direct guidance.

The exclusive reliance on the office session is in sharp contrast to the new approach. In sex therapy the experiences suggested by the therapist and conducted by the patient and his partner while they are alone together are considered to be a vital factor and indeed an essential change-producing agent of the therapeutic procedure. The rational use of these therapeutic experiences amplifies the power of psychotherapy enormously.

However, dynamically oriented sex therapists do not rely exclusively on prescribed sexual interactions. Rather we employ an *integrated combination* of sexual experiences and psychotherapy. This combination constitutes the main innovation of sex therapy and holds the secret of its power. Psychotherapeutic intervention alone, both individual and conjoint, helps sexual problems to some extent. Highly stimulating and concomitantly reassuring sexual experiences probably can help some persons overcome sexual difficulties. However, the judicious combination of prescribed sexual interactions between the sexual partners which are systematically structured to relieve specific sexual difficulties, employed synergistically together with psychotherapeutic sessions which are designed to modify the unconscious intrapsychic and transactional impediments to sexual functioning and to create a free and secure sexual system between the partners, is the most effective and far-reaching approach to the treatment of sexual difficulties yet devised and constitutes a major advance in the behavioral sciences.

The sessions and experiences mutually reinforce each other to reveal and resolve impediments to the couple's free and healthy sexual expression and also to reveal and resolve personal and marital difficulties. On the basis of our initial evaluation we formulate a provisional concept of their manifest sexual problem and also of the deeper structure beneath this. In prescribing the initial sexual tasks, we are guided by this formulation. The couple's responses to these tasks then further clarify the dynamics of the difficulty. For example, the case presented was formulated as follows: the chief complaint was the husband's ejaculatory incontinence. The immediate cause of this problem was his avoidance of the experience of high surges of erotic sensations premonitory to orgasm. The deeper structure beneath this problem was presumably his unconscious hostility toward women which made him ambivalent about giving his wife pleasure and distracted him from sexual abandonment. A contributory factor which reinforced the premature ejaculation pattern was the destructive sexual system that was created by his wife's fear that a sexually adequate man would abandon her and prefer another more desirable woman.

The strategy adopted in this case was to attempt to modify the immediate causes of the dysfunction and to circumvent the deeper conflict to the extent that this was possible. Thus, the initial sig.* was the Semans exercises. After they conducted the prescribed experiences at home, they returned and discussed their experiences in detail with me. As is usual, a wealth of psychodynamic material was evoked by these experiences. These data were used to correct and refine my concept of the deeper structure of the couple's problem, and so enable me to devise and prescribe further sexual tasks. At the same time this process also made psychodynamic material available for psychotherapeutic intervention during the sessions.

In the case cited above, the wife's dormant abandonment anxiety was mobilized by her husband's rapidly growing control over his ejaculatory reflex. This took the form of an unpleasant mood, and was

*Sig. stands for *signa*, a term used in medicine to designate "prescription."

also acted out in her reluctance to carry out the assigned sexual task. Although these resistances impeded treatment temporarily, they also provided the therapist with an opportunity to deal with this significant material during the sessions. The wife's fears of abandonment had to be dispelled before the couple's sexual functioning could be secure. Resolution of this long-standing problem was extremely helpful to her, apart from the improvement in sexual functioning.

THE TREATMENT FORMAT

The formats used by different sex therapy clinics and therapists all share one feature in common: they make possible the combined use of prescribed sexual experiences and psychotherapeutic sessions. Beyond this general principle, the specific formats employed by the various groups differ considerably. Because the Masters and Johnson program served as the prototype for the sex therapy treatment format, it will be described in some detail. The program used by Masters and Johnson, and by most of the clinics directed by clinicians trained by them, provides treatment for a limited period, usually two weeks. Treatment is conducted by a mixed-gender team of cotherapists, one of whom must be a physician. Initially, each partner is interviewed separately by each therapist. Each spouse also receives a medical examination as part of the intake procedure. All four then meet for a "round table" discussion of the couple's problem and the treatment objectives. Thereafter, the couple is seen every day (including Sundays) in sessions which vary in duration. The couple is usually seen in joint session by both cotherapists, unless separate sessions are specifically indicated, in which event each partner is seen individually by one or the other cotherapist.

As a general rule, only couples are accepted for treatment. However, if the patient has no partner, or if the partner is not available for treatment, Masters and Johnson and other therapists have provided the patient with a surrogate partner, a stranger who, for a fee, will spend two weeks with the patient and participate in the prescribed sexual tasks.

During the treatment period, the couple does not live at home. Arrangements are usually made for them to stay at a pleasant motel near the clinic.

The treatment formats used at other sex therapy clinics differ from the Masters and Johnson program in various respects. Cotherapists are not always used. Therapists trained by Masters and Johnson, as well as the sex clinics patterned on the Masters and Johnson model, are all deeply committed to the mixed-gender, dual-therapist approach, and usually require that one team member be a physician. Other clinicians do not consider it essential that treatment be conducted by a physician. Hartman and Fithian, on the West Coast, who also employ mixed-gender cotherapists, do not require that either be a physician (although they give their patients medical examinations). In contrast to these clinics, others, including our own at Cornell, use individual therapists of either gender. The time-limited approach is also not universal and patients are not always seen every day in other programs. At some clinics, patients are seen from once to three times a week, and no time limit is set on the duration of treatment. The locus of the prescribed sexual experiences varies. Some Masters and Johnson type programs require patients to leave their homes, take up residence near the clinic, and devote two weeks exclusively to treatment. The rationale behind this practice is that rapid sexual therapy requires the patient to be free of the usual pressures of home and business, and this can only be accomplished if the patient changes his environment. Some even provide private rooms in the treatment complex where the couple can carry out their prescribed erotic tasks and then immediately discuss their reactions with their therapists. Recent attempts to combine erotic experiences with group process constitute a further modification in format. Various programs are experimenting with sex therapy groups and marathons. At Cornell, for example, we are treating premature ejaculation in couples' groups. It is too early to evaluate this and similar experiments conducted by other clinicians. However, on the basis of our limited experience, we believe that the combined use of group modalities with sex therapy holds considerable promise.

It is important to experiment with new forms and variations in order to improve our clinical techniques and also because we need to identify the "active ingredients," i.e., the essential change-producing factors of sex therapy, if the field is to advance. Unfortunately, because of the great needs in this area, some "therapists" seem to be exploiting the current interest in sexual therapy by initiating poorly conceived and sensational quasi-orgy "therapeutic" procedures.

Another difference in treatment format centers on the medical examination, which is required of all couples by some programs but required only when specifically indicated by others. Similarly, some sex therapists require all prospective clients to submit to a psychiatric examination in order to rule out high-risk patients, while others, including Masters and Johnson, rely on the psychiatric findings of the referring professional.

With regard to therapeutic technique, almost all programs rely on initial coital or orgastic abstinence and some form of systematic tactile stimulation. Usually, therapy tries to get the couple to substitute the

giving and receiving of pleasure for the exclusive goal of achieving orgasm. Open discussion between the partners of previously avoided sexual material is also an important aspect of most programs. Programs
differ somewhat in the methods they use to implement these objectives.
They prescribe somewhat different sexual tasks for their patients, and
also differ in the sequence and application of these tasks. In addition,
individual therapists and clinics have developed special techniques for
the treatment of specific syndromes. These are described in the chapters
which deal with these syndromes.

Masters and Johnson and their disciples employ the same routine
and sequence of tasks for all their patients. Regardless of diagnosis, the
Masters and Johnson treatment begins with coital abstinence and sensate focus exercises. After the couple reports an increase in erotic pleasure, they are instructed to proceed to the specific sexual tasks which are
indicated for their particular sexual disorder, e.g., the "squeeze" technique in cases of premature ejaculation and erectile dysfunction, the fe-
male-controlled nondemand thrusting in the orgastic dysfunctions, etc.

In our own program we do not employ a specific sequence, but
prescribe tasks only when they seem specifically indicated. For example,
in the case described earlier in this chapter, the Masters and Johnson
model was not followed and sensate focus exercises were not prescribed
initially. It was felt that these preliminary exercises were not necessary;
instead, this couple proceeded directly to the use of the Semans "stop-
start" technique.

THEORETICAL ORIENTATION

Finally, the most significant differences between programs arise
from differences in the *conceptualization of the therapeutic process*, which
are ultimately reflected in the conduct of treatment. Some of the clinicians who practice sex therapy are not trained in the theory of psychopathology, nor are they skilled psychotherapists. Consequently, they appear to conduct sex therapy without any theoretical concept. They work
empirically and deal only with surface causes. They rely primarily on sex
education and counseling and the prescription of erotic tasks to achieve
their therapeutic objectives. In sharp contrast, my own psychodynamically oriented approach conceptualizes sex therapy as a form of psychotherapy. Although the sexual experiences are crucial to treatment, they
constitute just one aspect of the total therapeutic process. At Cornell,
although the goal of sex therapy is limited to improvement of sexual
functioning, treatment is conducted within a psychodynamic conceptual
framework. We attempt to understand the causes of the patient's problem, and to relate treatment to this formulation. Both the immediate and

the deeper causes are considered, and each task, as well as each therapeutic maneuver, is based on a rational consideration of its impact on the couple's psychopathological structure. Each spouse's intrapsychic resistances and unconscious motivations, as well as the pathological dynamics of the couple's relationship, are among the factors which are considered and dealt with within therapeutic process.

The basic conceptual framework upon which our clinical work is based is multicausal and eclectic. I feel that many determinants may produce the sexual dysfunctions. However, the immediate causes of the sexual dysfunctions seem to be much more specific for each of the dysfunctions than the remote causes. It is these deeper causes which vary tremendously from patient to patient and couple to couple.

These deeper etiologic factors may primarily involve one spouse's unconscious intrapsychic conflict which may entail an oedipal problem, religiogenic guilt, fear of intimacy and commitment, unresolved dominance and submission struggles, etc. Interpretation varies with the specific problem presented by the patient. This eclecticism is not confined to intrapsychic issues. I am also eclectic with regard to a systems versus an intrapsychic approach. While one mate's intrapsychic problem is clearly the crucial pathogenic variable in one case of impotence, in other cases it is clearly the couple's sexually destructive system which is the critical cause of the man's erectile difficulty and also the optimal point of therapeutic intervention. Many couples create sexual and marital systems in which it is impossible for a sensitive person to function. When the system is destructive, the rational method of proceeding is not primarily to attempt to change the patient's psyche, but rather to work to modify the system to which he is responding. I see no dichotomy between the intrapsychic model which seeks cure by changing the patient and the systems model which attempts to help by changing the environment which has produced the patient's abhorrent response. In actual clinical practice, therapeutic emphasis in a particular case is on one or the other, but both intrapsychic and ecological factors are dealt with to some extent in virtually all cases. At any rate, even when the therapeutic focus is largely intrapsychic, when sex therapy has been successful, the couple's sexual system has invariably changed to a freer, more humanized ambience.

The counterpoint between the prescribed sexual interactions and the psychotherapeutic experience is exploited fully in our program. The sexual tasks reveal individual conflicts and marital pathology far more rapidly and dramatically than mere discussion, and this material is worked with extensively and intensively in the psychotherapeutic sessions.

Essentially, I view sex therapy as a task-centered form of crisis intervention which presents an opportunity for rapid conflict resolution. Toward this end the various sexual tasks are employed, as well as the methods of insight therapy, supportive therapy, marital therapy, and other psychiatric techniques as indicated.

A review of the practices of others and of our own experiences yields the impression that the format in which sexual therapy can be conducted successfully may vary considerably as long as the basic and essential principles which underlie this approach are adhered to. Any format is potentially effective if it provides the opportunity to combine conjoint and individual psychotherapy with the systematic prescription of sexual experiences.

Within this framework, our program is adapted to the resources and limitations of an outpatient psychiatric clinic and/or private psychotherapeutic practice. It is also geared to the reality problems of patients who differ widely in terms of socioeconomic status, etc. Some flexibility in format is essential for this highly diverse population. Such a flexible treatment format does not seem to impair the effectiveness of treatment. On the contrary, this approach seems to have certain therapeutic advantages.

All couples who seek help for their sexual problems at Cornell have a psychiatric examination before they are accepted for treatment. This procedure alerts us to the possibility that one partner or the other may develop adverse reactions to rapid treatment. It also provides the therapist with information about the dynamics of the couple's problem. In addition, we take a medical history, and refer those patients whose sexual problem might be related to physical factors for a medical, gynecological, and/or urological examination as indicated.

In our program couples continue to live at home and are seen once or twice a week. This spacing of visits gives the couple sufficient time to carry out the prescribed sexual tasks and to discuss their reactions to these experiences with the therapist in a systematic manner. The instructions and tasks have been modified to accommodate to this treatment format. In other words, during a session the couple may receive instructions for several sequential experiences. Telephone contact is available if specific questions arise in the interval between scheduled sessions.

No time limit is placed on treatment. Therapy is terminated when good sexual functioning has been established, with some indication that this will be relatively permanent. In general, the duration of treatment varies with each dysfunction. For example, on the average, premature ejaculation is relieved in 6.5 sessions conducted over a period of three to six weeks, while the mean for vaginismus is 10 visits over a six-week period. However, after treatment has been terminated, some of our couples request additional individual or conjoint therapy for nonsexual problems which come to light during sex therapy.

Since a crucial ingredient of successful therapy is the participation of two individuals in the sexual exercises which are required to improve the previously destructive sexual system, we consider the use of couples indispensable. However, we are flexible with respect to the extent to which we require both partners to participate in each of the psychotherapeutic sessions. Usually, the couple is seen together during the initial evaluation and in most subsequent sessions. But the therapist remains alert to situations which require that the spouses be seen individually, e.g., evidence that sexual "secrets" exist, or when material must be dealt with which may have a deleterious effect on the other or on their relationship. In addition, apart from such considerations, some disorders require that treatment focus primarily on one or the other partner. When such a situation exists, we do not insist on the couple's joint attendance at therapeutic sessions, nor do we insist that both participate in the sexual exercises. This "splitting" is especially useful, for example, in treating the woman who suffers from severe orgastic inhibition. In such cases the initial tasks, which are designed to enable the patient to achieve her first orgasm, are often best conducted by the patient alone because the partner may find them so tedious that requiring him to perform these exercises might be destructive to the couple's sexual relationship.

The format described above which is used at Cornell has been found by us to be effective and practical. However, any flexible and psychodynamically oriented treatment format can meet the needs of the wide variety of patients who suffer from sexual dysfunctions if it retains the essential ingredients of sex therapy, i.e., the combined and integrated use of prescribed, systematically structured sexual experiences and psychotherapeutic intervention within a basic psychodynamic context.

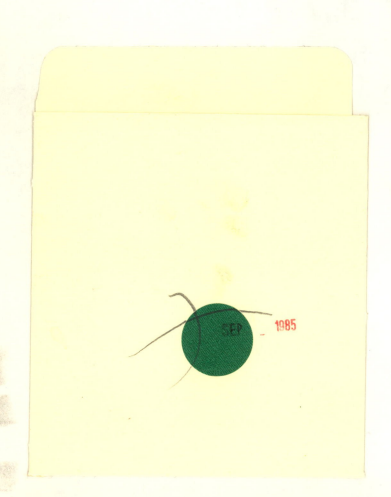